Measuring and Valuing Health Benefits for Economic Evaluation

Measuring and Valuing Health Benefits for Economic Evaluation

SECOND EDITION

Professor John Brazier

Professor of Health Economics

School of Health and Related Research,
University of Sheffield, UK

Professor Julie Ratcliffe

Professor of Health Economics

Flinders Health Economics Group

School of Medicine

Flinders University, Adelaide, Australia

Professor Joshua A. Salomon

Professor of Global Health

Department of Global Health and Population

Harvard T.H. Chan School of Public Health,
Harvard University, USA

Professor Aki Tsuchiya

Professor of Health Economics

School of Health and Related Research,
and Department of Economics

University of Sheffield, UK

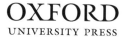

OXFORD
UNIVERSITY PRESS

OXFORD
UNIVERSITY PRESS

Great Clarendon Street, Oxford, OX2 6DP,
United Kingdom

Oxford University Press is a department of the University of Oxford.
It furthers the University's objective of excellence in research, scholarship,
and education by publishing worldwide. Oxford is a registered trade mark of
Oxford University Press in the UK and in certain other countries

First Edition published in 2007
Second Edition published in 2017

Published in the United States of America by Oxford University Press
198 Madison Avenue, New York, NY 10016, United States of America

British Library Cataloguing in Publication Data
Data available

Library of Congress Control Number: 2016949678

ISBN 978–0–19–872592–3

Preface

There has been an increasing use of economic evaluation to assist policy makers concerned with the health impact of their programmes. Major users include agencies such as the National Institute for Health and Care Excellence (NICE) in England and similar bodies around the world (Scotland, Australia, Canada, the Netherlands, and Sweden). In North America, there is also an increasing interest in the potential role of cost-effectiveness analysis in the evaluation of non-health care as well as health care interventions that impact on health. This has resulted in a corresponding increase in the need for data on costs and benefits of these interventions for use in economic evaluation. This book is concerned with the measurement and valuation of health benefits.

This book is aimed to complement those that currently exist on economic evaluation and health outcome measures. The valuation of health benefits is a central concern in economic evaluation that raises different types of problems from those conventionally addressed in the psychometric literature on health and quality of life assessment. Our philosophy in writing this book has been to draw on these two fields and to forge a book that is comprehensive and above all useful to the practitioner in this field, whether they are academics, students, consultants, or policy makers.

The writing of this book has been a collective enterprise, drawing on our different expertise in measuring and valuing health. Like many textbooks, it began life as teaching material delivered on courses, including Masters Degrees for health economists, health services researchers, and public health physicians, and a commercial course delivered to pharmaceutical companies. It soon evolved into something much larger to take into account such a large and diffuse area of research. We hope this proves to be a useful source book for the wide range of readership to which it is aimed.

J.E.B
J.R
J.A.S
A.T

Acknowledgements

We owe a considerable debt to colleagues, particularly those at the Universities of Sheffield and Harvard, with whom we have worked with in this field over the years. The first edition benefited from the comments of Chris McCabe, Chris Murray, Jennifer Roberts, Paul Dolan, Jim Hammitt, Tony O'Hagan, and Milt Weinstein. We are particularly grateful to those who kindly agreed to comment on sections of this book as it emerged in various draft forms. We would specifically like to thank: Simon Dixon, Richard Edlin, Enrico de Nigris, Jennifer Roberts, Katherine Stevens, Isabel Towers, and Yaling Yang. For the second edition we would also like to thank Donna Rowen, Katherine Stevens, and Clara Mukuria for their comments; Liz Metham for her administrative support; Aurialiano Finch for providing early access to his review of generic measures; and to Louis Matza for making substantive suggestions on the section about vignettes. Any remaining errors or omissions are the responsibility of the authors alone.

Finally, we would like to acknowledge our collective intellectual debt to Alan Williams, who was one of the pioneers in measuring and valuing health and has been such an inspiration to many of us working in this field.

Contents

Chapter 1

The purpose and scope of this book

1.1 Purpose, scope, and outline of this book

The measurement and valuation of health benefits form a substantial component of economic evaluation in health care. It continues to be a major source of contention, and yet in the last three decades there have been significant advancements in its methods. The number of tools has expanded considerably from the early notion of a 'health index' (Fanshel and Bush 1970). At the same time there have been important debates in the literature on a range of key issues, such as: the definition of health; the techniques of valuation; who should provide the values; approaches to modelling health state values; the appropriateness of valuation tools in children and vulnerable groups; cross-cultural issues; and the problems of selecting instruments from the ever growing number available. These raise normative issues and technical problems that are essential to the practice of economic evaluation. By addressing these issues in depth, this book aims to supplement a range of more general texts on economic evaluation in health care (e.g. Drummond *et al.* 2015).

The issues addressed in this book are also important to health services research and to the field of quality of life research (sometimes known as patient-reported outcomes or patient-reported outcome measures) in general, to which health economics is but one contributing discipline. This field has seen contributions from different disciplines, including psychology and psychometrics, sociology, statistics, philosophy, and the many health professions. The field of measuring health status and health-related quality of life already has a number of classic texts (Streiner and Norman 1989; McDowell and Newell 1996; Bowling 2004). These texts are primarily concerned with what economists would regard as measurement rather than valuation, and are not concerned with the very specific requirements of economic evaluation. This book aims to help bridge the gap between conventional psychometric approaches to *measuring* health and *valuing* health, both of which are needed for economic evaluation.

We hope our book provides the reader with an in-depth knowledge of one of these two key elements of economic evaluation in health care. It is written as a textbook which aims to include a comprehensive coverage of topics, while also being up-to-date at the time of going to press. We believe that it helps meet an important need that has been generated by the establishment of the National Institute for Health and

Care Excellence (NICE) and similar bodies around the world, which require cost-effectiveness evidence in the form of incremental cost per quality-adjusted life year (QALY). It is aimed at: academics and students of health economics and other areas of economics concerned with the valuation of intangible benefits such as health; practitioners from economics and other disciplines engaged in generating economic evaluations for research bodies; governmental agencies in health care (such as NICE) and non-health care agencies whose programmes affect health (e.g. human services, environment, and transport); pharmaceutical companies; and private research consultancies. The book should appeal to professional economists and comparative novices alike. The measurement and valuation of health is a multidisciplinary endeavour, and this book seeks to be inclusive and accessible to a wide audience.

Chapter 2 is an introduction to the topic, and experienced health economists may already be familiar with this content. It provides a justification for why health economists have entered an already crowded field. It presents the basic economic problem of scarcity and choice, and an overview of the techniques developed to assess the relative efficiency of different programmes. The chapter then considers the role and limitations of clinical and health-related quality of life measures in economic evaluation. These limitations provide the rationale for developing an alternative measure of the value of health, namely the QALY. One of the best-known examples of an instrument to calculate QALYs is the generic preference-based measure, the EQ-5D (Brooks 1996). Underpinning the EQ-5D and similar instruments are a number of core questions: what should be the measure of value; how should it be described; how should health states be valued; who should provide the values; how should the values be used in economic evaluation; and how should these values be aggregated? The remainder of this book examines these questions from a number of different perspectives and explores the various methods used to address them.

Chapter 3 examines the welfare economic foundation of valuing health benefits and the appropriate measure of value. It starts with a review of the conditions of a perfect market, and how a health care market fails to satisfy them, which opens the way to government intervention and planned resource allocation. It considers in some detail the theoretical foundation for assessing programmes using the Kaldor–Hicks compensation criteria and cost-benefit analyses. It then considers why the method of willingness to pay, which is often the preferred approach in economics to valuing intangibles, has not been as widely used in health care. The chapter offers alternative justifications for the concept of QALY, including welfarist and non-welfarist approaches.

Chapter 4 turns to the issue of how to value health states. It describes the range of techniques that are currently used and considers the arguments for and against each of them. It looks in some detail at the theory behind the methods and how they compare. A more neglected topic has been the impact of different variants on the values obtained, which has been shown to be more important in some cases than the differences between techniques, as is also considered here.

Chapter 4 goes on to examine the question of those values. Values have been shown to differ systematically by a number of personal characteristics such as age and illness experience. It has also been shown that patients valuing their own state give different values from those given by members of the general population trying to imagine the state. The reasons for these differences are examined, with interesting parallels to the notion of response shift from the psychometric literature. In this chapter, we review the normative arguments for and against using patient experiences compared with the hypothetical preferences of members of the general population.

Most descriptive systems give rise to a larger number of possible health states than can be feasibly valued in a valuation survey, and so values are usually elicited for a subset. The problem then becomes how to model from this subset in order to value all possible states defined by the instrument's descriptive system. Chapter 5 addresses this problem. Two main approaches have been used to estimate health state values for all states: methods based on multiattribute utility theory, and those based on statistical inference. This chapter considers the technical issues in applying these approaches and reviews some of the latest developments in the field, including the use of a nonparametric Bayesian approach.

Chapter 6 follows this in examining the rapidly developing field of using ordinal data generated from ranking and discrete choice experiments (DCEs) to estimate health state values. Given the complexity of conventional cardinal valuation techniques, there has been interest in using apparently simpler tasks such as ranking and DCEs to estimate mean health state values. While ordinal methods, especially DCEs, have been used for a number of years in health economics, it is only recently that they have been used to value health states for use in economic evaluation. Ordinal methods offer a promising approach to obtaining valuation data from more vulnerable groups, such as children and the very elderly. This chapter presents the theoretical basis for using ordinal data and their analysis, and reviews recent empirical work.

Chapter 7 reviews the six main generic preference-based measures (GPBMs) of health including EQ-5D, HUI2, HUI3, SF-6D, QWB, and AQoL (assessment of quality of life instrument). It examines the latest versions of these measures including the five-level EQ-5D-5L, QWB-SA, AQoL-8D, and SF-6Dv2. These six measures are compared in terms of the health state values they generate and their validity across different patient populations. It offers a useful checklist for deciding on the most appropriate GPBMs for a given population. This chapter also presents a description and review of preference-based measures in children.

Chapter 8 reviews alternatives to the use of GPBMs for obtaining health state values. It begins by looking at situations where the preferred measure has not been used in a key study. One method for addressing this problem has been to map from other health or clinical measures used in the study onto GPBMs. This chapter examines the methods for estimating these mapping functions. It then reviews the alternatives where GPBMs of health are considered inappropriate. Firstly, it discusses the development and use of condition-specific measures, including the problems of achieving comparability between QALYs calculated using different measures. Next, we examine the approach of developing extra or 'bolt-on' dimensions for GPBMs. Then the chapter examines the use of health vignettes or scenarios that do not require patient-reported outcome data, but can be constructed by experts following consultation with patients or clinicians. It also looks at the use of health state values directly obtained from patients (e.g. they value their own health using time trade-off). Finally, this chapter reviews the role of well-being measures as alternatives to the health-based measures in economic evaluation.

Chapter 9 considers the practical issues surrounding the use of health state values in assessing cost-effectiveness, in terms of cost per QALY, using two vehicles: alongside clinical trials and decision analytic models. Their use in assessing cost-effectiveness alongside clinical trials raises important issues of design, such as the method of data collection, mode of administration, whom to ask, and how frequently to administer the measure. It also raises important analytical problems of dealing with missing data and uncertainty. The second, and increasingly the more important application, is in the context of decision analytic modelling. These models are typically driven by a number of health states that patients live in for a specified duration of time. The analyst must consider the best place to obtain the relevant data (e.g. from the literature, observational studies, or clinical trials) and how to adapt or modify the data to make them suitable for use in the model (e.g. dealing with co-morbidities). There is also the important problem of how to characterize the uncertainty around health state values for use in sensitivity analyses.

Having calculated the size of net QALY gains from treatment using one of the methods described in this book, Chapter 10 addresses the question of whether the social value of a QALY gain to a group with one set of characteristics is the same as that to another group, which differs in terms of their socio-demographic variables, health status, or even the extent to which they have brought the condition upon themselves.

Interest in using cost per QALY to inform resource allocation has mainly come from developed countries. Low- and middle-income countries have shown less interest, but it is arguably more important for them given the more severe resource constraints. Chapter 11 reviews the attempts to apply the ideas described in this book through the particular lens of lower-income countries' perspective. There is a brief introduction to the disability-adjusted life year (DALY), which is an alternative to the QALY that has been favoured in much of the cost-effectiveness work in developing countries. It provides specific answers to the questions raised in this book about the issues of definition, description, and valuation in the context of the added considerations demanded by cross-cultural applications of the methods.

The final chapter concludes with a discussion of the way forward in light of the substantial methodological differences, the role of normative judgements, and where further research is most likely to be productive in taking the field forward (at least in our opinion!).

References

Bowling A (2004). *Measuring health: a review of quality of life and measurement scales*. Open University Press, Milton Keynes, UK.

Brooks RG (1996). Euroqol: the current state of play. *Health Policy* **37**:53–72.

Drummond MF, Sculpher M, Claxton K, O'Brien B, Stoddart GL, Torrance GW (2015). *Methods for the economic evaluation of health care programmes*. Oxford Medical Publications, Oxford, UK.

Fanshel S, Bush J (1970). A health status index and its application to health service outcomes. *Operations Research* **18**:1021–66.

McDowell I, Newell, C. (1996). *Measuring health: a guide to rating scales and questionnaire*. Oxford University Press, Oxford, UK.

Streiner DL, Norman, GR (1989). *Health measurement scales: a practical guide to their development and use*. Oxford University Press, Oxford, UK.

Chapter 2

Introduction to the measurement and valuation of health

2.1 Introduction

The purpose of this chapter is to set the scene for the remainder of the book and it has been written in a non-technical style, designed to be accessible to non-economists and economists alike. The chapter begins by considering the trade-offs implied by the resource allocation decisions made by policy makers, particularly regarding different aspects of health. It then provides an introduction to the techniques of economic evaluation that are used by economists to help generate the information required to inform such decisions. This is followed by a description of health status measures (which will be very familiar to quality of life researchers) and the problems with using them in economic evaluation. We then provide a basic introduction to the quality-adjusted life year (QALY), followed by a discussion of the key issues in the construction of measures used to calculate them, which are addressed in the rest of the book.

2.2 The rationale

It has long been recognized that health care is faced with the common problem that the resources available to spend are insufficient to meet all demands. The resources used to provide health care, including staff, facilities, equipment and knowledge, are scarce. Decisions about what services to provide, to whom, where, and when, usually have resource implications. For example, pursuing one course of action, such as offering screening for a particular condition to a defined population in a given location at a given frequency, means that other possible approaches for that and other conditions are not taken. Therefore, the resource costs will mean that fewer resources are available to provide for other services for that and other conditions—in other words, there will be lost opportunities (known as opportunity costs).

In a publicly funded health care system with a limited budget, or even in an insurance-based system where premiums have to be capped in order to be competitive, such decisions have implications for health. The overall aim of economic evaluation is to aid decision makers to make efficient (and equitable) decisions by comparing the costs and benefits of health care interventions (Drummond *et al.* 2015). There has been an increasing use of economic evaluation to inform policy making in health over the last decade through the establishment of organizations such as the National Institute for Health and Care Excellence, the Scottish Medicines Consortium (2014), and similar agencies in Australia (Commonwealth Department of Health 2002), Canada (Canadian Agency for Drugs and Technologies in Health 2006), and the Netherlands (CVZ 2004). In the USA, there has been interest in the potential role of cost-effectiveness analysis in health care (Gold *et al.* 1996) and in the evaluation of non-health care interventions through the impact on health (Miller *et al.* 2006). This has resulted in a corresponding increase in the need for data on the benefits of these interventions for use in economic evaluation.

While it may seem quite obvious how to cost the direct resource consequences and even the less direct ones, such as any impact on productivity from illness and its treatment, the health consequences are not as tangible and it is much less obvious how to assess them. This must be considered because the health consequences are just as important; indeed, they are the main reason why health services are provided.

The health effects of interventions are difficult to assess since they are uncertain and multidimensional, changing over time. A person's life expectancy might be extended and/or the quality of their health may improve in terms of various dimensions such as mobility, dexterity, sensory perception, social activities, pain relief, and mental health. However, there is no natural metric for these types of outcomes. Traditional clinical and biomedical measures define health in natural units such as blood pressure or respiratory function, but these do not provide a measure of what it is like for the patient. Therefore, measures have been developed that focus on the concerns of the recipient of the service, such as their ability to function, their social functioning, and their psychological well-being (Bowling 2004).

The outcomes of health care interventions are usually uncertain. Most interventions cannot guarantee any given outcome, so there is a probability associated with a range of outcomes. Furthermore, medical knowledge is limited by the available evidence on effectiveness, which leads to further uncertainty. The existence of uncertainty has potentially important implications for the valuation of health outcomes. In addition, the outcomes may fall on different people at different points in time, and this has implications for equity.

The way in which benefits are measured and valued is fundamental to economic evaluation in health care and ultimately for informing the decision maker. The next section looks at the different techniques of economic evaluation.

2.3 Techniques of economic evaluation in health care

Economic evaluation is the comparative assessment of the costs and benefits of alternative health care interventions (Drummond *et al.* 2015). The techniques of economic evaluation are: cost-minimization, cost-effectiveness, cost-utility, cost-benefit, and cost-consequence analysis. The unit for measuring the benefits of health care is the key feature that distinguishes the different techniques of economic evaluation (see summaries in Box 2.1). This section provides a brief overview of each technique to provide

Box 2.1 Techniques of economic evaluation

Cost-minimization analysis compares across interventions to achieve a fixed outcome, to identify the least costly option. This technique is only valid if it can be shown that the alternatives achieve identical outcomes. However, in practice this very rarely holds since there is always uncertainty surrounding the estimated outcome.

Cost-effectiveness analysis compares across different interventions that achieve an outcome measured in a common metric, to identify the one that is the least costly per unit outcome. The outcome is usually measured in 'natural' units, and presents results in terms of cost per unit of effect (e.g. cost per positive cancer detected or cost per symptom-free day).

Cost-utility analysis also compares across different interventions that achieve an outcome measured in a common metric, to identify the one that is the least costly per unit outcome. The outcome is measured in terms of quality-adjusted life years (QALYs).

Cost-benefit analysis compares all the costs and benefits of a given intervention, both measured in the same metric (usually money), to determine whether the outcomes are worth achieving given the costs.

the context for the rest of this book. (Readers wanting to learn more about these techniques are encouraged to read Drummond *et al.* 2015.)

2.3.1 Cost-effectiveness analysis

This technique compares the costs of alternative ways of achieving a given objective. Where two or more interventions are found to achieve the same level of benefits, the intervention with the least cost is the most cost-effective alternative. Under these circumstances, cost-effectiveness analysis (CEA) is equivalent to cost-minimization analysis; however, this situation seldom arises, in part because of the uncertainty that usually exists around the estimates of benefits (Briggs and O'Brien 2001) that require a full probabilistic analysis of cost-effectiveness (see Chapter 9).

When the benefits of competing interventions can be measured along a single dimension, CEA can be used to rank interventions in terms of their ratio of cost per unit of effect. These effects are usually measured in 'natural' units. Typical examples of 'natural' measures used in CEA include, for example, life years saved, or the number of gallstone episodes avoided. CEAs can consider a wide range of end-points such as detecting cancers, reductions in blood pressure, and improvements in bone mineral density. However, for any given analysis, only one measure of outcome can be used. The important features of the measures are that more of a good outcome is better than less, and that the measure lies on an interval scale over the range being examined: in other words, a scale that allows meaningful comparisons of differences. An important question addressed later in this chapter is whether it is possible to conduct a CEA using the scores generated by measures of health-related quality of life.

The key characteristic of CEA is that the objective implied by the measure (e.g. detecting cancers) is not being questioned, or its worth valued. In this sense, it is the most straightforward technique of economic evaluation. However, it is also very limited in terms of the questions it can address. It cannot be used to compare interventions that affect two or more outcomes, for example (1) where a treatment improves survival at the expense of a poorer quality of life; or (2) where an intervention improves two dimensions because we do not know how much cost to attribute to each, so we cannot attain the cost per unit health improvement. It is also unable to inform decisions on the efficient allocation of resources between disease groups or health care programmes with health outcomes across different dimensions. Nonetheless, it is a widely used technique that can be extremely helpful in addressing those questions where the objective is not being questioned and no trade-off between dimensions of health is required.

2.3.2 Cost-utility analysis

Cost-utility analysis (CUA) can be seen as a form of CEA as it is similar in that it compares interventions in terms of their cost per unit of effect (Drummond *et al.* 2015). Although much of the literature on economic evaluation, particularly in the United States, makes no distinction between CUA and CEA, the typology used by Drummond and colleagues regards CUA as a special case of CEA, in which the unit of effect is 'a year in full health'. The most widely used measure of years in full health is the QALY. The number of QALYs is calculated by multiplying a person's life expectancy by the value of the health-related quality of life in each period, measured on a scale between zero (dead) and one (full health). Being on hospital renal dialysis, for example, may be assigned a quality adjustment value or weight of 0.8. A 20-year period on renal dialysis is then 16 QALYs, and this is assumed to be equivalent to someone living for 16 years in full health. If being on dialysis affects more than one dimension of health (e.g. restricted activities and physical discomfort), then the 0.8 reflects two pieces of information: the value of the two dimensions of health relative to each other, and the relative value between the dialysis state and full health. For more complex time profiles of health, involving transitions between states of health, the number of QALYs is calculated by summing the product of the time spent in each state and the value attached to that state.

There are two components to the procedure for estimating the quality adjustment values for QALYs. The first is the *description* of the state or time profile of a person's health and the second is the *valuation* of these descriptions. An important class of measures is the generic preference-based measure of health (e.g. EQ-5D, HUI3, or SF-6D). These measures have health state descriptive systems that are accompanied by a set of health state utility values (or 'health utilities'), elicited using preference-based valuation techniques.

CUA has several advantages compared with CEA. First, interventions affecting more than one dimension of health, including any side effects, can be analysed as the preference-based measure will combine changes in multiple dimensions of health into a single number. Secondly, interventions for the same condition that impact upon different dimensions of health can be compared against each other. Thirdly, interventions for different conditions affecting different dimensions of health can be compared. The results are reported in terms of the incremental cost per QALY. Although some authors have used the term CUA to represent this kind of analysis, for the rest of this book the term CEA with QALYs, or cost per QALY analysis, will be used instead. The reason for avoiding the term cost 'utility' analysis will become clear towards the end of Chapter 3.

Health care interventions can be compared in terms of their effectiveness or incremental cost per QALY (i.e. the extra cost of an intervention over the next best alternative divided by the extra QALY gain) within and between programmes (Williams 1985). It even permits comparisons between programmes primarily concerned with increasing survival and those which mainly improve health-related quality of life. The earliest application of the QALY measure was undertaken in North America by Torrance *et al.* (1972) and Weinstein and Stason (1977), and in the United Kingdom by Williams (1985).

A collection of CEAs with QALYs can be brought together to form an ordering of various alternatives, ranked in terms of cost-effectiveness. This league table may be able to assist in determining the best way to spend a limited health care budget, but CEAs cannot help in the more fundamental questions about how much to spend on health care. One practical solution to this shortcoming is the introduction of a 'threshold' cost per unit outcome. For example, an intervention with a cost per QALY above the threshold (say £25,000) would not be funded, but one below would (all else being equal). This ensures that the total health measured in QALYs generated from a given budget is maximized.

An important challenge, then, is the determination of the threshold cost per QALY. In England, the National Institute for Health and Clinical Excellence (NICE) established a range of £20,000–£30,000 per additional QALY (NICE 2004, 2008). Interventions below £20,000 would probably be funded, those within the range would be considered alongside other factors (such as uncertainty and innovation), and when above £30,000 the case for these other factors must be stronger.

The threshold value could be set to reflect society's valuation of a QALY of health and there has been work to obtain this value by asking which individuals are willing to pay for a 1 QALY gain as *private consumers* or as *citizens*. These methods have resulted in a range of possible estimates in different countries (Baker *et al.* 2010). By using this approach, the budget is set to fund all interventions below the societal threshold value. However, the budget for many publicly funded health care systems is determined politically without explicit consideration of people's willingness to pay for a QALY and is fixed in any given year. In a situation where the budget is less than that required to fund all interventions below the societal cost per QALY threshold, then to apply this threshold would result in inefficiency. Supposing the societal threshold cost per QALY is £60,000 but the marginal decision implied by the budget has a cost per QALY of £25,000, then to agree to fund the new intervention at a cost per QALY of £50,000 would displace more health than it creates, resulting in a net health loss (e.g. if the treatment costs of 1,000 patients is £1m then it generates 20 QALYs, but the number of displaced health would be 40 resulting in a net loss of 20 QALYs).

It has been argued that in the context of a fixed budget the threshold value for cost per QALY is a factual matter and not one of preferences or judgements (Claxton *et al.* 2013). The threshold value is determined by the interaction of the fixed budget, the needs of the population, and the production possibilities. The threshold should be set so that the marginally adopted technologies have a better incremental cost per QALY ratio than any technologies not adopted. In the past, the threshold used by NICE was based on informal judgement. A more empirically based method would be to try to find the specific activities that have been displaced, but in the context of a large and complex health system like the National Health Service (NHS) this has proved to be a major challenge. An alternative methodology proposed by Claxton and colleagues (2013) in the context of the NHS has been to estimate the relationship between changes in expenditure and outcomes across local health authorities. The 'York threshold project' has used natural variation in expenditure and outcomes (i.e. mortality) across the health authorities by broad International Classification of Diseases groupings. This research had to overcome major technical challenges, including endogeneity in expenditure and outcomes, and translating the mortality data into QALY terms, which are detailed in their report (Claxton *et al.* 2013). The specific results are surrounded by considerable uncertainty (their best estimate is nearer £13,000) and not relevant to the discussion here. The main point is their approach of seeing the threshold as a technical fact, and not a matter of preferences or judgement.

2.3.3 **Cost-benefit analysis**

The key feature of cost-benefit analysis (CBA) is that all the benefits of an intervention, alongside the costs, are valued in monetary terms. This does not mean that only financial consequences are included, but that intangible outcomes, such as the effects on survival and health, have to be valued using money as the numeraire. An intervention is considered worthwhile if the monetary valuation of all the benefits exceeds the costs (i.e. positive net benefit). This technique can be used to address the question of whether a treatment/programme is worthwhile for society, rather than restricting it to the NHS budget or to a single objective. As for CUA, it is based on the notion that those who gain (i.e. enjoy the benefits) could compensate the losers (i.e. incur the costs) (see Chapter 3 for a review of this justification). A further advantage of CBA is that the measure of benefit encompasses a wider range, and in particular, non-health benefits.

There are a number of techniques for obtaining monetary valuations of health benefits. One is the human capital approach that values health changes in terms of their impact on productivity, such as through labour force participation and presenteeism. However, this is a very limited view of what constitutes the value of health, since it excludes the less tangible benefits. Another approach is to infer values from people's 'revealed preferences' in market settings. One example of this is using the extra wages of construction workers in risky jobs to infer a value for a life. However, applying revealed preference methods to the consumption of health care is difficult due to its well-documented features, including consumer ignorance and zero or subsidized price at the point of use (see Chapter 3). This can be overcome in some cases by obtaining revealed preference data from outside the health care sector (such as the value for life in the labour market suing differentials in risk of mortality). However, these methods assume that the labour market is free and unregulated, that workers are fully informed, make free choices to maximize utility, and that workers are representative of the rest of the population in terms of socio-demographics and other characteristics.

These difficulties have led to the adoption of a range of techniques in applied microeconomics under the broad heading of 'stated preference' methods or contingent valuation. These methods ask respondents to express how much they would be 'willing to pay' for an intervention, even though they are not required to pay.

The use of stated willingness to pay (WTP) has been popular in other areas such as transport and environment, but less so in health economics (Donaldson and Gerard 1993). WTP has not been widely used in health economics distributional implications, since it assumes the current distribution of income is appropriate (though there are ways of adjusting for this effect). Another problem arises from the use of WTP in CBA from the fact that many health systems, such as the NHS, have a fixed budget, and so the decision rule must be modified to examining the relative costs and benefits from different programmes. As we have seen here, the WTP technique is still used in health care as a means of valuing health and other benefits, but CBA has been used much less than CEA. This book focuses on the CEA using QALYs and does not have much on CBA, though the normative arguments for using CBA are reviewed in Chapter 3.

2.3.4 **Cost-consequence analysis**

Cost-consequence analysis (CCA) is founded on scepticism concerning the extent to which all the relevant considerations in an economic evaluation could be presented in one number, such as the monetary cost per unit outcome or net benefit of treatment. To give a few examples, these efficiency measures on their own do not tell us anything about: the size of the health gain; what severity of health the health improvement starts from; what happens to patients if they do not get the treatment; the age and life stage or socio-economic situation of typical patients; or the magnitude or rarity of the health problem. All these might be relevant considerations in determining the relative ranking of different interventions. Therefore, the results of CCA are reported in the form of a table, where all the relevant factors are presented, but do not have a single number to enable a unique and complete ranking of different treatment options. This last stage is left to the 'decision maker', for whom the analyses were carried out.

The advantage of this approach is that it retains the way of thinking and discipline of economic evaluation (Coast 2004). To the extent that the data are helpful, it can be seen within the decision-aiding tradition of economic evaluation (Sugden and Williams 1978). The disadvantages are that the basis for a decision can often be unclear and will not be based on explicit values. More recently, health economists have been looking into the use of multicriteria decision making, to help decision makers structure their consideration of the different consequences of a decision. It typically involves a more explicit elicitation of scores and weights (usually by an analyst) for the different types of consequences, with the aim of improving the transparency of decision making (Thokala and Duenas 2012).

2.4 Measures for describing health

2.4.1 What is health?

Health has been variously defined, but one of the most enduring and influential definitions is the statement in the Constitution of the World Health Organization (1948) that health is: 'A state of complete physical, mental and social well-being, and not merely the absence of disease and infirmity'. While this definition has been influential in the development of measures in this field, it is very broad and not easy to operationalize. It could be argued, for example, that social well-being is not health *per se*, but an aspect of quality of life that is affected by health. Some developers have chosen to take a much narrower definition of health in the construction of their measure. Consequently, measures of health, or health-related quality of life often differ considerably in their content. To add to the potential for confusion, some measures claim to measure quality of life, and yet their content is narrowly focused on health.

In the health literature terms such as health, health status, health-related quality of life, and quality of life are used to mean different things by different instrument developers. In a sense the terminology itself does not matter, but underlying this issue of semantics is an important implication for policy in terms of what should be counted as a benefit and what might be ignored for the purpose of informing health policy. Whether or not social activities are counted as health, health-related quality of life, or quality of life does not matter—the important question is whether impact on social activities should form part of the description of the benefits of health care (see Chapter 7 for a review of the content of generic preference-based measures).

An important feature of health is that it includes domains (such as pain, feelings, or various symptoms) that are experienced by an individual. It is difficult to measure these domains by external observation. There is evidence of significant differences between what professionals report on a patient and what the patients say themselves, particularly for psychosocial domains (Jachuck *et al.* 1982). It is becoming increasingly recognized in clinical and health services research that descriptions of the experience of a health state should be elicited from the patients themselves or, where this is not possible, from others on their behalf, in order to best reflect the actual experience of the disease and its treatment (Fitzpatrick *et al.* 1998).

2.4.2 What are patient-reported outcome measures of health?

A common method for describing an individual's health is to obtain the reports from the individuals themselves. This method has been named 'patient-reported outcomes' (PROs) or patient-reported outcome measures (PROMS). PROMS obtain the individual's own report of their health on various health dimensions and apply a numerical scoring system to provide numeric descriptions of their health. The domains in PROMs do not include biomedical measures (such as blood pressure, forced expiratory volume, cholesterol levels, etc.) or relate to specific diagnostic instruments used in clinical practice. While both of these are important in the clinical management of a patient and potentially important in predicting a person's future health, they are less pertinent to understanding the health experience of a patient.

Self-reported measures of health have been available since the 1940s (Karnofsky and Burchenal 1949), but did not become widely used until the 1960s and 1970s. However, by 1987, there were over 200 measures of health identified by Spilker and colleagues (1990). They can assess symptoms, function, or well-being depending on the specific definition of health being used. They can be 'generic' and hence designed for use across different conditions, or specifically designed for a particular disease.

PROMS are increasingly being used to assess the efficacy and effectiveness of health care interventions. The use of (non-preference-based) PROMS in economic evaluation is limited because they do not have the necessary properties to undertake CEA. However, such measures will continue to be widely used in clinical trials and other studies due to their popularity with clinicians and health services researchers who are seeking to gather evidence for other purposes. It is therefore important to understand how health status measures could be used in economic evaluation.

2.4.3 **The content of instruments**

Measures of health vary widely in terms of content, format, and scaling. The principal features of a sample of five measures are presented in Table 2.1. They have been selected to demonstrate the diversity of measures in terms of their size, coverage of health domains, method of administration and sources of values, not for being typical, or even representative.

The content varies considerably between the measures. They cover generic concepts of functioning (such as physical functioning) through to specific symptoms (e.g. dyspnoea for respiratory disease, dexterity for arthritis, and so forth). The methods of completing the questionnaires include clinical interview, professional assessment, researcher interview, and self-completion, either in the clinic or at home. While most of these measures are self-reported, we note that the Barthel Index is an exception, being completed by the health professional. The Chronic Respiratory Questionnaire incorporates a further development, where patients are asked to identify the important activities which make them breathless, as well as providing the assessment. The developers have argued that this approach has the advantage of generating a score that is more responsive to health change (Guyatt et al. 1987), though it reduces interpersonal comparability. Responses to items are combined into either a single index or a profile of several subindices of scores.

Most measures of health have a simple 'summative' scoring system. The SF-36 health survey, for example, is a questionnaire used to assess patient health across eight dimensions (Ware et al. 1993). It consists of items or questions which present respondents with choices about their perception of their own health (see Table 2.2). For example, the physical functioning dimension has 10 items to which the patient can make one of three responses: 'limited a lot', 'limited a little', or 'not limited at all'. These

Table 2.1 Characteristics of five health status measures

Measure	No. of dimensions	Description of dimensions/items	No. of items	Source of responses	Method of administration	Source of values	Score(s)
Condition-specific St George's Respiratory Questionnaire	4	Symptoms (e.g. shortness of breath and wheezing), activity (e.g. walking and playing games), impacts (e.g. embarrassment)	50	Patient	Interview or self-completion	Patients (using VAS)	By dimension and index
Chronic Respiratory Questionnaire	4	Dyspnoea, fatigue, emotional function, mastery	20	Patient	Interview	Summative	By dimension
Barthel	1	Mobility, grooming, dressing, continence	10	Professional	Professional assessment	Summative	Index
Generic SF-36 health survey	8	Physical functioning, role limitations (physical and emotional problems), social functioning, pain, mental health, general health perception	36	Patient or proxy	Self-completion, interviewer administration	Summative	By dimension
Nottingham Health Profile	6	Mobility, social isolation, pain, emotional reactions, energy	38	Patient	Self-completion	Thurston's method	By dimension

Reprinted by permission of Sage Publications Ltd from Andrew Stevens et al. (eds.), *The Advanced Handbook of Methods in Evidence Based Healthcare*, Sage Publications Ltd., London, UK, Copyright © 2001. Editorial arrangement, Introduction, and Part Introductions © Andrew Stevens, Keith R. Abraham, John Brazier, Ray Fitzpatrick, and Richard J Lilford 2001. Chapters 1–27 © the Contributors 2001.

Table 2.2 An example of a measure of health status—the SF-36 health survey

Dimension	No. of items	Summary of content	No. of response choices	Range of response choice
Physical functioning	10	Extent to which health limits physical activities such as self-care, walking, climbing stairs, bending, lifting, and moderate and vigorous exercises	3	'Yes limited a lot' to 'no, not limited at all'
Role limitations–physical	4	Extent to which physical health interferes with work or other daily activities, including accomplishing less than wanted, limitations in the kind of activities, or difficulty in performing activities	2	Yes/No
Bodily pain	2	Intensity of pain and effect of pain on normal work, both inside and outside the home	5 and 6	'None' to 'very severe' and 'not at all' to 'extremely'
General health	5	Personal evaluation of health, including current health, health outlook, and resistance to illness	5	'All of the time' to 'none of the time'
Vitality	4	Feeling energetic and full of life versus feeling tired and worn out	6	'All of the time' to 'none of the time'
Social functioning	2	Extent to which physical health or emotional problems interfere with normal social activities	5	'Not at all' to 'extremely' and 'All of the time' to 'none of the time'
Role limitations–emotional	3	Extent to which emotional problems interfere with work or other daily activities, including decreased time spent on activities, accomplishing less, and not working as carefully as usual	2	Yes/No
Mental health	5	General mental health, including depression, anxiety, behavioural–emotional control, general positive affect	6	'All of the time' to 'none of the time'

Reproduced with permission from Brazier J et al., A review of the use of health status measures in economic evaluation, *Health Technology Assessment*, Volume 3, Issue 9, Copyright © 1999 NETSCC.

responses are coded 1, 2, and 3, respectively, and the 10 coded responses are summed to produce a score from 10 to 30. The same procedure is used for all eight dimensions. These raw dimension scores are transformed linearly onto a 0–100 scale. The eight dimension scores of the SF-36 are not comparable across dimensions. This procedure has been misleadingly described in the psychometric literature as being 'unweighted' (Jenkinson 1991), yet implies an *equal* weighting.

Scoring can be more sophisticated, such as with the use of statistical techniques like factor analysis for the SF-36 (Ware *et al.* 1993). More recently, Rasch models have been suggested to take into account the degree of difficulty, or severity, of an item in relation to the underlying, unobserved (latent) scale that the item is presumed to measure. Some instruments, such as the St George's Respiratory questionnaire and the Sickness Impact Profile weight items using explicit valuation procedures. This involves asking people to rate the importance of each item using a visual analogue scale (VAS) (see Chapter 5). Other instruments ask the patients to record how bothersome they find the attribute described by the item, and this is then used to weight the item.

2.5 The use of non-preference-based measures of health in economic evaluation

2.5.1 Criticisms of non-preference-based health status measures

2.5.1.1 Scoring by dimension

The simple summative scoring algorithms described in the previous section have been used by most measures of perceived health. These measures are designed to produce scales that claim to measure the severity of health dimensions, but not their relative importance. The latter aspect requires the assumption that there are equal intervals between the response categories and that the items are of equal importance. However, there is no reason to suppose that, for example, patients value the intervals of the responses to items of the SF-36 physical functioning dimension, 'not limited at all' and 'limited a little', to be equivalent to the interval between 'limited a little' and 'limited a lot'. To take another example from the SF-36, the intervals for an item on how much bodily pain a person has had in the last 4 weeks are 'none' to 'very mild', 'very mild' to 'mild', 'mild' to 'moderate', 'moderate' to 'severe', and 'severe' to 'very severe'. This would imply that in a trial, a reduction in pain from 'mild' to 'very mild' would be equivalent to a reduction from 'severe' to 'moderate'. Yet evidence using visual analogue and standard gamble valuation techniques suggests that, on average, people do not value 'very mild' significantly better than 'mild', but there is a very large and significant difference between the values for 'moderate' and 'severe' (Brazier *et al.* 1998, 2002).

The summing of scores will also not necessarily reflect the value people would place on different items. In the physical functioning scale of the SF-36, the item 'limitations in climbing one flight of stairs' is assumed to be of equal importance to 'limitations in walking more than one mile'. For someone living in a single storey building, limitations in walking would probably be regarded as a far worse problem. Given the lack of any empirical basis for these assumptions, there must be doubts about even the ordinal properties of these scales as indicators of people's preferences, particularly over small changes in the dimension scores.

The equal interval assumptions underlying most measures of health have been defended by some researchers. It has been claimed that the relative importance of the different health concepts (as perceived by the instrument developers) is in part accounted for by the number of items used to represent them. It has also been claimed that it makes little difference in practice whether or not equal interval weighting is used (Jenkinson 1991). However, the numerous valuation studies with the EQ-5D, SF-6D, and HUI3 have all shown that intervals between response choices are not equal and that items do not have the same weight (see Chapter 8 for a review of these measures). Furthermore, studies have found only a low to moderate correlation between health status measures and various preference- or value-weighted measures (Brazier *et al.* 1999).

Some instruments have adopted psychometric methods such as factor analysis or Rasch modelling to improve their scoring as measures of severity. Factor analysis weights items according to the extent to which they contribute to some underlying latent variable. The stronger the correlation, the larger the weight of an item or dimension (depending on the unit of analysis). This has been used to re-score the SF-36 dimensions into two summary scores, one for physical health and the other for mental health (Ware *et al.* 1993). The scores have also been transformed so that a score of 50 represents the mean level in the general population and each movement of 10 points from this score represents a standard deviation of the score in the general population. While this scoring system offers a better statistical basis for understanding score differences between populations, there is no reason why weights based on correlation between items should reflect their relative importance to people in their daily lives.

There has been interest in using item response theory models such as Rasch to re-score instruments based on item response theory (Tennant *et al.* 2004). This technique was originally developed in education to provide a way of estimating how difficult different questions are against a uni-dimensional latent variable, for example numeracy (Rasch 1960). In health, the analysis will estimate the degree of severity for a latent health variable represented by different items, where the underlying construct can be dimensions such as physical functioning or pain. It is claimed that Rasch models result in a linear interval scale against which any item, regardless of the instrument from which it came, can be calibrated. One example of its application was a re-scoring of the 10 item physical functioning of the SF-36 (Raczek *et al.* 1997).

While Rasch models provide a useful technique for understanding the position of items within a construct, they do not provide an appropriate method for valuing health for economic evaluation (such as in a cost per QALY analysis). The fact that one item is found to be more difficult to do, say against the construct mobility, does not mean that it is more or less important in people's lives. While it may represent an improvement on summative scoring and has an important role in constructing measures (this is discussed in the context of constructing preference-based measures in Chapter 8), it does not provide the preference-based weights needed for cost per QALY analyses.

Box 2.2 The difference between measuring and valuing health

A common source of confusion between economists and other health researchers is the distinction between measuring and valuing health. While many psychometricians are seeking to measure or numerically describe health along its different dimensions, economists want to know the *relative value that patients or others* place on the dimensions and their components in order to undertake more than the most rudimentary form of economic evaluation. The value of a health improvement will be related to a measure of the size of the change, but these two concepts will not be perfectly correlated. For example, someone may regard a large health improvement (such as the ability to walk upstairs) as being of little or no benefit if they live in a single storey building. Conversely, an apparently small improvement in pain may be highly valued by the patient.

Over the years, there have been a number of interesting debates between psychometricians and economists. The main source of confusion seems to arise from the distinction between measuring the construct or constructs of health and the value of health. This difference is summarized in Box 2.2. While the dichotomy may seem rather simplistic, since measures of health do contain some degree of evaluation of the importance of the item, the distinction provides a useful way to understand the difference between the two approaches.

2.5.1.2 Score profile

Most health status measures present a profile of scores. The generation of a single index score for health has been opposed by many developers of measures of health. The developers of the Nottingham Health Profile, for example, have argued: 'The simple addition of affirmative responses gives misleading results because of the features of pain, social life, emotion, and so on are qualitatively distinct and made up of different facets which cannot have common denominators' (Hunt *et al.* 1986). This view is understandable when the purpose is to derive a descriptive *measure* of different aspects of health, but this is not sufficient for use in economic evaluation. To undertake economic evaluation, it will often be necessary to be able to combine the dimensions into an overall indicator of health. For example, in a comparison of the surgical and medical management of a condition, one might perform better against one dimension but worse against another. At the end of a clinical trial, it would not be possible to determine which treatment was most effective, let alone whether it was cost-effective. A trade-off needs to be made between dimensions in order to determine effectiveness, and for assessing cost-effectiveness some means of *valuing* the difference between interventions needs to be found.

Some measures of health combine dimensions to form a single index (e.g. St George's Respiratory questionnaire, the Sickness Impact Profile, and the Barthel Index). As for the aggregation of items, many assume an equal weighting between dimensions (e.g. Barthel), while others combine the items using item weights estimated using valuation techniques such as the VAS (a critique of VAS as a measure of preference is provided in Chapter 5). In addition to the criticisms of these methods of valuing, the scoring systems make an assumption of simple additivity between dimensions, where the value of one dimension is assumed to be unaltered by the level of another dimension. This rules out the prospect of any interaction between dimensions.

2.5.1.3 Health status and survival

Many health care interventions have implications for survival as well as health-related quality of life, but conventional measures of health cannot be combined with survival and so cannot be used to assess the overall cost-effectiveness of such interventions. Another limitation is through a statistical artefact known as the 'survivor' effect. In a clinical study, a lower survival rate in one arm of the trial can increase its mean health status score(s) compared with the other arms of the trial. This arises because the patients who have died probably have a lower than average health status. Assuming that increased survival is regarded as a good thing, the analyst is without any means for deciding which treatment is better. There are some statistical solutions to this problem, but they fail to address the central problem that these outcomes need to be combined in some way (Billingham *et al.* 1999).

There are some additional problems with the way scores from non-preference-based PROMS tend to be used. The effect of a treatment is often estimated as the mean difference between health scores before and after the treatment of patients in the trial. A more sophisticated approach to analysing repeated measures is to estimate the health change as the difference between the mean pre-treatment scores and a weighted average of mean scores across the post-treatment assessments, with the weights proportional to the time between each assessment. In other words, it is the 'area under the curve' where levels of health are plotted against time along the horizontal axis (Matthews *et al.* 1990). However, these methods of analysis ignore the fact that individuals may have time preferences over the occurrence of outcomes; for example, they may prefer to delay bad outcomes.

2.5.1.4 Uncertainty in outcomes

Outcomes in health care are rarely certain. Even common interventions such as cholecystectomy are associated with a wide dispersion of outcomes, such as in the relief of pain (Nicholl *et al.* 1992) and mortality. Most interventions come with some risks, including mortality in some cases, and numerous complications and side effects. When treatment begins, neither the doctor nor the patient knows the outcome for certain. Conventional analyses of measures of health assume people are risk-neutral (i.e. their decision is unaffected by the degree of uncertainty around the mean value). Yet, in health care, there is evidence that many people are averse to risk (Loomes and McKenzie 1989). Patients may choose a treatment that achieves a lower expected or mean improvement in the health than another, but which is associated with less variance (next we will consider how this concern also pertains to health measured in QALYs).

2.5.2 Limitations to using health status measures in economic evaluation

The usefulness of non-preference-based health status measures in assessing the relative efficiency of interventions depends on the results of the study. In Table 2.3 we present seven scenarios of costs and outcomes in a comparison of a new intervention

Table 2.3 Assessing the relative efficiency of two interventions given different cost and health outcome scenarios

Scenario	Cost	Health status measure	Can relative efficiency be evaluated?
1	Lower	Better in at least one dimension and no worse on any other	Yes, by dominance[1]
2	Same	Better in at least one dimension and no worse on any other	Yes[1]
3	Lower	Same across all dimensions	Yes, by cost minimization[1,2]
4	Lower	Better on some dimensions and worse on others	No
5	Same	Better on some dimensions and worse on others	No
6	Higher	Better in at least one dimension and no worse on any other	No
7	Higher	Better on some dimensions and worse on others	No

[1] Assuming the scale at least indicates ordinal preferences over the range being considered (see discussion in text).

[2] It has been argued that cost minimization is rarely achievable, given the uncertainty that exists around most estimates (see discussion in text).

Reproduced with permission from Brazier J *et al.*, A review of the use of health status measures in economic evaluation, *Health Technology Assessment*, Volume 3, Issue 9, Copyright © 1999 NETSCC.

with the existing one, and consider whether it is possible to assess cost-effectiveness using health status measures.

The limitations of conventional non-preference-based measures are most apparent where there are trade-offs, and these are shown in Table 2.3 as scenarios 4–7. In scenarios 4 and 5 the new treatment performs better on some dimensions but worse on others, hence it could have a lower cost per unit of health gain on some dimensions but higher on others. Furthermore, it is the incremental cost-effectiveness ratio that is important for resource allocation purposes. Therefore, where the less cost-effective intervention costs more and yields a higher benefit, the greater benefit could still be worth the extra cost, according to the threshold.

For multiple outcomes, one approach is to present the costs and benefits of the alternatives in a CCA. This type of presentation is unlikely to be helpful since scores on health status measures have no obvious intuitive meaning. Score differences cannot be compared between dimensions, nor can scores from non-preference-based health measures be compared with other outcomes like survival or cost. Non-preference-based health status measures cannot be used to assess the efficiency of interventions in these circumstances.

Overall, health status measures have a very limited role in economic evaluation in their usual form, if any at all. While clinical measures using natural units have some role in cost-effectiveness, these are also limited in terms of the questions that can be addressed (see section 2.3.1). For this reason, a different class of health status measures has been developed, known as preference-based measures of health or multiattribute utility scales, for calculating QALYs. However, this is not to say that the descriptive data collected by these non-preference-based health measures could not be used in other ways. In Chapter 8 we review a range of methods for using these data in an economic evaluation, including mapping onto preference-based measures and constructing new preference-based measures from them (as has been done with the SF-36 and a number of condition-specific measures). The next section provides an introduction to QALYs and to preference-based measures of health.

2.6 **An introduction to quality-adjusted life years**

One of the great innovations in the subdiscipline of health economics has been the development of a new method for valuing health benefits for use in economic evaluation, namely the QALY. The QALY values health in terms of a measure that combines longevity with quality of life into the common numeraire of a year in full health. The use of the QALY is a major departure from mainstream economics (see Chapter 3 for a review of theoretical foundation of the QALY measure and why it has gained prominence over the more conventional approaches used by mainstream economists). This section introduces the reader to the QALY and preference-based health status measures that provide the quality adjustment.

2.6.1 **Basic description**

The QALY has been developed in an attempt to combine the value of these attributes into a single index number. It has been defined as 'a measure of health outcome which assigns to each period of time a weight, ranging from 0 to 1, corresponding to the health-related quality of life during that period, where a weight of 1 corresponds to optimal health, and a weight of 0 corresponds to health state judged to be equivalent to being dead' (Gold *et al.* 1996). The basic idea is that, for any individual, the prospect of living Y years in less than full health, or 'optimal health', may be equated to a prospect of living X years in full health where X<Y. If different 'Ys' can be converted into equivalent 'Xs' (i.e. QALYs), and if more QALYs are preferred to fewer, then QALYs can be used to inform resource allocation decisions.

The idea of the QALY is represented graphically in Figure 2.1, which presents an example of the expected quality and length of life of patients with severe angina and left main vessel disease (Williams 1985). The graph shows the length of life along the horizontal axis and the quality of life, measured on the zero to one scale, along the vertical scale. Profile A is the expected profile following surgery where the patient lives for 11 years at different levels of quality of life. Profile B represents medical management and profile C the consequences of operative mortality from surgery. The number of QALYs associated with each profile is represented by the area under each curve. The net benefit of surgery over medication is profile A minus profile C and profile B. This is one of the oldest representations of the QALY measure and it is worth saying that the expected survival and

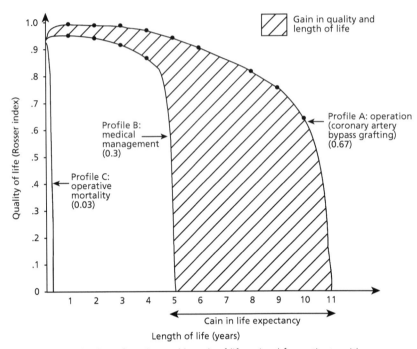

Fig. 2.1 Expected value of quality and length of life gained for patients with severe angina and left main vessel disease.

Reproduced from *The British Medical Journal*, Williams A, 'Economics of coronary artery bypass grafting', Volume 291, Issue 6491, pp. 326–9, Copyright © 1985 British Medical Journal Publishing Group, with permission from the BMJ Publishing Group Ltd.

quality of life data come from a very low level of evidence (the opinion of three clinicians!), but there are more robust methods described in this book (see Chapter 9).

More generally, the QALY measure is constructed as follows. The number of QALYs relating to a health outcome is expressed as the value given to a particular health state, multiplied by the length of time spent in that state. Since the outcomes of any given intervention are uncertain, the expected value of each possible outcome can be represented by the value weighted by its probability. Then, the expected outcome of the treatment itself can be represented by the sum of the expected value of the possible individual outcomes.

The benefit of the treatment is not the same as the outcome of the treatment, because the patient may recover even without treatment. So the net benefit of treatment is the difference between the expected outcome with and without treatment. The benefit of an intervention at the population level is then the aggregate of net benefits to individual patients. So, if the expected benefit of an average patient is obtained, the aggregate benefit to the population of a health care programme can be derived by multiplying the individual benefit by the number of patients expected. Thus, the QALY algorithm is a combination of value of health states (Q), durations (T), probabilities (P), and the

Box 2.3 The QALY algorithm

In the simplest case, with no uncertainty, no temporal discounting, and no changes in health over time, the value of a health gain from treatment for an individual, $QALY_G$, can be represented as:

$$QALY_G = T_1 Q_1 - T_0 Q_0,$$

where T is the number of years of survival, Q represents health state values, and the subscripts 1 and 0 represent health with and without treatment, respectively.

Alternatively, introducing uncertainty and temporal discounting, and assuming discrete time so that changes in health occur only when moving from one period to the next, the expected net gain of a treatment to any one individual can be expressed as:

$$QALY_G = \sum_h \sum_t p_{1ht} Q_{ht} - \sum_h \sum_t p_{0ht} Q_{ht},$$

where p_{1ht} and p_{0ht} represent the probabilities of an individual finding himself in health state h in time period t with and without treatment, respectively. Q_{ht} is the value of health state h at time t (the subscript t here allows for constant rate temporal discounting so that $Q_{ht} = Q_h/(1 + r)^t$ where r is the discount rate).

number of patients. This is expressed more formally in Box 2.3. Some simple exercises to calculate QALYs are provided in Drummond *et al.* (2015).

The QALY measure is used widely in economic evaluation to evaluate the cost-effectiveness of interventions. It also can be used at the *individual level* to inform clinical decisions between medical interventions for the same condition, as more QALYs are assumed to be better (see Chapter 3).

2.6.2 Assumptions underlying the preference-based QALY

Health is experienced as a profile of states occurring at different points in time, lasting for different periods of time, and occurring in different sequences. For the QALY to represent individual preferences over time, then a number of assumptions need to be made about the nature of these preferences. At this point it is sufficient to observe that in order for QALYs to represent individual preferences over health profiles, health state values must be independent of the duration of the states, when they occur and in what sequence, and in most applications it must be discussed that people are risk-neutral. These are very restrictive assumptions, but they would equally apply to the use of conventional health status measures. These assumptions of the QALY model are examined in detail in Chapters 3 and 11.

Table 2.4 EQ-5D questionnaire
Here are some simple questions about your health in general.
By ticking one answer in each group, please indicate which
statements best describe your own health state TODAY

Please tick one

1. **Mobility**
    I have no problems in walking about
    I have some problems in walking about
    I am confined to bed

2. **Self-care**
    I have no problems with self-care
    I have some problems washing or dressing myself
    I am unable to wash or dress myself

3. **Usual activities**
    I have no problems with performing my usual activities
        (e.g. work, study, housework, family or leisure activities)
    I have some problems with performing my usual activities
    I am unable to perform my usual activities

4. **Pain/discomfort**
    I have no pain or discomfort
    I have moderate pain or discomfort
    I have extreme pain or discomfort

5. **Anxiety/depression**
    I am not anxious or depressed
    I am moderately anxious or depressed
    I am extremely anxious or depressed

2.6.3 Putting the 'Q' into the QALY

To calculate the number of QALYs, it is necessary to represent health on a scale where the states of being dead and full health are assigned values of 0 and 1, respectively. Therefore, states rated as better than dead have values between 0 and 1, and states rated as worse than dead have negative scores which, in principle, are unbounded. The key task is to estimate the value of the 'Q' in the QALY, and this forms the focus of the remainder of this book.

How this can be done will be demonstrated by presenting one of the most widely used instruments for estimating the value of 'Q', the generic preference-based measure of health the EQ-5D (Brooks 1996). This instrument has a structured health state descriptive system with five dimensions: mobility, self-care, usual activities, pain/discomfort, and anxiety/depression. Each dimension has three levels: no problem (level 1); moderate or some problem (level 2); and severe problem (level 3). Together these five

Table 2.5 UK TTO EQ-5D tariff

Dimension	Level	Decrement
Constant		0.081
Mobility	2	0.069
	3	0.314
Self-care	2	0.104
	3	0.214
Usual activity	2	0.036
	3	0.094
Pain/discomfort	2	0.123
	3	0.386
Anxiety/depression	2	0.071
	3	0.236
N3		0.269

Reproduced from Dolan P, 'Modelling valuations for EuroQol health states', *Medical Care*, Volume 35, Issue 11, pp. 1095–108, Copyright © 1997, with permission from Lippincott, Williams and Wilkins.

dimensions define a total of 243 health states formed by different combinations of the levels (i.e. 3^5), and each state is described in the form of a five-digit code using the three levels (e.g. state 12321 means no problems in mobility, moderate problems in self-care, and so on). A new five-level version describes 3,125 health states (Dolan 1997; see Chapter 7). EQ-5D can be administered to patients or their proxies using a short one-page questionnaire with five questions (Table 2.4).

The five-digit EQ-5D data generated this way can be converted into preference-based single indices in a number of ways with different methods of valuation and source country, but the most widely used to date is the UK York time trade-off (TTO) algorithm (Dolan 1997) shown in Table 2.5. This 'population value set' provides an algorithm to the value of all 243 states. For all health states other than 11111, there is a constant decrement of 0.081, followed by the decrement associated with each level 2 or 3 that appears in the state; finally, for those states with a level 3, there is an additional decrement (the 'N3' term). For example, the value for the EQ-5D state 11223 is $1.0 - (0.081 + 0.036 + 0.123 + 0.236 + 0.269) = 0.255$.

This algorithm was estimated by valuing a sample of 42 health states defined by the EQ-5D using the TTO method with a sample of around 3,000 members of the UK general population. This asks people to imagine that they will be in an EQ-5D state for 10 years (t), and then asks them to consider a number of shorter periods in full health (for states better than dead; i.e. at level 1 in each dimension). At the point where respondents are unable to choose between t years in the state and x years in full health, the value of the state is given as x/t. Different valuation methods are reviewed in Chapter 4. These health state valuation data were then analysed by regression in order to estimate the decrements shown in Table 2.5. The different methods for modelling health state preference data are described in detail in Chapter 6.

One advantage of using generic preference-based measures like the EQ-5D is that they are easy to use. They can be incorporated into most clinical trial and routine data collection systems comparatively easily, with little additional burden for respondents. All are self-completed, though they can be administered through carers or other proxies. They are generic and so should be relevant to all patient groups. This last feature is important to those health economists seeking to standardize all aspects of methods in order to achieve comparability between patient groups. The arguments for and against this degree of standardization are reviewed in Chapter 8.

The aim of this book is not to promote one or other of the generic preference-based instruments, but to provide an in-depth understanding of the technical and normative judgements involved in their construction. The field has been developing rapidly in recent years, and now is not the time to call a halt to such developments.

2.7 The questions addressed in this book

The EQ-5D provides a useful starting point for the rest of this book, since it demonstrates the key features of any method for measuring and valuing health. Underpinning this and similar instruments are a number of core questions: what is the unit of value? What is being valued? How is it valued? Who values it? How it is used in economic evaluation? And finally, how should it be aggregated? (Box 2.4).

The first of these core questions is the unit of value. To be able to make cross-programme comparisons, it is necessary to have a numeraire or some means of valuing benefits in a common currency. This can be money, as used in CBA. The QALY is another unit and forms the main subject of this book. A unit of value must allow cross-programme comparisons, so a QALY estimated for an intervention in one group of patients is comparable with QALYs estimated for another intervention for a different medical condition in a different group of patients.

Having decided to use the QALY to capture outcomes, the next question concerns what should be included in the description of health or quality of life. Some measures for quality of life adjustment cover quite narrowly defined aspects of impairment and symptomology associated with medical conditions, while others take a higher level and broader conception of quality of life. There are questions as to whether the measure should be generic like the EQ-5D or more specific, and indeed whether it should be based on a structured classification at all, or rather use a bespoke vignettes approach.

The next set of questions all relate to how health should be valued, or how to quantify the quality adjustment. The most commonly used techniques are time trade-off,

Box 2.4 Core questions to address in the measurement and valuation of health for use in economic evaluation

What should be the measure of value?

To be able to make cross-programme comparisons, it is necessary to have a numeraire or some means of valuing benefits using a common currency. This can be money, as used in cost-benefit analyses. Another that has become widely used is the QALY.

How should it be described?

Having decided to use the QALY, a key question is what should be valued, and for generic preference-based measures of health what aspects of health should be included in the health state classification system. Some cover quite narrowly defined health domains of impairment and symptomology associated with a medical condition, while others look at health-related quality of life. Some are intended to be generic across patient groups and others are more specific to a condition.

How should it be valued?

There are a range of techniques for valuing health (including cardinal techniques such as standard gamble, time trade-off, and visual analogue scales, and ordinal ones like discrete choice experiments and ranking) and their different variants.

Who should provide the values?

A number of different people could provide the values, including the patients themselves, their carers and medical professionals, or members of the general population.

How should values be used in economic evaluation?

The use of health state utility values in economic evaluation raises issues about where, how, and when they should be collected; how they should be analysed; and how they need to be modified for use in decision models.

How should QALYs be aggregated?

The value of a QALY may depend on when it arises or who receives it.

standard gamble and visual analogue scales, and more recently ordinal techniques such as discrete choice experiments. A related issue is the *variant* of technique that should be used, since major differences have been found across variants for the same technique, mostly due to framing effects. There are also important issues around how such data should be analysed. The second question concerns the source of values, and whether they should be obtained from patients themselves, their carers and medical professionals, or members of the general population. The third issue is about the more technical concerns of how health state values should be used in economic evaluation. This includes issues of how and when preference-based measures should be administered to patients and how the data should be analysed. Economic evaluation is increasingly being undertaken alongside mathematical decision models and these often require additional modifications to the values. Another question is how to aggregate numbers of QALY gains across populations. Can we assume that a QALY is a QALY regardless of who receives it, or does the value of a QALY depend on when it arises or on who receives it? Finally, there is an international perspective to measuring and valuing health covering all these issues.

2.8 Concluding remarks

The impact of health care interventions on a person's perceived health is an important benefit. Many of the existing health status measures used in clinical trials and health services research in general are not suitable for use in economic evaluation. These instruments were not designed for this purpose and have little role in the assessment of cost-effectiveness in their current form. For this reason, preference-based measures have been developed in order to generate QALYs. These instruments directly incorporate preferences and values, and produce a measure that in principle enables cross-programme comparisons, at least within health care. Underpinning these instruments are a number of core questions that are addressed in this book: what should be the measure of benefits in health care (Chapter 3)? How is it to be described (Chapters 7, 8, and 11)? How is it to be valued (Chapters 4, 5, and 6)? Who is to value it (Chapter 5)? How to use them in economic evaluation (Chapter 9)? Finally, how should the measure be aggregated (Chapter 10)? Addressing these questions forms the main focus of this book.

References

Baker R, Bateman I, Donaldson C, Jones-Lee M, Lancsar E, Loomes G, Mason H, Odejar M, Pinto Prades JL, Robinson A, Ryan M, Shackley P, Smith R, Sugden R, Wildman J (2010). Weighting and valuing quality-adjusted life-years using stated preference methods: preliminary results from the Social Value of a QALY project. *Health Technology Assessment* **14**:27.

Billingham LJ, Abrams KR, Jones DR (1999). Methods for the analysis of quality of life and survival data in health technology assessment. *Health Technology Assessment* **3**(10):1–152.

Bowling A (2004). *Measuring health: a review of quality of life and measurement scales.* Open University Press, Milton Keynes, UK.

Brazier J, Usherwood T, Harper R, Thomas K (1998). Deriving a preference-based single index from the UK SF-36 Health Survey. *Journal of Clinical Epidemiology* **51**:1115–28.

Brazier JE, Deverill M, Green C, Harper R, Booth A (1999). A review of the use of health status measures in economic evaluation. *Health Technology Assessment* **3**(9):1–164.

Brazier J, Roberts J, Deverill M (2002). The estimation of a preference-based single index measure for health from the SF-36. *Journal of Health Economics* **21**:271–92.

Briggs AH, O'Brien B (2001). The death of cost-minimisation analysis? *Health Economics* **10**:179–84.

Brooks R & the EuroQol Group (1996). EuroQol: The current state of play. *Health Policy* **37**:53–72.

Claxton K, Martin S, Soares M, Rice N, Spackman E, Hinde S, Devlin N, Smith PC, Sculpher M (2013). *Methods for the estimation of the NICE cost-effectiveness threshold*. Centre for Health Economics Research Paper 81, University of York, UK. Available at: http://www.york.ac.uk/media/che/documents/papers/researchpapers/CHERP81_methods_estimation_NICE_costeffectiveness_threshold_(Nov2013).pdf

Coast J (2004). Is economic evaluation in touch with society's health values? *British Medical Journal* **329**:1233–6.

Commonwealth Department of Health, Housing and Community Service (2002). *Guidelines for the pharmaceutical industry on the submission to the Pharmaceutical Benefits Advisory Committee*. Australian Government Publishing Service, Canberra, Australia.

Canadian Agency for Drugs and Technologies in Health (CADTH) (2006). *Guidelines for the economic evaluation of health technologies*: Canada. 3rd edn. CADTH, Ottawa, Canada.

Dolan P (1997). Modelling valuation for EuroQol health states. *Medical Care*, **35**(11):1095–108.

Donaldson C, Gerard K (1993). *Economics of health care financing: the visible hand*. Macmillan, London, UK.

Drummond MF, Sculpher M, Claxton K, O'Brien B, Stoddart GL, Torrance GW (2015). *Methods for the economic evaluation of health care programmes*. Oxford Medical Publications, Oxford, UK.

Fitzpatrick R, Davey C, Buxton M, Jones DR (1998). Evaluating patient-based outcome measures for use in clinical trials. *Health Technology Assessment* **2**(14):1–74.

Gold MR, Siegel JE, Russell LB, Weinstein MC (1996). *Cost-effectiveness in health and medicine*. Oxford University Press, Oxford, UK.

Guyatt GH, Berman LB, Townend M, Pugsley SO, Chambers LW (1987). A measure of quality of life for clinical trials in chronic lung disease. *Thorax* **42**:773–8.

College voor zorgverzekeringen (CVZ) (2004). *Guidelines for pharmacoeconomic research in the Netherlands April 2006*. (Dutch version, 2004).

Hunt SM, McEwen J, McKenna SP (1986). *Measuring health status*. Croom Helm, London, UK.

Jachuck SJ, Brierley H, Jachuck S, Willcox PM (1982). The effect of hypotensive drugs on quality of life. *Journal of the Royal College of General Practitioners* **32**:103–5.

Jenkinson C (1991). Why are we weighting? A critical examination of the use of item weights in a health status measure. *Social Science and Medicine* **27**:1413–6.

Karnofsky DA, Burchenal JH (1949). The clinical evaluation of chemotherapeutic agents against cancer. In: McLeod CM (ed.) *Evaluation of chemotherapeutic agents*. Columbia University Press, New York, pp. 191–205.

Loomes G, McKenzie L (1989). The use of QALYs in health care decision making. *Social Science and Medicine* **28**:299–308.

Matthews JNS, Altman DG, Campbell MJ, Royston P (1990). Analysis of serial measurements in medical research. *British Medical Journal* **300**:230–5.

Miller W, Robinson LA, Lawrence RS (2006). *Valuing health for regulators cost-effectiveness analysis*. The National Academic Press. Washington.

National Institute for Health and Clinical Excellence (2004, 2008). *NICE guide to the methods of technology appraisal*. NICE, UK.

Nicholl J, Brazier JE, Milner PC, Westlake L, Kohler B, Williams BT, Ross B, Frost E, Johnson AG (1992). Randomised controlled trial of cost-effectiveness of lithotripsy and open cholecystectomy as treatments for gallbladder stones. *Lancet* **340**:801–7.

Raczek AE, Ware JE, Bjorner JB, Gandek B, Haley S, Aaronson NK, Apolone G, Bech P, Brazier JE, Bullinger M, Sullivan M (1997). Comparison of Rasch and summated rating scales constructed from the SF-36 physical functioning items in seven countries: results from the IQOLA project. *Journal of Clinical Epidemiology* **51**:1203–14.

Rasch G (1960). *Probabilistic models for some intelligence and attainment tests*. University of Chicago Press Chicago, IL.

Scottish Medicines Consortium (2014). *Guidance to manufacturers for completion of new product assessment form*. NHS Scotland. Available at: http://www.scottishmedicines.org.uk/Home

Spilker B, Molinek FRJr, Johnston KA, Simpson RLJr, Tilson HH (eds.) (1990). Quality of life bibliography and indexes. *Medical Care* **28**:DS1–77.

Sugden R, Williams A (1978). *The principles of practical cost-benefit analysis*. Oxford University Press, Oxford, UK.

Tennant A, McKenna SP, Hagell P (2004). Application of Rasch analysis in the development and application of quality of life instruments. *Value Health* 2004; 7 Suppl 1:S22–6.

Thokala P, Duenas A (2012). Multiple criteria decision analysis for health technology assessment. *Value in Health* **15**: 1172–81

Torrance GW, Thomas WH, Sackett DL (1972). A utility maximization model for evaluation of health care programs. *Health Services Research* **7**:118–33.

Ware JE, Snow KK, Kolinski M, Gandeck B (1993). *SF-36 health survey manual and interpretation guide*. The Health Institute, New England Medical Centre, Boston, MA.

Weinstein MC, Stason WB (1977). Foundations of cost-effectiveness analysis for health and medical practices. *New England Journal of Medicine* **296**:716–21.

Williams A (1985). Economics of coronary artery bypass grafting. *British Medical Journal* **291**:326–9.

World Health Organization (1948). *Constitution of the World Health Organization. Basic documents*. World Health Organization, Geneva, Switzerland.

Chapter 3

Foundations in welfare economics and utility theory: what should be valued?

3.1 Chapter overview

This chapter examines the first of the questions identified in the previous chapter (Box 2.4): what is to be valued? It starts by reviewing the economics of health care resource allocation through the market. It then presents the alternative of resource allocation by government intervention and the implications this has for the use of economic evaluation and the measure of benefit. This is followed by a consideration of the welfarist foundation for a measure of health, and finally some non-welfarist arguments.

3.2 Economic theory and economic evaluation

3.2.1 Resource allocation through the market

Modern micro-economics is built on a theory of competitive markets, between free sellers and buyers. The good in question can be raw materials, equipment, labour hours and skills, various services, and final consumption goods. Economic theory explores the assumptions under which, with minimal external regulations and interventions from the government (limited to those enforcing property rights and background law and order), 'market equilibria' are achieved. The quantity the sellers want to sell is increasing in price, whereas the quantity the buyers want to purchase is decreasing in price. When the price is 'right', a market equilibrium is achieved so that the total quantity the sellers want to sell at that price exactly matches the total quantity the buyers want to purchase at the price, and the market 'clears' with no leftovers or shortages. Modern economic theory has demonstrated that free competitive market equilibria are 'Pareto efficient'. Pareto efficiency is satisfied when there is no wastage: it is impossible to improve further the situation of anybody involved without making worse the situation of at least one other person. If a fully functioning, competitive market would achieve Pareto efficiency without government intervention, there would be no need for economic evaluation or any other means of valuing benefits.

A significant part of modern micro-economic theory is about predicting what happens to different markets when the conditions for such perfect markets are not met, and/or about exploring ways to achieve Pareto efficiency in the absence of these conditions.

There are several conditions for a perfect market: the four most important ways in which the health care market fails are discussed next.

3.2.1.1 Lack of certainty

Health and health care have several layers of uncertainties associated with them (Arrow 1963). For many types of illness people do not know when they will become ill, and what treatment they will require. This, combined with 'risk aversion', means that there is scope for health care insurance (see Box 3.1).

However, full coverage insurance has its own side effects (Pauly 1968). The first of these is *ex ante* consumer moral hazard. '*Ex ante*' means that this happens *before* the illness incident. Once consumers are covered by insurance, this makes the risk of possible health care expenditure less of a concern to them. If so, individuals may take less precaution and care to avoid illnesses, potentially leading to increased levels of risk (and thus, higher incidence, service use, costs, and premiums). The second is *ex post* consumer moral hazard. '*Ex post*' indicates that this concerns the stage *after* the incidence of illness. The effect of insurance on individual consumers is that they no longer have to pay for medical bills out of pocket at the point of health care consumption, while the actual cost required to produce that health care remains unaffected. So when rational individuals decide the amount of health care to consume, they overconsume relative to the socially optimal level. (These can also interact with information asymmetry between the insurer and consumer; see section 3.2.1.2.)

3.2.1.2 Lack of symmetry of information

Symmetry of information between two parties means that both parties have the same information. When individuals have different levels of risk of ill health, and there is an asymmetry of information and common knowledge about this in the health care

Box 3.1 Actuarially fair premium and risk aversion

The *actuarially fair premium* for health care insurance is calculated as the product of the size of the possible health care expenditure and the probability that this need arises. So, for example, if the expenditure, should it be required, is £500, and if the chances of it being required is 1 per cent, then the actuarially fair premium is £5.

An individual who is *risk-averse* prefers the 'certain' prospect of paying this £5 insurance premium upfront and not facing the £500 medical bill, even if they become ill, to the 'uncertain' prospect of having no insurance and possibly having to pay the £500 medical bill out of pocket should they become ill. The degree of *risk aversion* determines how much more than the actuarially fair premium the individual is willing to pay as an insurance premium. On the other hand, an individual who is indifferent between having insurance coverage at an actuarially fair premium and not purchasing the insurance is *risk-neutral*.

insurance market so that individuals know their own risk level but the insurer only knows the population average risk, and the existence of the asymmetry is known to both parties, this may lead to 'adverse selection' (Akerlof 1970). One extreme case is the situation where whatever premium the insurer sets, those with lower risks relative to it will leave the risk pool. The premium then needs to be adjusted upwards in order to cover the higher average risk among the policy holders, leading to more relatively lower risk individuals leaving. Eventually, either the premium for the higher risks becomes too expensive for them or the risk pool becomes too small for the insurer, and the market itself collapses. This is a 'market failure' for the lower risks, since there is an insurer willing to insure them at a premium they are willing to pay, but the transaction does not take place because the insurer cannot tell the lower risks apart from the higher risks. This is not a market failure for the higher risks, since for them it simply means that either the price of what they want is beyond their means or that the service they want is not on offer. (However, there may be associated equity issues.) One way to counter this is to introduce a compulsory insurance system that redistributes from the lower risks to the higher risks.

In another context, lack of symmetry of information between the doctor and patient in the health care market means that the consumer is not independent from the supplier. Because the doctor (supplier) has more information than the patient (consumer) about the health problem and available health care interventions, he often acts as the 'agent' for the patient who then becomes the 'principal'. This imperfect or dual agency, where the doctor is both the supplier and the agent of the consumer at the same time, may lead to supplier-induced demand (Green 1978). This is the case where the supplier manipulates the preference and demand of the consumer, causing overconsumption of health care, which can be exacerbated by health care insurance where the patient does not pay the full cost of health care. This is also called supplier moral hazard.

3.2.1.3 Existence of externalities

An externality is present when production activities or consumption behaviour affects third parties. For instance, the effect of consumption may spill over to those beyond the consumer. A positive externality in consumption means that one individual's consumption not only improves the consumer's own utility, but also improves other people's utility. There are two different kinds of externalities in health care (Culyer 1989). One is called *selfish externality*. This is when the benefit of health care consumption is not restricted to the consumer alone: if one individual gets vaccinated, not only is she protected from the infectious disease, but those around her are exposed to one fewer possible route of infection. The other is called *caring externality*. This is when an individual's utility is directly affected by the well-being of others (not through reduced risk of her own ill health). For example, people may find it uplifting to know that those who previously could not purchase health care are provided for. The existence of positive externalities will lead to underconsumption of health care in the market.

3.2.1.4 The efficiency of a health care market

While in reality most actual markets fail to satisfy some conditions for a perfect market, a special characteristic of the market for health care is that a whole series of these conditions are unmet, which interact with each other with potentially large and disruptive implications for individuals and society. However, it does not automatically follow that, just because a given free unregulated market will lead to highly ineffi-cient outcomes, therefore there should be government regulations and public policy interventions. The beauty of the idea of a free competitive market mechanism is that it is a completely decentralized system: each individual player will make decisions for himself based on information that is locally and readily available to him. Compared with this, resource allocation by policy intervention implies centralization, which is a high-cost process requiring large amounts of information to be gathered and analysed in order for collective decisions to be made. There are two things to consider before introducing major government regulations to the market: the size of the efficiency loss, and whether government interventions will do more good than harm.

On the other hand, government intervention may be justified independently of the market mechanism. Even where Pareto efficient outcomes are achieved by non-intervention, if the equity of the distribution of the good is a policy concern, then gov-ernment may be required to intervene (provided intervention does more good than harm). Indeed, most people agree that health is special, since being healthy is funda-mental to individual well-being and flourishing (Culyer *et al.* 1992). If this puts *health* and its equity implications on the policy agenda, then, to the extent that *health care* contributes to the upkeep and improvement of health, this should also be regarded as an equity concern.

Thus, the market for health care resource allocation is highly likely to be distorted without regulation, leading to inefficiencies, and with potential implications for equity. Effective evidence-based planned resource allocation is called for in order to achieve more efficient and equitable results, than leaving the process to an unregu-lated market.

3.2.2 **Resource allocation by planning**

Once the judgement has been made that health care resource allocation should not be left to unregulated market forces, a need for decision criteria arises. The starting point may be to go back to the Pareto efficiency criterion, and to aim to design a resource allocation system that will achieve such efficiency. However, the Pareto efficiency cri-terion is not very practical, because it is rarely the case that a programme will make at least one person better off without making anybody else worse off. In reality, most programmes are likely to affect at least one person negatively; and in such cases, the Pareto criterion is inconclusive.

The Kaldor and the Hicks criteria address this inconclusiveness. The Kaldor crite-rion claims that, if, after the change, the 'winners' (i.e. those whose situations improve due to the programme) could jointly 'compensate' all the 'losers' (i.e. those whose situ-ations worsen) so that at least one person is better off and nobody is worse off with the change, then the programme improves total efficiency (Kaldor 1939). The Hicks criterion is similar to this and asks whether, before the change, the losers-to-be could jointly 'bribe' all the winners-to-be, so that without the change, at least one person is better off and nobody is worse off, and if so, dropping the programme improves total efficiency (Hicks 1939).

There are two related things to note. One is that *actual* compensations or bribes are not required, and therefore the Kaldor or Hicks criteria will inevitably result in actual losers and violate the Pareto criterion. The losers in the Kaldor scenario, who need compensation from the winners to be at least as well off as they were before the implementation of the programme, will be made worse off with the change, because the compensation is not actually paid to them when the programme is implemented. Similarly, the winners-to-be in the Hicks scenario, who need the bribe from the losers-to-be in order to be at least as well off without the programme as they would be with the programme, will be made worse off, because the bribe is not actually paid to them when the programme is withdrawn. The customary practice of referring to the Kaldor and Hicks criteria as 'potential Paretian' is misleading in this respect: in practice they *always* violate the Pareto criterion. The other, related, point to note is that the Kaldor and Hicks criteria only relate to efficiency, or the total good and wealth in an economy, and have no regard for distribution or fairness (and that is why it does not matter if the compensation or bribe are not actually paid, because they are transfers and do not affect total efficiency).

What the winners gain from a decision can be called 'benefits' of the programme, and what the losers bear can be called 'costs'. Then, the cost-benefit analysis (CBA) becomes the operationalization of the Kaldor criterion. The basic idea of CBA is to sum up all costs and benefits associated with a given programme and, if the 'net benefit' is positive (i.e. the sum of benefits is larger than the sum of costs), then the total gains to the winners are larger than the total losses to the losers. This implies that should the winners be called upon to jointly compensate the losers, their gains are large enough to compensate the losers for their losses, and thus satisfy the Kaldor criterion. This is the welfare economic foundation of CBA. Since CBA is founded on the Kaldor criterion, it has no regard for distribution or fairness. (For further details on this topic, see Boardway and Bruce 1984.)

There are (at least) two concerns regarding the use of CBA in publicly funded health care resource allocation. First, there is strong resistance within the medical community, some parts of the health economics community, and among the general public towards attaching a monetary value to the health (and life) of a person. If economic evaluation can be carried out without representing health benefits directly in monetary terms, then policies based on such an analysis may become more widely acceptable. Second, CBA requires an individual level valuation of the benefits (and the costs) in monetary terms, which means that the value of a unit of health benefit is affected by whether it is a unit of health benefit to, for example, a rich person or to a poor person, because rich people can afford to pay more for a given health benefit. Indeed, this is the intended effect: other things being the same, it is more efficient to improve the health of somebody who values their health more rather than less, and how much one is willing to pay for a good is a measure of the value. However, this may have equity implications.

One way to deal with such equity implications is to aggregate the costs and benefits with appropriate 'distributional weights' applied to them, to correct for the difference in the ability to pay by income (see Box 3.2). Its main difficulty is in determining the actual weights. The essence of welfarism is that the only information that goes into the

Box 3.2 The marginal social welfare of individual income and inequality aversion

Where social welfare is represented by W and individual i's income by y_i, marginal social welfare of individual income is the partial derivative of the former by the latter: $\partial W/\partial y_i$. This concept can be further broken down into two factors: the marginal social welfare of individual utility, $\partial W/\partial u_i$, where u_i represents individual i's utility; and the marginal individual utility of own income, $\partial u_i/\partial y_i$.

The latter of these, the extent to which one derives additional utility from one's own income increase ($\partial u_i/\partial y_i$), is a factual matter (which in practice may, or may not, be measured accurately). If all individuals had diminishing marginal utility of income so that they derived less and less pleasure out of each additional unit of money, then the social welfare impact of additional money is maximized when it is given to the poorest person—but note that this is a matter of efficiency, not fairness.

In contrast, the former notion, marginal social welfare of individual utility ($\partial W/\partial u_i$), is a matter of normative judgement: it depends on the degree of *inequality aversion* represented in the particular social welfare function. Aversion to inequality in distribution means that if the total across the population is the same, then a more even distribution across the population is preferred to a less even distribution. The implication is that a smaller total with a more even distribution can be equally preferable to a larger total with a less even distribution. The issue here is: preferable to whom?

assessment of social welfare is based on the choices (real or hypothetical) that individuals make for themselves. Nevertheless, distributional weights cannot be based on selfish preferences that people have for themselves, or on externalities that ultimately serve their own utility. Instead, they need to be based on distributional judgements that reflect normative views on what constitutes a fair distribution within a society. A practical way forward would be for researchers or policy makers simply to impose some 'reasonable' level of *aversion to inequality* (with appropriate sensitivity analyses). However, strictly speaking, this is no longer welfarist, because the judgement of social welfare now includes information other than individuals' self-regarding preferences.

On the other hand, there are also three possible concerns regarding the use of cost-effectiveness analysis (CEA) in public resource allocation. The first is that cost per quality-adjusted life year (QALY) analysis struggles to capture 'non-health benefits', such as the value of improved productivity of patients and/or informal carers, the reassurance of having information, being treated with respect, and so on. CEA is based on the intuitively attractive idea that efficiency is the ratio of inputs to outputs. However, if inputs are converted to money terms and outputs are represented in health terms, where do such non-health benefits fit in? Non-health benefits that cannot be converted to units of health gain could be either converted into monetary terms and processed as negative costs, or used to adjust the size of health gains (see Box 10.1 in Chapter 10 for an example), or simply ignored (which is often the case). Nevertheless, either way, the analysis no longer represents the ratio of all inputs to all outputs. (Note that the ratio of health *and* non-health benefits to costs is not the same as the ratio of health benefits to costs *minus* non-health benefits.) In contrast, with CBA, since all inputs and all outputs are measured in the same unit, and the results are reported in terms of net benefits, there are no ambiguities about the treatment of non-health benefits: they can be treated as positive benefits, or as negative costs, and the results are not affected.

As a second concern, even when there are no benefits beyond improved patient health, (as was noted in Chapter 2), CEAs on their own cannot recommend whether or not a given health care intervention should be taken up, unless the analysis is combined with the concept of a threshold to reflect the opportunity cost of the displaced activities, which is introduced from outside the study. This means that while CBAs can be used to analyse allocative efficiency (i.e. is the treatment worthwhile?), CEAs can only be used to analyse technical or operational efficiency (is the treatment more or less efficient relative to those activities that are being displaced in the context of a fixed budget?), and not allocative efficiency.

The third concern surrounding cost per QALY analysis is that it is inefficient, because an efficient system needs to allocate resources according to 'effective demand' or, in other words, according to how much people are willing to pay for the good. The amount of money people are willing to pay for a unit of health can vary enormously both by income and by preferences, and this variation needs to be exploited to achieve efficiency. On the other hand, allocating resources according to CEAs with QALYs, where everybody's unit of health is counted the same, does not achieve maximum efficiency.

How to balance these concerns is linked to two schools of thought. One is often referred to as the 'welfarist' approach, and holds that CBA is the theoretically correct method of economic evaluation, and cost per QALY analysis is a poor substitute for it, merely tolerated because it avoids the thorny issue of monetary valuation of health. An important topic within this school is the identification of the conditions under which the two types of analysis will become identical (e.g. Johannesson 1995b; Garber and Phelps 1997; Bleichrodt and Quiggin 2003; see also Dolan and Edlin 2002; Hansen *et al.* 2004). The other school of thought, referred to as the 'extra-welfarist', 'non-welfarist', or 'decision maker's' approach, holds that cost per QALY analysis is the preferred type of analysis not because it is a practical second-best, but because it is the type of analysis that is more relevant to policy, where equity is a main concern alongside efficiency. The equivalence or otherwise of CBA and CEA with QALYs is not an issue (Tsuchiya and Williams 2001). Furthermore, to the extent that the objective of publicly funded health care is to improve population health, it becomes appropriate to leave out non-health benefits.

3.3 **The measure of benefit**

The aforementioned description of going from CBA to cost per QALY analysis involves not only the change in the way outcomes are presented, but also a possible change in the underlying philosophy regarding the measure of health benefits. CBA builds on welfarism: what matters in the measurement of social welfare is the well-being of constituent individuals *as assessed by themselves*. Applied to the economic evaluation of health care interventions, it means that assessment of the benefit of the medical intervention should be based on the extent to which individual patients are affected and how they, as consumers, value this impact. This is why CBAs are typically based on how people value changes in their own health. The methods of eliciting monetary preferences for health programmes are beyond the scope of this book, and the interested reader is referred to, for example, Johansson (1995), Johannesson (1996), Pauly (1996), or Drummond *et al.* (2015). However, to give a simplified explanation, people can be asked to specify how much additional tax they are willing to pay in order to introduce a particular health care programme—the question should spell out the probability of the respondents themselves needing this service and the expected benefit they will receive as a result of the additional payment. It would then be equivalent to a private insurance scenario, which is welfarist.

On the other hand, CEA with QALYs is usually regarded as building on a non-welfarist approach, where the measurement of social welfare is based on external assessments of the well-being of affected individuals. While the *description* of the relevant health states come from the patients themselves, the *valuation* of these states come from elsewhere, typically from a representative sample of the wider public (for further details, see Chapter 5).

Nonetheless, there can also be welfarist CEAs with QALYs, and there can be non-welfarist CBAs as well. Welfarist cost per QALY analyses base the concept of the QALY upon utility theory, and this is one of the approaches explained next. Conversely, non-welfarist CBA would rely on monetary valuation of benefits, but this valuation would be drawn from a non-welfarist perspective. For example, respondents can be asked to imagine they are the local policy maker and to allocate public resources across competing health programmes (Schwappach 2003). Since CBAs based on such information are no longer underwritten by individual utility theory, rather than calling them CBAs that carry welfarist connotations, it may perhaps be more appropriate to call them 'CEAs with monetized benefits'. An interesting issue is the assumed policy objective. Welfarist economic evaluation aims to maximize the sum of individual utility. Non-welfarist CEA with QALYs has population health as the desideratum. However, non-welfarist CEA with monetized benefits can include non-health benefits, and if it does, it would no longer make sense to say population health is the desideratum. It would need some concept of the 'good', to be distributed across the population.

The next section looks at welfarist foundations of the concept of the QALY, followed by non-welfarist foundations (see Table 3.1 for a summary).

3.3.1 The welfarist theory of the QALY

The welfarist theory of the QALY assumes that the number of QALYs represents the level of (cardinal) utility of an individual concerning their own health. A simple case is where the health status stays constant throughout the survival, so that there is only one health state between 'now' and 'death'. This is usually referred to as a 'chronic' state. If the utility associated with this constant state survival is to be represented by the number of QALYs, that is, by the number of years of survival multiplied by the health

Table 3.1 Cost-benefit analysis (CBA) and cost-effectiveness analysis (CEA): welfarism and non-welfarism

	Welfarist		Non-welfarist	
	CBA	**CEA with QALYs**	**CEA with monetized benefits**	**CEA with QALYs**
Measure of health benefit	Monetary value	QALYs	Monetary value	QALYs
Perspective of valuation of benefit	The potential patient/consumer/ insurance policy holder	The potential patient/ consumer/ insurance policy holder	The citizen	The citizen
Measure of efficiency	Net benefit	Cost per QALY	Net benefit	Cost per QALY
Concept of efficiency	Allocative efficiency	Technical efficiency	Allocative efficiency	Technical efficiency
Treatment of non-health benefits	Yes	No	Yes	No
Concern for equity	Low	Low	Mild	Moderate
The desideratum	Sum of individual utility	Sum of individual utility as captured by QALYs	Sum of social good	Sum of population health

state value corresponding to that state, then 'mutual utility independence between quantity and quality of life', 'constant proportional time trade-off', and 'risk neutrality with respect to life years' need to be satisfied (Pliskin *et al.* 1980). The derivation of these conditions is based on expected utility theory, a theory of choice under uncertainty. Box 3.3 gives examples of what these conditions mean, and of subsequent developments. The interested reader should consult the original papers referenced there.

In addition to these conditions, if more than one 'temporary' health state is involved to form a 'health profile' followed by death, and if the number of QALYs associated with the whole health profile over time is to be equal to the sum of individual temporary health states, then the 'additive separability' condition is also required. Additive separability assumes that the utility of a state is unaffected by states that precede it or follow it, which might be unrealistic. An alternative approach that does not require additive separability is to treat multistate health profiles themselves as the unit of valuation, and to value these directly. This will allow interactions between the value of health states, their duration, and their profiles over time. The obvious disadvantage is that the number of outcomes that need to be valued will multiply, making it impossible to have any kind of off-the-shelf preference-based measure. The approach is associated with the healthy year equivalent (HYE), explained in Box 3.4. (This is also related to the vignette approach reviewed in Chapter 8.)

Box 3.3 When is a QALY a representation of individual utility over health?

The adjective 'mutual' in the first condition of Pliskin *et al.* (1980) implies two elements: (1a) utility over durations is independent of the quality of life associated with the survival; and (1b) marginal utility, or the health state value, associated with survival in a given health state is independent of the duration. Suppose individuals are asked to make a choice over two alternatives, after which they will die:

alternative 1: to live in health state h for *2 years for certain*

alternative 2: a lottery with a 50–50 chance to live in health state h for *either 1 year or for 4 years.*

There are no right or wrong answers, and individuals can prefer either alternative. Condition (1a) means that the individual's choice over the two alternatives is not affected by what health state h is. So, if one prefers alternative 1 over alternative 2 when health state h is 'constant mild depression', then one should also prefer alternative 1 to 2 when state h is replaced with 'constant severe depression'.

Condition (1b) means that the individual's choice over alternatives 3 and 4 are not affected by the duration t (after which they will die):

alternative 3: to live for t years for certain *in constant moderate pain*

alternative 4: a lottery with a 50–50 chance to live for t years *either in constant mild pain or in constant severe pain.*

So, if one prefers alternative 3 over alternative 4 when duration t is 2 years, then one should continue to prefer alternative 3 over 4 when duration t is increased to 20 years, or reduced to 2 months.

The second condition, constant proportional time trade-off, means that, suppose an individual is indifferent between alternatives 5 and 6:

alternative 5: to live for T years for certain *in constant severe depression*

alternative 6: to live for t years for certain *in constant mild depression* $(t < T)$;

this indifference is not affected by changing the values of t and T proportionately. So, if one is indifferent between the two alternatives when $T = 3$ years and $t = 2$ years, then one should continue to be indifferent when these figures are changed to $T = 30$ years and $t = 20$ years, or to $T = 3$ months and $t = 2$ months.

The third condition, risk neutrality over years of life, means that the individual is indifferent between:

alternative 7: to live in health state h for *2 years for certain*

alternative 8: a lottery with a 50–50 chance to live in health state h for *either 1 year or for 3 years,*

because the expected duration of alternative 8 (the sum of the years weighted by the respective probabilities: $0.5 \times 1 + 0.5 \times 3 = 2$) is the same as the expected duration of alternative 7: to live for 2 years in state h.

Subsequently, Bleichrodt *et al.* (1997) demonstrated that the number of assumptions could be reduced to two: risk neutrality in life years, and the 'zero condition'. The latter implies that where the duration of survival is zero life years, all health states have the same utility level.

For the case of risk aversion, Miyamoto *et al.* (1998) further demonstrated that the requirement becomes the zero condition and 'standard gamble invariance'. Suppose the individual is indifferent between:

alternative 7': to live in health state *h* for *2 years for certain*

alternative 8': a lottery with a 40–60 chance to live in health state *h* for *either 1 year or for 3 years*,

then standard gamble invariance means that this 40–60 chance is not affected by the health state *h*, as long as it is a health state worth living in.

Box 3.4 Two proposals to make the QALY better reflect actual individual preferences

Healthy years equivalent

The first proposal is to define the measure of benefit as the number of years in full health that is equivalent to the expected health outcome (which may consist of multiple health states). This number is defined as the healthy years equivalent (HYE; Mehrez and Gafni 1989). The concept does not impose any conditions on individual preference between life years and quality of life. It was subsequently proposed that this concept can be operationalized through the use of a two-stage standard gamble (Mehrez and Gafni 1991), which led to a major debate (Buckingham 1993; Culyer and Wagstaff 1993; Gafni *et al.* 1993; Bleichrodt 1995; Johannesson 1995a; Loomes 1995; Culyer and Wagstaff 1995; Wakker 1996; Morrison 1997). The conclusion reached is that HYE measured by two-stage standard gambles is theoretically equivalent to a time trade-off exercise of multistate profiles, but with a larger margin for error at the practical level. For a review of the HYE debate, see Towers *et al.* (2005). For the valuation of multistate profiles, see the vignette approach in Chapter 8.

Enhancing the QALY model

A more recent proposal is to re-build the QALY model based on generalizations of expected utility theory developed in theoretical economics, for example rank-dependent expected utility theory (Wakker and Stiggelbout 1995: Miyamoto 1999; Doctor *et al.* 2004; Bleichrodt and Pinto 2005; Bleichrodt and Quiggin 2005). The essence of this proposal is to allow for the fact that people seem to overestimate very small and very large probabilities, and to underestimate mid-range probabilities. By introducing the notion that subjective probability (based on which people make choices) is not the same as objective probability, the theory provides a more accurate account of individual choice under uncertainty.

At an empirical level, there are numerous studies demonstrating that expected utility theory does not have descriptive validity regarding individual choice under uncertainty. In the context of choice over health outcomes, individual preferences are frequently found to violate the conditions mentioned here in a non-systematic way (for a review, see Tsuchiya and Dolan 2005). This has two implications: first, there is no systematic way to correct the violations at the individual level; but, secondly, the conditions are often satisfied at the aggregate level.

There are two approaches to this. One is to generalize or adapt utility theory so that it can accommodate individual behaviour that amounts to violations of the original theory (see Box 3.4). The aim of such research is to reconstruct the QALY concept based on relaxed utility foundations, and then to explore whether or not actual individual choice behaviour will satisfy the associated conditions for the new QALY concept to hold, as a measure of individual utility. The objective of this first approach then is to identify a theory that successfully represents actual individual choice under uncertainty. The alternative approach is to accept that real individual choice under uncertainty violates axioms of expected utility theory, but to continue to use the theory as the normative basis on which to build policy decisions, since such violations do not diminish the normative validity of the theory. If individual choice in the real world is found to be irrational by whatever definition of rationality, arguably, it makes little sense for public policy to emulate such irrational choices, nor does it make sense to abandon the definition of rationality because of it (Tsuchiya and Dolan 2005). Alongside the exploration of theories of individual choice that have improved descriptive validity, there needs to be a normative discourse on what should be the basis on which to make policy decisions, and how this should be determined.

3.3.2 The non-welfarist theory of the QALY

An altogether different approach is a 'non-welfarist theory' of the QALY. Non-welfarism challenges the welfarist notion of the social good as a function of individual utility as assessed by the individuals themselves, and allows for the notion of the social good which is a function of, for example, total population health as assessed by the citizenry at large. This leads to an alternative approach to the value of the QALY, where it is not a representation of individual utility, but a measure of health as a social desideratum. The reason why producing 10 QALYs of health is twice as good as producing five QALYs at the same cost is not because it generates twice as much individual utility, but because it generates twice as much social good. So, under this approach it is awkward to refer to cost per QALY analysis as cost 'utility' analysis.

One basis for this approach can be traced back to the theory of capabilities and functionings, first proposed by Amartya Sen (1982, 1985; also see Sugden 1993), as an alternative to welfarism. Sen's proposal is to involve a much wider information base than utility to capture how well an individual is doing, and to extend it to the set of opportunities the individual has beyond the particular outcomes they would choose for themselves. Note that the set of desirable basic opportunities for individuals does not necessarily come from the individuals themselves, because it is based on the notion of what 'personal advantage' everybody ought to have. The approach was adopted in the area of health care by Culyer (1989) under the banner of 'extra-welfarism'—which regards the generic preference-based measures of health such as the EQ-5D as ways of incorporating this wide notion of 'personal advantage', or characteristics of people as Culyer termed it (also see Brouwer and Koopmanschap 2000; Cookson 2005).

Actual patient utility may or may not change proportionally to the size of QALY gains, but under non-welfarism, this is no longer relevant (Tsuchiya and Williams 2001). The difficulty of this approach is that the process by which the social desideratum is determined is not clear, and possibly beyond the remit of economic analysis. However, note how similar this non-welfarist approach is in some respects to the argument here on the normative status of expected utility theory; and there, too, the difficulty would be the issue of who decides what constitutes rationality, and how.

3.4 **Conclusion**

The aim of this chapter was to examine what is to be valued for use in economic evaluation and specifically the place of the QALY measure. It started with a brief review of the economists' default position, the market mechanism, how its failure leads to health care resource allocation by government intervention, followed by the distributional implications of using CBA, and the cost per QALY analysis as an alternative to CBA. The next section looked at two different theories of the QALY: one that interprets the QALY as a representation of individual utility, and another that interprets the QALY as a measure of social good in health policy. Despite coming from different normative foundations, both of them provide a theoretical basis for cost per QALY analyses as a form of economic evaluation for health care interventions.

References

Akerlof GA (1970). The market for "lemons": Quality uncertainty and the market mechanism. *The Quarterly Journal of Economics* **84**:488–500.

Arrow KJ (1963). Uncertainty and the welfare economics of medical care. *American Economic Review* **53**:941–73.

Bleichrodt H (1995). QALYs and HYEs—under what conditions are they equivalent? *Journal of Health Economics* **14**:17–37.

Bleichrodt H, Pinto JL (2005). The validity of QALYs under non-expected utility. *The Economic Journal* **115**:533–50.

Bleichrodt H, Quiggin J (2003). Life-cycle preferences over consumption and health: when is cost-effectiveness analysis equivalent to cost-benefit analysis? *Journal of Health Economics* **18**:681–708.

Bleichrodt H, Quiggin J (2005). Characterizing QALYs under a general rank dependent utility model. *Journal of Risk and Uncertainty* **15**:151–65.

Bleichrodt H, Wakker P, Johannesson M (1997). Characterizing QALYs by risk neutrality. *Journal of Risk and Uncertainty* **15**:107–14.

Boardway R, Bruce N (1984). *Welfare economics*: Basil Blackwell, Oxford, UK.

Brouwer W, Koopmanschap M (2000). On the economic foundations of CEA: ladies and gentlemen, take your positions! *Journal of Health Economics* **19**:149–67.

Buckingham K (1993). A note on HYE (healthy years equivalent). *Journal of Health Economics* **12**:301–9.

Cookson R (2005). QALYs and the capabilities approach. *Health Economics* **14**:817–29.

Culyer AJ (1989). The normative economics of health care finance and provision. *Oxford Review of Economic Policy* **5**:34–58

Culyer AJ, van Doorslaer E, Wagstaff A (1992). Access, utilisation and equity: A further comment. *Journal of Health Economics* **11**(2):207–10.

Culyer AJ, Wagstaff A (1993). QALYs versus HYEs. *Journal of Health Economics* **12**:311–23.

Culyer AJ, Wagstaff A (1995). QALYs versus HYEs—a reply to Gafni, Birch and Mehrez. *Journal of Health Economics* **14**:39–45.

Doctor JN, Bleichrodt H, Miyamoto J, Temkin NR, Dikmen S (2004). A new and more robust test of QALYs. *Journal of Health Economics* **23**:353–67.

Dolan P, Edlin R (2002). Is it really possible to build a bridge between cost-benefit analysis and cost-effectiveness analysis? *Journal of Health Economics* **21**:827–43.

Drummond MF, Sculpher MJ, Claxton K, Torrance GW, Stoddart GL (2015). *Methods for the economic evaluation of health care programmes*, 4th edn. Oxford University Press, Oxford, UK.

Gafni A, Birch S, Mehrez A (1993). Economics, health and health economics—HYEs versus QALYs. *Journal of Health Economics* **12**:325–39.

Garber AM, Phelps CE (1997). Economic foundations of cost-effectiveness analysis. *Journal of Health Economics* **16**:1–31.

Green J (1978). Physician-induced demand for medical care. *Journal of Human Resource* **13**:21–34.

Hansen BO, Hougaard JL, Keiding H, Østerdal LP (2004). On the possibility of a bridge between CBA and CEA: comments on a paper by Dolan and Edlin. *Journal of Health Economics* **23**:887–98.

Hicks JR (1939). *Value and capital*, 2nd edn. Clarendon Press, Oxford, UK.

Johannesson M (1995a). Quality-adjusted life-years versus healthy-years equivalents—a comment. *Journal of Health Economics* **14**(1):9–16.

Johannesson M (1995b). The relationship between cost-effectiveness analysis and cost-benefit analysis. *Social Science and Medicine* **41**:483–9.

Johannesson M (1996). *Theory and methods of economic evaluation of health care*. Kluwer Academic Publishers, Dordrecht, the Netherlands.

Johansson P-O (1995). *Evaluating health risks: an economic approach*. Cambridge University Press, Cambridge, UK.

Kaldor N (1939). Welfare propositions of economics and interpersonal comparisons of utility. *The Economic Journal* **49**:549–52.

Loomes G (1995). The myth of the HYE. *Journal of Health Economics* **14**:1–7.

Mehrez A, Gafni A (1989). Quality-adjusted life years, utility-theory, and healthy-years equivalents. *Medical Decision Making* **9**:142–9.

Mehrez A, Gafni A (1991). The healthy-years equivalents—how to measure them using the standard gamble approach. *Medical Decision Making* **11**:140–6.

Miyamoto J (1999). Quality-adjusted life years (QALY) utility models under expected utility and rank dependent utility assumptions. *Journal of Mathematical Psychology* **43**:201–37.

Miyamoto JM, Wakker PP, Bleichrodt H, Peters HJM (1998). The zero-condition: a simplifying assumption in QALY measurement and multiattribute utility. *Management Science* **44**:839–49.

Morrison GC (1997). HYE and TTO: what is the difference? *Journal of Health Economics* **16**:563–78.

Pauly MV (1968). The economics of moral hazard: comment, *The American Economic Review* **58**(3):531–7.

Pauly MV (1996). Valuing health care benefits in money terms. In: Sloan FA (ed.) *Valuing health care: costs, benefits, and effectiveness of pharmaceuticals and other medical technologies.* Cambridge University Press, Cambridge, UK, pp. 99–124.

Pliskin JS, Shepard DS, Weinstein MC (1980). Utility functions for life years and health status. *Operations Research* **28**:206–24.

Schwappach DL (2003). Does it matter who you are or what you gain? An experimental study of preferenes for resource allocation. *Health Economics* **12**:255–67.

Sen A (1982). *Choice, welfare, and measurement.* Basil Blackwell, Oxford, UK.

Sen A (1985). *Commodities and capabilities.* North-Holland Publishing, Amsterdam, the Netherlands.

Sugden R (1993). Welfare, resources, and capabilities: a review of inequality reexamined by Amartya Sen. *Journal of Economic Literature* **31**:1947–62.

Towers I, Spencer A, Brazier J (2005). Healthy year equivalents versus quality-adjusted life years: the debate continues. *Expert Review of Pharmacoeconomics and Outcomes Research* **5**:245–54.

Tsuchiya A, Dolan P (2005). The QALY model and individual preferences for health states and health profiles over time: a systematic review of the literature. *Medical Decision Making* **25**:460–7.

Tsuchiya A, Williams A (2001). Welfare economics and economic evaluation. In: Drummond M, McGuire A (eds). *Theory and practice of economic evaluation in health care.* Oxford University Press, Oxford, UK, pp. 22–45.

Wakker P (1996). Criticism of healthy-years equivalents. *Medical Decision Making* **16**:207–14.

Wakker P, Stiggelbout A (1995). Explaining distortions in utility elicitation through the rank-dependent model for risky choices. *Medical Decision Making* **15**:80–6.

Chapter 4

Valuing health

4.1 Introduction to valuing health

The key question addressed in this book is how to adjust life years to reflect health levels experienced during those years (i.e. putting the 'Q' into QALYs). This chapter explores the methods for valuing health, sometimes known as preference elicitation techniques. It begins by describing and reviewing the main cardinal techniques used in the health economics literature for valuing health states (i.e. those methods that produce responses that are already on some interval scale). Ordinal or ranking techniques are considered in Chapter 6. Different techniques can generate different values, and so this chapter also addresses the question of which technique should be used. It goes on to examine the variants of each technique and the resulting implications of these for the values obtained. Finally, this chapter addresses the question of who should be asked to value health states, and considers whether values should be based on preferences (as is usually the case in economics) or experiences.

4.2 Health state valuation techniques: a description

The standard gamble (SG), time trade-off (TTO), and the visual analogue scale (VAS) are three main techniques for valuing health states, often called preference elicitation techniques. However, VAS is not strictly preference-based, and so the more general term of valuation is used to describe these techniques. The use of ordinal approaches, including ranking and discrete choice experiments (DCE) to value health states, is considered separately in Chapter 6. The person trade-off (or PTO) approach, a technique that has been used less frequently to value health states, is also considered here but rather more briefly than the three main techniques. This section describes how each technique can be used to value chronic states that are considered to be better than being dead, states worse than being dead, and temporary states.

4.2.1 The visual analogue scale

The VAS, sometimes referred to in the literature as the category rating scale, or just the rating scale, is simply a line that usually has well-defined end-points on which respondents are able to indicate their judgements, values, or feelings (hence it is sometimes called a 'feeling' thermometer). The distances between intervals on a VAS should reflect a person's understanding of the relative differences between the concepts being measured. VAS is intended to have interval properties, so that the difference between 3 and 5 on a 10-point scale, for example, should equal the difference between 5 and 7.

VAS was first identified as a possible measure for use in economic evaluation over four decades ago (Patrick *et al.* 1973) and has become one of the most widely used measures for this purpose, whether directly with patients or as a means of valuing health state classifications, including: the Quality of Well-being Scale (QWB) (Kaplan and Anderson 1988); Health Utilities Index (HUI) (Feeny *et al.* 2002); 15-D (Sintonen 1994); and the EQ-5D (Brooks *et al.* 2003).

To successfully use VAS in economic evaluation, it is essential that comparability between respondents is ensured. To achieve this, clear and unambiguous end-points are required such as 'full health' at the top end (in the case of a vertical scale) and 'dead' at the lower end. It is important to define 'full health' in order to minimize the risk of between-respondent variation, although there inevitably remains some variation in the interpretation of 'full health' no matter how it is defined by the researchers. For generic preference-based measures, there is a question as to whether the best imaginable health state should be defined as full health, or as the best state according to the classification system (e.g. state 11111 for the EQ-5D). The use of terms such as 'best imaginable' health state and 'worst imaginable' health state as end-points (traditionally utilized by the EuroQol group) arguably provide less definitive meaning and interpretation than the best EQ-5D state (i.e. 11111), or even 'full health' and 'dead'; they leave more scope for variation in meaning between respondents, and hence potentially reduce comparability between them (Feng *et al.* 2014) (see Fig. 4.1).

4.2.1.1 Visual analogue scale for states considered worse than dead

For use in economic evaluation, it is desirable to ensure that health state valuations can be placed on a zero to one scale, where zero represents states regarded as equivalent to dead, and one is for a state of full health. It is also necessary to allow for states that could be valued as worse than being dead. For these reasons, it is important for respondents to be asked to value being dead on the same scale as their own health, or the various hypothetical states they are being asked to value. Having obtained a value for dead, all health state valuations then need to be transformed using the following formula:

$$A_i = R_i - R \text{ (dead)} / R \text{ (best)} - R \text{ (dead)},$$

where A_i = adjusted VAS rating for health state h_i; R (being dead) = raw rating given to being dead; R_i = raw rating given to health state h_i; R (best) = raw rating given to the best health state.

This transformation results in the value 1.0 for the best (or full) health state and zero for being dead. The value of A_i would lie within this range, or assume a negative value for states valued as worse than being dead. This adjustment is claimed to allow interpersonal comparisons (Torrance 1986; Measurement and Valuation of Health Group 1994) and more arguably transforms the VAS values on to the zero to one scale used for quality-adjusted life years, or QALYs (Kaplan *et al.* 1979). However, it should be noted that this transformation is unbounded below zero. It is also helpful

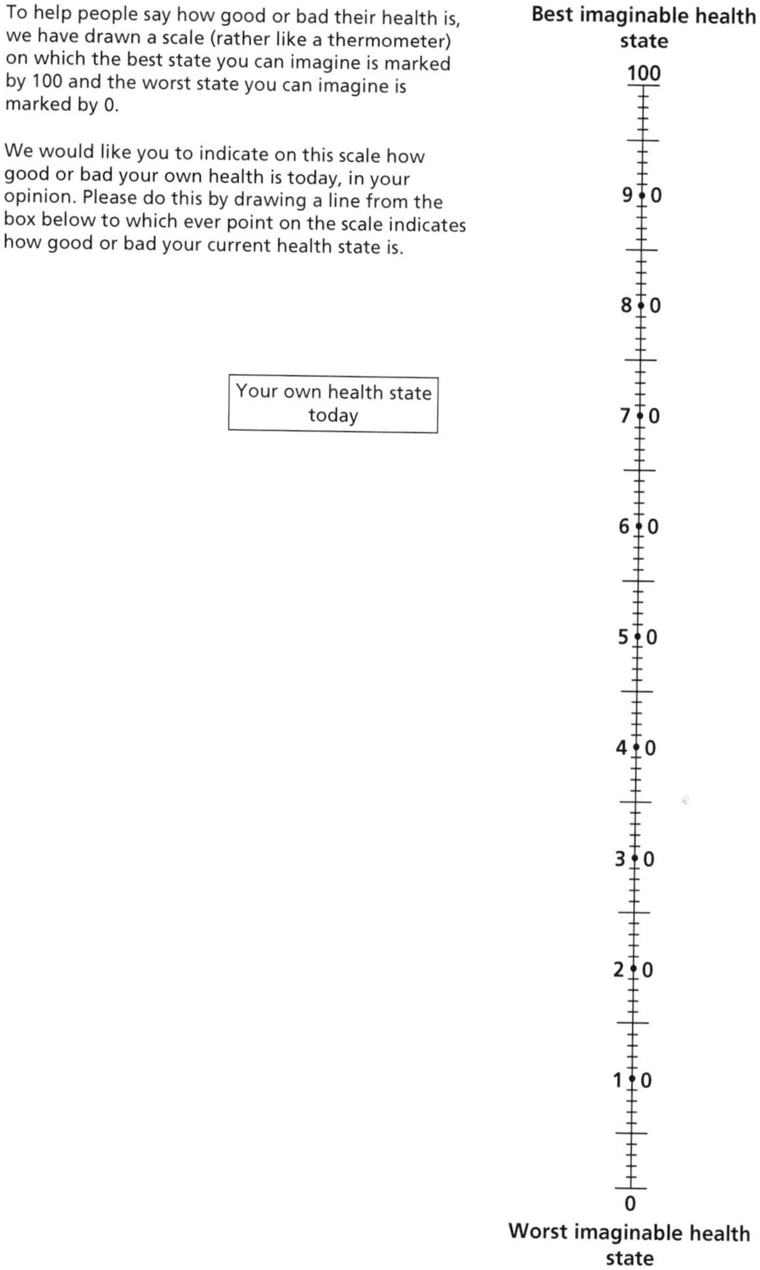
To help people say how good or bad their health is, we have drawn a scale (rather like a thermometer) on which the best state you can imagine is marked by 100 and the worst state you can imagine is marked by 0.

We would like you to indicate on this scale how good or bad your own health is today, in your opinion. Please do this by drawing a line from the box below to which ever point on the scale indicates how good or bad your current health state is.

Your own health state today

Best imaginable health state
100
90
80
70
60
50
40
30
20
10
0
Worst imaginable health state

Fig. 4.1 Example of a visual analogue scale (EQ-5D VAS)—own health.

Reproduced by permission of EuroQol Research Foundation from Oemar M and Oppe M, *EQ-5D-3L User Guide: Basic information on how to use the EQ-5D-3L instrument*, EuroQol Research Foundation, the Netherlands, Copyright © EuroQol Research Foundation 2015, available from http://www.euroqol.org/fileadmin/user_upload/Documenten/PDF/Folders_Flyers/EQ-5D-3L_UserGuide_2015.pdf for respondents completing the VAS if there is a clear calibration on the scale, such as 0 to 10 or 0 to 100, although it is not clear whether the refinement of the latter really produces greater accuracy in the scale since respondents tend to opt for multiples of 10 or 5 on a 100-point scale. Figure 4.1 presents an example of the VAS developed by the EuroQol group.

4.2.1.2 Visual analogue scale for temporary health states

Temporary health states are defined as states lasting for a specified period of time after which there is a return to good health, whereas chronic health states last for the rest of a person's life (Torrance 1986). The duration of temporary health states may be specified in terms of weeks, months, or years, the only requirement being that the duration is less than life expectancy. Preferences for temporary health states can be measured using a VAS by instructing the respondent that the health states will last for a specified period of time, after which the person will return to full health. The respondent is asked to place the best state (healthy) at one end of the scale and the worst temporary state at the other end. As with the valuation of chronic health states, the remaining temporary health states are then placed along the line, so that their location reflects their relative ratings by the respondent. To encourage elicitation of interval scale values, respondents must be instructed to place the temporary health states on the line in such a way that the relative distance between the locations reflects the differences they perceive between the health states.

4.2.1.3 Variants of the visual analogue scale

There are many variants of the VAS technique. The lines can vary in length, be vertical or horizontal, and may or may not have intervals marked out with different numbers. For example, the QWB multiattribute utility scale (MAUS) was valued by asking respondents to place health states into one of 15 numbered slots, where zero was dead and one was optimum health. The EQ-5D was valued using interval markings of 0–100, where 0 corresponds to the worst imaginable health and 100 corresponds to the best imaginable health (Fig. 4.1). Respondents may be asked initially to place the best and worst health states at the end-points of the scale, or they may be asked to place the states on the scale in any order. Feeny and colleagues (2002) also developed a feeling thermometer on which the respondent places cards describing different health states. Alternatively, respondents may be asked to indicate the position of their own or hypothetical health state/s by placing a line from the health state to the VAS (Feng *et al.* 2014).

4.2.2 The standard gamble

The SG method gives the respondent a choice between a certain intermediate outcome and the uncertainty of a gamble with two possible outcomes, one of which is better than the certain intermediate outcome, and one of which is worse. The SG task for eliciting the value attached to health states considered better than dead is displayed in Figure 4.2 (based on Drummond *et al.* 2005). Essentially, the respondent is offered two alternatives. Alternative 1 is a treatment with two possible outcomes: either the patient is returned to normal health and lives for an additional t years (probability P), or the patient dies immediately (probability $1 - P$). Alternative 2 has the certain outcome of

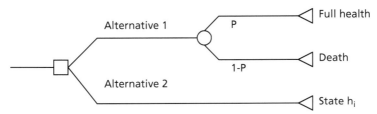

Fig. 4.2 Standard gamble for a chronic health state preferred to dead.
Source: data from Drummond MF *et al.*, *Methods for the Economic Evaluation of Health Care Programmes,* Third Edition, Copyright © 2005 Oxford University Press.

chronic state h_i for life (*t* years). The probability *P* of the best outcome is varied until the individual is indifferent between the certain intermediate outcome and the gamble. This probability *P* is the utility for the certain outcome, state h_i. This technique is then repeated for all intermediate outcomes. The SG can also be applied to elicit the value attached to health states considered worse than dead and temporary health states, as described in the next section.

4.2.2.1 Standard gamble for states considered worse than dead

For chronic health states considered worse than dead, the standard gamble question has to be modified to that shown in Figure 4.3. Sometimes in the literature, states are described as being better or worse than death, but it is not the process of death that is relevant here rather the state of being dead. Again, the respondent is offered two alternatives. Alternative 1 is a treatment with two possible outcomes: either the patient is returned to normal health and lives for an additional *t* years (probability *P*), or the patient remains in the chronic health state h_i for life (*t* years) (probability $1 - P$). Alternative 2 has the certain outcome of death. Torrance (1986) suggests that one way to present such a choice is to ask the respondent to imagine that they have a rapidly progressing terminal disease that will lead quickly to death if no intervention takes place. However, there is a treatment with a probability *P* of a complete cure and probability $1 - P$ of remaining in chronic state h_i. The probability *P* is varied until the individual is indifferent between the certain outcome of death and the gamble, at which the preference value for health state $h_i = -P/(1 - P)$.

This formula for translating SG responses to health state values results in a scale ranging from $-\infty$ to $+1$, which gives greater weight to negative values in the calculation of mean scores and presents problems for the statistical analysis. Therefore, it has

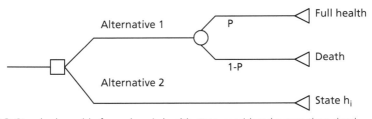

Fig. 4.3 Standard gamble for a chronic health state considered worse than dead.

been suggested in the literature that states valued worse than dead should be simply the negative of the indifference probability of the best outcome (Patrick *et al.* 1994). This has the effect of bounding negative values at –1. This transformation has no theoretical support and is only one of a number of possible ways of dealing with the problem, but it is one that has become widely used elsewhere in the literature (Brazier *et al.* 2002; Feeny *et al.* 2002).

4.2.2.2 Standard gamble for temporary health states

There is a concern that temporary states also represent an unusual situation where the imminence of death in the task might distort respondents' valuation of the state. One solution suggested by Torrance (1986) is a two-stage process, of which stage 1 involves an SG where all outcomes last for an additional *t* weeks, months, or years followed by full health (though it could be another state). Alternative 1 is a treatment with two possible outcomes: either the patient is returned to normal health (probability *P*), or the patient lives for time period *t* in the worst temporary health state followed by full health (probability 1 – *P*). Alternative 2 has the certain outcome of the intermediate temporary health state h_i for an equivalent amount of time (*t* weeks, months, or years) after which the patient is returned to full health. The probability *P* of the best outcome is varied until the individual is indifferent between the certain intermediate outcome and the gamble. If more than one temporary health state is being valued relative to the worst temporary health state, then this procedure is repeated for each health state.

Using this format, the formula for the utility of state h_i for time *t* is: $h_i = P + (1 - P) h_j$, where h_i is the state being measured and h_j is the worst state. Here h_i is measured on a utility scale where full health for time period *t* is 1.0. In order to relate these utilities to the full health–dead scale used to derive QALYs, there needs to be a second stage that involves valuing the worst temporary health state. This can be achieved by redefining it as a short duration chronic state for time *t* followed by death, and valuing it relative to being dead and full health using the same technique as that described here for valuing chronic health states. This gives the value for h_j for time *t*, which can then be inserted into the aforementioned formula to find the value for h_i for time *t* (see Fig. 4.4).

Some health economists have viewed the standard gamble as the 'gold standard' for the measurement of the 'utility' associated with particular health states; it is based on the axioms of expected utility theory (EUT), which offers a normative framework for describing how individuals would make decisions under conditions of risk and uncertainty if they adhered to a set of basic axioms (von Neumann and Morgenstern 1944).

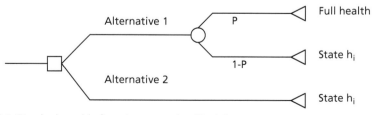

Fig. 4.4 Standard gamble for a temporary health state.

The SG has also been advocated on the basis that almost all decisions about health care are made under conditions of risk and uncertainty (Mehrez and Gafni 1993). The SG technique has been widely applied in the decision-making literature (Keeney and Raiffa 1976). It has also been extensively applied to medical decision making, including the valuation of health states, where it has been used (indirectly via a transformation of VAS) to value the HUI2, HUI3, and SF-6D, and also to value numerous condition-specific health state scenarios or vignettes.

4.2.2.3 Variants of the standard gamble

There are many variants of the SG technique, which differ in terms of the procedure used to identify the point of indifference, the use of props, and the method of administration (e.g. by interviewer, computer, or self-administered/paper questionnaire).

A widely used variant has been developed by Torrance and colleagues which addresses the problem of explaining probabilities to respondents through the use of a visual aid, known as the probability wheel (Torrance 1986; see Appendix 4.1 for an example of a probability wheel). This helps respondents to determine their point of indifference between the certain outcome and the gamble by iterating between values for the probability of success P (i.e. the 'ping–pong' method). The probability wheel is an adjustable disc with two sectors, each a different colour. It is constructed so that the relative size of the two sectors can be readily changed. The two alternatives are presented to the individual on cards and the two outcomes of the gamble alternatives are colour coded to match the two sectors of the probability wheel. The individual is informed that the probability of each outcome is proportional to the similarly coloured area of the disc. An example interview script for this variant of SG is reproduced in Appendix 4.2.

An alternative SG variant that does not require the use of a visual aid (titration method) was developed by Jones-Lee and colleagues (1993). It uses a titration procedure with a list of values for the chances of successful treatment. The chances of success may be specified in terms of 'bottom-up' titration (i.e. 0, 5, 10 per cent, etc.) or 'top-down' titration (i.e. 100, 95, 90 per cent, etc.). Choosing from this list, respondents are asked to indicate all the values of P at which they are confident they would opt for treatment and all the values of P at which they would reject treatment. Finally, they are asked to indicate the value of P where they find it most difficult to choose between treatment and remaining in a hypothetical health state (see Appendix 4.3 for an example of the titration method for SG). This variant has been adapted for use on the computer by Stein *et al.* (2006*a*) and Lenert *et al.* (2002).

The process of 'chaining' described for temporary states can be used to value mild states where there is a concern that respondents might not be willing to trade the risk of being dead for an improvement in health. The worst state h_j is some state better than being dead. The validity of such chaining is discussed next in section 4.2.3, which focuses upon the impact of different variants.

4.2.3 The time trade-off

The time trade-off technique (TTO) was developed specifically for use in health care by Torrance (1976) as a less complex alternative to the SG that overcomes the problems

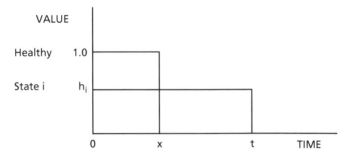

Fig. 4.5 Time trade-off for a chronic health state preferred to dead.

of explaining probabilities to respondents. In common with the SG, TTO presents the respondent with a choice. However, in TTO the respondent is asked to choose between two alternatives of certainty, rather than between a certain outcome and a gamble with two possible outcomes. The application of TTO to a chronic state considered better than dead is illustrated in Figure 4.5.

The conventional TTO technique involves presenting individuals with a paired comparison. For a chronic health state preferred to being dead, alternative 1 involves living for period t in a specified but less than full health state (state h_i). Alternative 2 involves full health for a time period x where $x < t$. Time x is varied until the respondent is indifferent between the two alternatives. The score given to the less than full health state is then x/t.

4.2.3.1 Time trade-off for states considered worse than dead

For a chronic health state considered worse than dead, the TTO task can be modified. In the Measurement and Valuation of Health (MVH) study, states considered worse than dead were valued using a procedure which involved respondents choosing between alternative 1, immediate death (being dead), and alternative 2, spending a length of time (y) in state h_i followed by x years in full health, where $x + y = t$. Time x is varied until the respondent is indifferent between the two alternatives. The value for state h_i is then given by $h_i = -x/(t - x)$. Hence, the more time that is required in full health to compensate for the time spent in state h_i, the lower the score for state h_i (see Fig. 4.6).

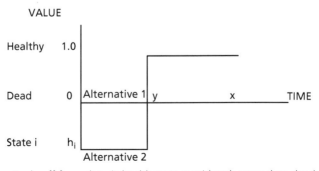

Fig. 4.6 Time trade-off for a chronic health state considered worse than dead.

One practical difficulty with the SG technique is that despite imposing an upper limit of 1.0 on chronic health states preferred to being dead, it poses no comparable lower limit on health states that are considered worse than dead. This results in a scale ranging from minus infinity to + 1.0, thereby giving greater weight to negative values in the calculation of mean scores and presenting problems for statistical analysis. Therefore, it has been recommended that the preference values of states considered worse than dead are rescaled so that the worst possible state is assigned a preference value of –1.0 (Dolan 1997; Shaw *et al.* 2005). Although this represents a convenient transformation, as noted previously with the SG technique, it has no theoretical support and the transformed scores cannot be interpreted as values measured on the same utility scale as states considered better than dead (Patrick *et al.* 1994; Rowen and Brazier 2011).

4.2.3.2 Lead-time and lag-time time trade-off

Three alternative approaches have recently been proposed to handle values for states considered worse than dead. The first approach involves modelling the data using a different economic or mathematical model (Craig and Busschbach 2009; Craig and Oppe 2010) (see Chapter 5). The second and third approaches involve changes to the TTO procedure, first introduced by Robinson and Spencer (2006). Lead-time TTO (LT-TTO) involves the introduction of a 'lead time' whereby a period in full health is added to the start of the conventional TTO (Devlin *et al.* 2011). In lag-time TTO, the period in full health follows the time period spent in the impaired health state, rather than preceding it (Augustovski *et al.* 2013).

LT-TTO represents an alternative choice task to conventional TTO, which involves using the same TTO task regardless of whether the state being valued is considered better or worse than being dead. The lead-time TTO presents respondents with a choice between two alternatives: alternative 1, full health for f years followed by state h for $t - f$ years; and alternative 2, full health for g years whereby $g > f$ for states considered better than dead and $g < f$ for states considered worse than dead. The time spent in full health g is varied until the respondent is indifferent between the two alternatives. The value for state h_i is then given by $h_i = (g - f)/(t - f)$. Hence, the same method, props, and formula are used to calculate the TTO values for all states and the only difference is that the value is negative for states worse than dead and positive for states better than dead (Devlin *et al.* 2011) (see Figs 4.7 and 4.8). A version of this has been adopted by the EuroQol group to value EQ-5D health states considered worse than dead, with the conventional TTO approach being maintained for EQ-5D health states considered better than dead (Devlin *et al.* 2015).

Lag-time TTO is similar to lead-time TTO except for the temporal repositioning of the time spent in state h so that the period in full health f follows rather than precedes it. In a comparison of values for the EQ-5D-5L using both choice tasks, Augustovski *et al.* (2013) found no meaningful or systematic differences, which suggests that the two variants may be equivalent. However, it was noted that differences between the two choice tasks may have been obscured by other aspects of the study design. In addition, given that the two approaches differ in the placement of the time spent in state h relative to being dead, time preferences regarding health at the end of life may lead to a difference in values (Tilling *et al.* 2010) (Fig. 4.9).

Lead Time TTO (state happens to be better than dead)

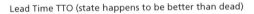

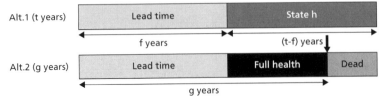

Lead Time TTO (state happens to be worse than dead)

Alt.1 (t years) — Lead time — State h

Alt.2 (g years) — Lead time — dead

g years

Fig. 4.7 'Lead time' time trade-off for a chronic health state better than dead.

A recent study by Pinto-Prades and colleagues (Pinto-Prades and Rodríguez-Míguez 2015) investigated the influence of lead-time TTO for health states considered better than dead in a sample of the Spanish general population (N = 500). A split sample compared conventional TTO and lead-time TTO for a set of 24 health states reflecting six dimensions relating to physical and emotional dependency. A total of 188 participants were interviewed with lead-time TTO and the remainder with conventional TTO.

Lead-time TTO values were found to be higher on average, with the differences in values between methods increasing with the severity of the health state under consideration (lead-time TTO was found to add about 0.14 to the average value for mild states, 0.23 to the intermediate states, and 0.28 points to the more severe states). Hence, health problems are perceived as less severe if a lead period in full health is added upfront, implying that there are interactions between disjointed time periods. These findings imply a violation of the assumption of additive separability, which represents one of the cornerstones of the QALY model. Pinto-Prades and colleagues concluded by noting that the advantages of this method have to be compared with the cost of modelling the interaction between periods.

4.2.3.3 Time trade-off for temporary health states

Figure 4.10 illustrates how temporary health states can be valued using the conventional TTO method. As with the SG, intermediate states are measured relative to the

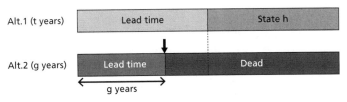

Fig. 4.8 'Lead time' time trade-off for a chronic health state considered worse than dead.

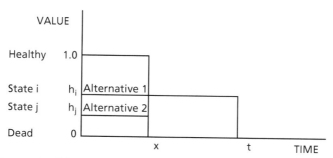

Fig. 4.9 Time trade-off for a temporary health state.

best state (healthy) and the worst state (temporary state h_j). The respondent is offered a choice between two alternatives. Alternative 1 involves living in temporary health state h_i for time period t (the time period specified for the temporary health states), followed by a return to full health. Alternative 2 involves living in temporary health state h_j for time x where $x < t$, followed by full health. Time period x is varied until the respondent expresses indifference between the two alternatives, at which point the required preference value for state $h_i = 1 - (1 - h_j)x/t$. If h_j is set to 0, this reduces to $h_i = 1 - x/t$. To transform the values onto the full health–dead scale, the worst temporary health state must be redefined as a short duration chronic state (as for SG) and valued using the same conventional TTO technique as that already described for valuing chronic health states.

4.2.3.4 Variants of the time trade-off

Similarly for SG, there are numerous variants of TTO using different elicitation procedures, props (if any), and modes of administration. As in common with SG, TTO values can be elicited using the ping–pong or titration search procedures. Visual aids have been developed to assist the respondent in the TTO elicitation task, including props comprising a set of health state cards and a moving sliding scale to represent life years (see for example Torrance 1976; Dolan *et al.* 1996). The widely used variant developed by the York EQ-5D team for interviewer administration and using props is included in the appendix (Appendices 4.4–4.6). The conventional TTO approach was administered to value the first version of the HUI1 (Horsman *et al.* 2003), the EQ-5D-3L (Dolan *et al.* 1996) and the assessment of quality of life instrument, or AQoL (Hawthorne *et al.* 1999), as well as numerous condition-specific health states. Lead-time and lag-time TTO approaches have also been administered more recently as part of the EQ-5D-5L Multinational Pilot Study (Augustovski *et al.* 2013). The data for this study were collected in group interviews using an interview script and digital aids developed to present each variant of the TTO (Figure 4.9). The conventional TTO approach has also been adapted for online administration and utilized in the development of Australian and Canadian general population value sets for the EQ-5D-3L (Viney *et al.* 2011; Bansback *et al.* 2012). The EuroQol group has also recently developed variants of the TTO which incorporate different routing procedures to the conventional TTO. The variants incorporate different starting points and iteration sizes in an effort to reduce the clustering of EQ-5D health state values at −0.5, 0, and 0.5, which was evident when applying the original and widely used variant developed by the York EQ-5D team (Rand-Hendriksen *et al.* 2014).

4.2.3.5 **The person trade-off**

The PTO is a technique for estimating the social value of different health states (Nord *et al.* 1999; Schwarzinger *et al.* 2004; Petrou *et al.* 2013; Robinson and Bryan 2013). As with TTO and SG, the PTO technique asks the respondent to make a choice between two alternatives. The respondent is asked to make a choice in the context of social decision making, which involves groups of other people rather than asking the respondent to value her own state or imagine being in the state herself. The PTO is an adaptation of the method of adjustment or equivalent stimuli described in the psychometrics literature (Patrick *et al.* 1973). It was first applied within the health care field by Patrick and Erickson (1973), in the valuation of levels of well-being for a health status index.

Using this technique, the respondent is asked to indicate how many people in health state B are equivalent to a specified number of people in health state A, by asking the following kind of question: 'If there are x people in adverse health situation A and y people in adverse health situation B, and you can only help (cure) one group, which group would you choose?' (Nord 1992, p. 569). The number of people in health state B (y) is then varied until the respondent finds the two groups equivalent in terms of needing help. The undesirability of health state B is then x/y times as great as that of health state A. This process is then repeated for all other health states to be valued.

PTO has attracted the interest of researchers who regard this approach as being more relevant for social choice contexts than the conventional individual perspective of the other methods of preference elicitation.

4.3 **Review of health state valuation techniques**

In an extensive review of outcome measures for use in economic evaluation, Brazier and colleagues advocated the three basic concepts of practicality, reliability, and validity as the criteria that should be used to compare the performance of alternative methods of preference elicitation (Brazier *et al.* 1999). The practicality of a method is dependent upon its acceptability to respondents, which is a function of the length and complexity of the task, as well as its ability to keep the respondents' interest. It may be the case that some tasks cause distress to respondents (e.g. where there is reference to an early death). These aspects of practicality can be assessed by examining the proportion of those individuals approached who agree to participate (i.e. the response rate) and the level of missing data (i.e. completeness). Reliability is the ability of a measure to reproduce the same quality adjustment values on two separate administrations, over which there is no difference in true health (or in whichever quantity is being measured, which may be the value placed on a hypothetical health state). The two measurements can be elicited from the same respondents at two points in time, and this is known as test–retest reliability.

The basis of the techniques in economic theory or 'theoretical validity' has been argued by some health economists to be the most important criterion in the assessment of the validity of a measure to be used in economic evaluation (Gafni 1996). The assessment of the theoretical basis of the techniques also helps identify the testable assumptions that underpin them. These provide a means of testing the empirical validity of the techniques. Tests of empirical validity also include consistency with other measures of stated preferences, such as ranking of states or other cardinal health state valuation techniques (although this does not greatly help to distinguish between them).

4.3.1 **Visual analogue scales**

There is general agreement that VAS represents the most feasible of the health state valuation techniques, demonstrating high response rates and high levels of completion (Froberg and Kane 1989; Drummond *et al.* 2005; Feng *et al.* 2014). Green *et al.* (2000) reported that completion rates for VAS-based surveys were typically in excess of 90 per cent. VAS methods tend to be less expensive to administer than other methods because of their relative simplicity and ease of completion. This practicality has contributed to the wide utilization of VAS. There is also a significant amount of empirical evidence to demonstrate the reliability of VAS methods in terms of inter-rater reliability and test–retest reliability (see for example O'Brien and Viramontes 1994; Gloth *et al.* 2001; Mannion *et al.* 2006). These studies cite test–retest correlation coefficients (intraclass correlation or Pearson correlation) ranging from $r = 0.61$ (O'Brien and Viramontes 1994) to $r = 0.95$ (Mannion *et al.* 2006).

Recently, some concerns have been raised in relation to the reliability of VAS methods for the assessment of an individual's own health state (as opposed to the assessment of hypothetical health states). A study to assess the performance of the EQ-VAS in the NHS PROMs programme (Feng *et al.* 2014) noted that while a large majority (95 per cent) of EQ-VAS responses were completed in an unambiguous way, only a minority (45 per cent) conformed strictly to the instructions given (by placing a line from their own health state today to the position on the VAS indicating how good or bad their health state is today). The different completion types posed challenges for data coding and interpretation. It was noted that the reliability of VAS data might be improved by providing better guidance and more precise instructions to respondents in the future as to how to complete the EQ-VAS.

The direct and choice-less nature of the VAS task has also given rise to concerns over the ability of this technique to reflect preferences on an interval scale (Bleichrodt and Johannesson 1997). A theoretical argument for VAS has been provided by Dyer and Sarin (1982) who argue that VAS offers a measurable value function that represents preferences under conditions of certainty, whereas utilities represent preferences under uncertainty. This enables a link to be made between the value and uncertainty in terms of an individual's relative risk attitude (Torrance *et al.* 1996). Dyer and Sarin suggest that this offers a stable relationship between SG and VAS, and hence a means of estimating SG values from VAS responses. However, research into the existence of a stable value function is inconclusive. Bleichrodt and Johanneson (1997) did not find evidence of a stable value function, although a re-analysis of their data by Schwartz (1998) found that after adjustment for range frequency bias in the VAS data, the results were consistent with the existence of a stable value function. Robinson and colleagues (2001) also found that adjusted VAS data were consistent with a stable value function, whereas unadjusted data were not. Schwartz, and Robinson and colleagues both used the Parducci–Weddell (PW) range frequency model to adjust the VAS data (Parducci and Wedell 1986), and Torrance and others have recommended that this model be routinely used for VAS data which are to be applied in economic evaluation (Torrance *et al.* 2001). McCabe and colleagues demonstrated that the application of the PW model may produce data that are not on the 0–1 scale required for estimating utility weights in the QALY model and cannot be translated on to this scale using a linear transformation because the true adjusted value of the upper anchor is unknown (McCabe *et al.* 2004). Obviously, data of this nature cannot readily be incorporated into economic evaluation.

There is also a concern that VAS methods are susceptible to response spreading, whereby respondents use all areas on the valuation scale when responding, especially where multiple health states are valued on the same scale. Response spreading can lead to similar health states being placed at some distance from one another on a valuation scale and health states that are essentially different being placed very close to one another, as the respondent seeks to place responses across the whole (or a specific portion) of the available scale. If response spreading does occur, then this implies that VAS techniques do not generate an interval scale and the numbers obtained may not be meaningful (in the cardinal sense).

More generally, VAS is prone to context effects where the average rating for items is influenced by the severity of other items being valued. Robinson *et al.* (2001) found that a series of core health states were given lower values when placed in a wider set of more severe health states than when placed in a wider set of milder health states. In addition, Torrance and colleagues (2001) found evidence of an end-point bias whereby health states at the top and bottom of the scale are placed further apart on the scale than would be suggested by a direct comparison of differences. It is not clear what interaction (if any) there might be between range frequency and end-point bias, or whether a simple adjustment for end-point bias followed by the application of the PW model would adequately remove bias from the data.

One economist, Broome (1993), has argued that VAS can be seen as better than SG and TTO because it is not contaminated by risk and time preference, respectively (discussed next). Broome is concerned with measuring some notion of 'good' rather than individual preferences that do not fall within the conventional welfarist framework. However, Broome's arguments may be viewed as consistent with a non-welfarist approach. There is also evidence to indicate that, in contrast to the TTO approach, VAS is not influenced by individuals' attitudes towards death and being dead. Augestad *et al.* (2013) conducted a study in the Norwegian general population study in which respondents were asked to rank eight hypothetical EQ-5D health states in addition to 'perfect health' and 'immediate death', and then to value each of the ranked states including 'perfect health' and 'immediate death' on a VAS. The sample was then split into two and respondents were instructed to value the eight hypothetical EQ-5D health states using either the conventional TTO or lead-time TTO. It was found that values for EQ-5D health states derived using either conventional or lead-time TTO were influenced by attitudes towards euthanasia (and the influence was more pronounced for the most severe EQ-5D health states presented), but this was not found to be the case for VAS. Augestad *et al.* indicate that whether or not health state values should be dependent on attitudes towards death is a normative question. To the extent that health state values are anchored on the zero to one scale used for QALYs and therefore should be dependent on attitudes towards death, it may be argued that the valuation of health states using the VAS does not capture an important aspect of health states preference.

Historically, the ordinal properties of VAS methods have been largely accepted, given their origins within psychometrics and psychophysics. Although they often correlate well with measures of health status (e.g. pain, functioning, and clinical symptoms), VAS techniques have generally been found to have only a weak correlation with SG and TTO (Jansen *et al.* 2000; Bryce *et al.* 2004; Joyce *et al.* 2012). VAS techniques appear to measure aspects of health status changes rather than the satisfaction or benefit conveyed by such changes. This hypothesis is supported by the qualitative evidence of respondents who see VAS methods as an expression of numbers in terms of 'percentages of the best imaginable state' (Nord 1991) or a 'percentage of functioning scale' (Robinson *et al.* 1997), rather than eliciting information about their preferences for health states. Given the evidence that VAS may not produce health state utilities that can be used directly in the calculation of QALYs, there has been interest in transforming VAS values to SG or TTO utility values

4.3.1.1 Mapping from VAS to SG and TTO

i. VAS to SG Torrance *et al.* (1996) and Feeny *et al.* (2002) pioneered the approach by using VAS to value single and multiattribute health states defined by the HUI2 and HUI3 and by transforming these values into SG utilities using a specially estimated power function. Torrance and colleagues suggested that this has the advantage of retaining the ease of use of VAS with the theoretical advantages of a choice-based measure of health.

The main theoretical argument for the relationship between VAS and SG is based upon the Dyer and Sarin (1982) argument that utilities are made up of a combination of the measurable value function and relative risk attitude. VAS is regarded as a technique for eliciting the measurable value function and SG as a technique for eliciting utilities. According to this theory, SG and VAS values will be the same for individuals who are risk-neutral. A risk-averse person would exhibit a concave relationship between VAS and SG, indicating that he/she would prefer a certain health state with value x to an expected equivalent value (calculated by summing two or more health state values by their probability). In contrast, a risk-loving person would exhibit a convex relationship between VAS and SG. Given that the majority of people have been found to be risk-averse over uncertain prospects involving health, this provides an explanation for the relationship presented in Figure 4.1.

A power function has been proposed to estimate this relationship represented by the following equation:

$$U = 1 - (1 - V)^b \quad \text{or} \quad U = V^b$$

where the power term b represents an individual's constant relative risk attitude, with b greater than 1 implying risk aversion and b equal to one implying risk neutrality. U is the SG utility and V is the VAS value for the health state in question.

Bombardier and colleagues (1982) have offered an alternative theoretical explanation for the relationship between VAS and SG based upon a general aversion to gambling with one's own health. This general aversion is fixed regardless of the level of risk and hence can be represented by a constant term for the difference between SG and VAS values. Bombardier and colleagues estimated a linear relationship between 35 VAS and SG mean health state values which explained 76 per cent of the variation. Torrance and colleagues as well as Loomes have subsequently fitted a power function to the same data with an estimated value for the power term of 2.16 and 2.27 (and explaining 80 per cent of the variation), respectively (Loomes 1993; Torrance *et al.* 1996). Torrance and colleagues estimated weights for the HUI2 using the relationship between mean SG and VAS values for four health states. They fitted a power function to the data, which explained 97 per cent of the variation and had a value of 2.29 for the power term. Stevens *et al.* (2006), in an examination of the relationship between SG and VAS values in a UK valuation study of the HUI2, question the reliance on mapping between values and utilities using only four data points with a limited number of observations and the assumption of a power curve relationship between VAS and SG data in the Health Utilities Index valuation framework. They found that the power function model tended to overfit the data. It was outperformed by all other model specifications in predictive performance (linear, quadratic, and cubic functions). Stevens and colleagues have since recommended further research to establish the most appropriate functional form for mapping between VAS and SG or a move towards the use of SG directly to avoid the problems inherent in the mapping approach (Stevens *et al.* 2007).

ii. VAS to TTO   The expected theoretical relationship between TTO and VAS has been the subject of rather less discussion in the literature, although an obvious source of any difference is time preference. For any rate of time preference other than zero, the time difference between the period in full health and the longer period in chronic health would influence the results. A constant positive time preference rate would reduce the value of time spent in the chronic state by a greater proportion than the time spent in full health, and so the corresponding TTO values would increase. A negative time preference rate would have the opposite effect. The duration of time spent in a health state may also impact upon TTO values. There is evidence to suggest that the prospect of longer periods of time spent in chronic health states may be considered worse than shorter durations (Attema and Brouwer, 2008; Sutherland *et al.* 1982), indicating that TTO values decline with time, the opposite effect of a positive time preference rate. These explanations do not predict a particular form of the relationship.

Studies mapping the relationship between VAS and TTO include work by Torrance who estimated a power function between VAS and TTO from 18 pairs of health state values, which explained 79 per cent of the variation and had a power term of 1.61 (Torrance 1976). Bombardier *et al.* (1982) estimated a linear model for the relationship between VAS and TTO for the 35 pairs of mean values, explaining 89 per cent of the variation. Similarly, Loomes estimated a power function of 1.82 explaining 88 per cent of the variation (Loomes 1993). Stiggelbout *et al.* (1994) have claimed to replicate Torrance's original findings on 183 cancer patients rating their own health. Unfortunately, none of these studies has presented standard econometric diagnostic information on the specification of the models, which means that it is not possible to compare the models or judge how well they actually fit the data.

Neither Torrance nor Stiggelbout *et al.* were able to fit satisfactory power functions to data at the individual level. Only Dolan and Sutton (1997) appear to have done this successfully. However, the linear models outperformed the power models once again, and the power models suffered from heterogeneity and misspecification. The mapping functions were also found to differ substantially between the two variants of TTO.

In conclusion, although there would be significant practical advantages to being able to map from VAS to one of these choice-based techniques, the evidence suggests that the relationships between studies are not stable in terms of the form of the relationship and size of the model parameters. More recently within the literature, there has been a move away from a reliance on mapping between VAS and choice-based techniques, in favour of direct elicitation using these approaches.

4.3.2 **Standard gamble**

The SG appears to be acceptable in terms of its practicality, since large numbers of empirical studies have reported good response and completion rates. Many studies, across different respondent groups, have reported completion rates in excess of 80 per cent, with some studies reporting completion rates as high as 95–100 per cent (see for example studies by Kharroubi *et al.* 2013; Luo *et al.* 2007; and Stewart *et al.* 2005). The SG has also been found to be feasible and acceptable among varied types of patient groups and clinical areas, including cancer, transplantation, vascular surgery, and spinal problems. Several studies have provided support for the reliability of the SG (Ross *et al.* 2003; Wasserman *et al.* 2005).

SG is rooted in expected utility theory (EUT). EUT has been the dominant theory of decision making under uncertainty for over half a century. Although there are now numerous alternative contenders, the simplicity and usefulness of EUT in constructing decision analytical models for use in economic evaluation have ensured its continued survival in applied work. Furthermore, the main preference-based QALY model is based in EUT (Chapter 3).

To recap, EUT theory postulates that individuals choose between prospects (such as different ways of managing a medical condition) in such a way as to maximize their 'expected' utility (von Neumann and Morgenstern 1944). Under this theory, for a given prospect such as having a surgical operation, a utility value is estimated for each possible outcome, good or bad. These values are multiplied by their probability of occurring and the result is summed to calculate the expected utility of the prospect. This procedure is undertaken for each prospect being considered. The key assumption made by EUT over and above conventional consumer theory is independence, which means that the value of a given outcome is independent of its context or how it was arrived at. In decision tree analysis, this is the equivalent of saying that the value of one branch of the tree is unaffected by the existence of other branches.

Due to its theoretical basis, the SG is often portrayed as the classical method of decision making under uncertainty, and due to the uncertain nature of medical decision making the SG is often classed as the 'gold standard' (Drummond *et al.* 2005). As medical decisions usually involve uncertainty, the use of the SG method would seem to have great appeal. However, Richardson (1994) notes that the type of uncertain prospect embodied in the SG may bear little resemblance to the uncertainties in various medical decisions, so this feature may be less relevant than others have suggested.

The status of SG as the gold standard has also been criticized given the existence of ample evidence that the axioms of EUT are violated in practice (Hershey *et al.* 1981; Schoemaker 1982). One response in health economics (as elsewhere) has been that EUT should be seen as a normative rather than a descriptive theory, in that it suggests how decisions should be made under conditions of uncertainty (Drummond *et al.* 2005). However, this still does not alter the concern that the values generated by SG do not necessarily represent people's valuation of a given health state, but incorporate other factors such as risk attitude, gambling effects, and loss aversion (Doctor *et al.* 2010; Van Osch *et al.* 2004; Richardson 1994). A respondent's attitude to risk, for example, may be risk-averse, risk-neutral or risk-seeking, and at times may be a mixture of all three (Doctor *et al.* 2010; Loomes and McKenzie 1989). Kahneman and Tversky (1979) have argued that respondents generally act as if they are risk-averse when choices are framed in terms of potential gains and as risk-seeking when choices are framed in terms of potential losses. Kahneman and Tversky found that individuals tend to overestimate small probabilities and underestimate large probabilities, and they also suggest that probabilities of less than 0.1 and greater than 0.9 present individuals with difficulties, which raises concerns in the context of health state valuation tasks. All these factors will 'contaminate' SG values in some way.

Empirical evidence relating to the consistency of SG responses with expected rankings is more promising. In a general population sample of 335 respondents, Dolan *et al.* (1996) examined the performance of the SG and TTO against 12 logically consistent comparisons (EQ-5D health states) and reported that SG produced high levels of consistency. Rutten van Molken *et al.* (1995) compared SG responses with hypothesized preferences based on the natural underlying order of health state descriptions used (fibromyalgia patients $n = 85$, anklyosing spondylitis patients $n = 144$) and found a high level of consistency. Llewellyn-Thomas *et al.* (1982) reported that the SG provided a high level of consistency against an expected rank ordering of health states (cancer patients, $n = 64$). They found that 54 (84 per cent) of 64 respondents ranked five health states via SG in accordance with *a priori* expectations, with nine of the remaining respondents providing a rank order with only one inconsistent pairing.

4.3.3 Time trade-off

A wide variety of empirical studies have demonstrated that the TTO technique is a practical, reliable and acceptable method of health state valuation (Green *et al.* 2000). The TTO has been used in a self-administered format (Stavem 1999), and several studies that are more recent have demonstrated that computer-based and online applications of TTO are practical and acceptable (Augustovski *et al.* 2013; Viney *et al.* 2011; Bansback *et al.* 2012).

The applicability of the TTO in medical decision making has been questioned by some commentators (e.g. Mehrez and Gafni 1991) due to the fact that the technique asks respondents to make a choice between two certain outcomes, when health care is characterized by conditions of uncertainty. Others have argued that it is possible to adjust TTO values to incorporate individuals' attitudes to risk and uncertainty

(Stiggelbout *et al.* 1994; Cher *et al.* 1997), though this is rarely done. Furthermore, adjusting for risk attitude is difficult when there are strong theoretical and empirical grounds for arguing that there is not a constant attitude to risk.

An underlying assumption of the TTO method is that individuals are prepared to trade-off a constant proportion of their remaining life years to improve their health status, irrespective of the number of years that remain. However, it seems reasonable to postulate that the valuation of a health state may be influenced by a duration effect relating to the time an individual spends in that state. A number of empirical studies have found evidence that the value of a heath state is related to its duration (Bleichrodt *et al.* 2003; Dolan and Stalmeier 2003; Spencer 2003). This body of work dates back to a study conducted over three decades ago by Sutherland and colleagues (1982), who identified a maximal endurable time for some severe health states beyond which they yielded negative utility. Furthermore, for short survival periods, it was observed that individuals were not willing to trade any survival time (measured in life years) for an improvement in quality of life, apparently suggesting that individuals' preferences are lexicographic for short time durations. Further work by Dolan (1996) and Dolan and Stalmeier (2003) found that poor states of health generated from the EQ-5D valuation system became more intolerable to a sample of the general population the longer their duration. If individuals do not trade-off a constant proportion of their remaining life expectancy in the valuation of health states, then values elicited using specific time durations (e.g. 10 years) cannot be assumed to hold for states lasting for different time periods. Craig and Busschbach (2009) notes that the findings from these previous studies re-emphasize the importance of developments in measurement and valuation techniques that account for duration dependence, for example, in discrete choice experiments, where survival duration is included as a separate attribute. Testing the impact of duration dependence with the TTO method requires experiments to be repeated with different numbers of remaining life years. In contrast, discrete choice experiments enable this assumption to be explored internally without repeating the experiment by modelling the remaining life year terms as categorical variables (Bansback *et al.* 2012).

The impact of *time preference* on valuations is another issue that causes theoretical concerns with the TTO. If individuals have a positive rate of time preference, they will give greater value to years of life in the near future than to those in the distant future. Alternatively, respondents may prefer to experience an episode of ill health immediately in order to eliminate 'dread' and move on. For instance, this hypothesis may explain why some women with a family history of breast cancer opt for mastectomy before any breast cancer is detected. In practice, there is considerable variability in procedures of eliciting discount values in the literature (see Mahboub-Ahari *et al.* 2014 for a recent overview). Therefore, it is difficult to conclude on the exact direction and size of the influence of time preferences on health state valuations. However, there is a body of evidence to suggest that, in general, individuals exhibit positive time preferences for health (Van der Pol and Cairns 2000; Chao *et al.* 2009; Attema and Versteegh 2013). However, empirically the validity of the traditional (constant) discounting model in health has been challenged in favour of alternative models that allow for decreasing time aversion (Cairns and Van der Pol 1997; Robberstad and Cairns 2007);

this implies that the longer the period of delay for the onset of ill health, the lower the discount rate. In practice, TTO values are rarely corrected for time preference.

Empirical evidence offers some support for the consistency of TTO responses. Dolan *et al.* (1996) reported high consistency for TTO responses generated from a large-scale UK general population study to value the EQ-5D-3L. Luo *et al.* (2014) examined the performance of the TTO against a logically consistent rank ordering of all 243 EQ-5D-3L health states in a Singaporean general population sample and reported that TTO generated logically consistent values. One concerning aspect of the empirical findings of TTO studies is the extent to which respondents have been unwilling to trade or sacrifice any of their remaining life expectancy for improvements in health in some studies. Robinson *et al.* (1997) refer to a 'threshold of tolerability' below which health states would have to fall before respondents would be willing to sacrifice even a few days. In a study to compare the feasibility of best–worst scaling, time trade-off, and standard gamble approaches to health state valuation in an adolescent sample, Ratcliffe *et al.* (2011) found that for CHU9D health impairment states the vast majority of adolescents were unwilling to trade any remaining life years for improvements in health. Evans and colleagues (2013) conducted a time trade-off study to assess the health status associated with daytime and nocturnal hypoglycaemic events in five countries. They reported that for the baseline diabetes health state, 22 per cent of the general population respondents (19–21 per cent for all the other health states) chose either not to trade any remaining life expectancy or to trade all remaining life expectancy, placing them at the distribution extremes. Other work conducted by the EuroQol group in valuing the EQ-5D has also indicated the possibility of a clustering of values at certain round numbers including the distribution extremes (1.0, 0.5, 0, −0.5, and −1.0) and this digit preference has been found to be associated with the routing procedure utilized with the conventional TTO approach using the original MVH protocol (see Shah *et al.* 2014, http://www.euroqol.org/uploads/media/EQ14-CH01_Shah.pdf).

Shah and colleagues found that using a starting point of 8 years, that is, close to a top-down titration approach, for the TTO procedure resulted in fewer inconsistent responses, substantially reduced the clustering of values and was generally well accepted by participants. While more research is needed, the work conducted by Shah and colleagues indicates a promising way forward in removing the inherent biases generated by the routing procedures that are traditionally adopted for the conventional TTO approach.

4.3.4 **Person trade-off**

In comparison with the other main health state valuation techniques, the PTO has not been widely used to value health states and hence the feasibility and acceptability of the PTO is relatively unknown. In an early examination of the technique, Patrick *et al.* (1973) report that it 'is too complex for use outside of a laboratory-like individual interview'. Nord (1995) reports that the PTO can be quite demanding, warns of possible framing effects, and advises the use of multistep procedures to introduce individuals to the issues involved. Nord suggests that self-administered formats may not be suitable, and also advocates the use of a reflective element within PTO to allow individuals to consider their responses. Pinto-Prades and Abellán-Perpiñán (2005) applied the PTO technique alongside several other health state valuation techniques to value five health states based upon the Modified Rankin Scale (a measure of physical functioning) with two random samples of the Spanish general population. The psychometric properties of PTO were assessed, including feasibility, test–retest reliability, and the consistency of the PTO values (in terms of the logical expected ordering of the five health states relative to the severity of health impairment). It was noted that while these properties have been studied for traditional methods like the SG, there is little evidence for the PTO. The results indicated that the PTO exhibited good feasibility, reliability, and consistency. In a more recent study, Robinson (2011) developed and applied a self-administered format for the PTO. It was found that the self-administered PTO exhibited good test–retest reliability. Robinson notes that these findings are encouraging because evidence on the reliability of PTO is limited.

Some studies employing PTO have included opportunities for group discussion, reflection, and deliberation as an important element of the process. For example, a study by Murray and Lopez (1997) reported on the use of the PTO technique to elicit health state preferences for the assessment of the severity of disability as part of a large multinational study. Although Murray and Lopez did not present information on the performance of the PTO technique, they reported that the PTO protocol was administered as a group exercise (nine groups) for between eight and 12 participants and group discussion was an important element of the process. In an exploratory mixed methods study to assess the impact of discussion and deliberation on health state values generated from PTO, Robinson and Bryan (2013) incorporated an open group discussion following the initial valuation exercise and gave the participants the opportunity to change their values. It was reported that 74 per cent of the participants changed their initial person trade-off valuations following the discussion, which also had an impact on the aggregate valuations. Robinson and Bryan highlight that these results challenge the notion that individuals have pre-existing health state preferences and call for further detailed research in this area.

Richardson (1994) supports the potential interval scale properties of the PTO due to the fact that there is a clear and comprehensible meaning to the PTO (where the numbers are specified). Pinto-Prades (1997) also comments that one of the hypothetical advantages of the PTO in the context of economic evaluation for health care is that it asks the right questions (i.e. trade-offs between people). There is some evidence to indicate that the PTO is better able to reflect social preferences than SG and VAS methods. Pinto-Prades (1997) assessed the techniques on the basis of strength of preference (cardinal) using a hypothetical voting exercise reflecting the treatment intervals of paired comparisons and found that the PTO (variant 3 used) was a better reflection of social preferences than other techniques used. Some would argue that such differences are unsurprising, since SG and VAS methods do not set out to measure social preferences. In a study to compare PTO with three other approaches (including a veil of ignorance approach, SG, and a variant of SG termed the 'double gamble') to measuring the health of populations, Pinto-Prades and Abellán-Perpiñán (2005) found that the PTO values were quite different from the veil of ignorance and double gamble values for identical health states. They note that individuals appear to be using different decision rules when employing the PTO approach. In the PTO there are no identifiable individuals, but it commonly compares life-saving treatments with treatments that mainly improve quality of life. Therefore, the responses to PTO questions may be influenced not only by health considerations, but also by the special consideration that life-saving treatments may have when individuals are asked to consider their preferences in a social decision-making context.

4.4 Overview and comparison of techniques

In the context of cost per QALY analysis, health economists have tended to favour the choice-based scaling methods of SG and TTO (Wisloff *et al.* 2014; Sonntag *et al.* 2013; Drummond *et al.* 2005). A choice-based method is also recommended by the National Institute for Health and Clinical Excellence (NICE) in its guide to the conduct of technology appraisals (2013). Each of the SG and TTO methods starts with the premise that health is an important argument in an individual's utility function. The welfare change associated with a change in health status can then be determined by the compensating change required in one of the remaining arguments in the individual's utility function, such that overall utility remains unchanged (Dolan *et al.* 1996). In the SG, the compensating change is valued in terms of the risk of immediate death. In the TTO, the compensating change is valued in terms of the amount of life expectancy an individual is prepared to sacrifice.

SG has the most rigorous foundation in theory, utilizing EUT theory of decision making under uncertainty. However, there are theoretical arguments against the use of SG in health state valuation and there is little empirical support for EUT. There are also concerns about the empirical basis of the TTO technique. There is evidence to suggest that duration effects and time preference effects can have an impact on the elicitation of TTO values (Sutherland *et al.* 1982; Dolan and Gudex 1995; Dolan and Stalmeier 2003; Spencer 2003).

In reality, SG and TTO valuations can both be seen as containing biases as measures of preference. A key review by Bleichrodt (2002) summarized each of these techniques in terms of four key possible sources of bias relating to utility curvature, probability weighting, loss aversion, and scale compatibility.

In terms of *utility curvature*, SG imposes no restriction on the utility function for the duration of the health state, whereas the TTO assumes that utility is linear in duration. If, as expected, the majority of individuals exhibit positive time preference for health, then this will result in TTO values being biased downwards. However, because SG imposes no restriction on the utility function for the duration of the health state, the existence of utility curvature does not lead to a bias in the SG utilities. Attema and Brouwer (2008) have developed and applied a new risk-free method to correct TTO scores for utility of life duration curvature. They note that the risk-free method appears to be useful to correct TTO scores for the influence of curvature in utility of life duration. In practice, TTO values are rarely adjusted to correct for utility curvature.

Probability weighting affects SG values but not TTO values, since these are elicited under conditions of certainty and no probabilities are involved. Empirical evidence suggests that the probability weighting function is most typically inverse S-shaped, implying that individuals tend to overweight small probabilities and underweight large probabilities. According to Bleichrodt (2002), the point where the function changes from overweighting probabilities to underweighting probabilities lies approximately at 0.35; given that the probabilities reported in SG elicitations tend to be over 0.35, this implies that SG values are generally biased upwards by probability weighting.

Loss aversion implies that individuals tend to be more sensitive to losses than to gains. If loss aversion holds, then this will make individuals more reluctant to give up healthy life years in the TTO, leading to an upward bias in TTO utilities. In the case of SG, loss aversion will tend to cause individuals to weight the certain outcome more highly than the gamble. They will tend to state a higher value of *P* at which they would be indifferent between the gamble and the certain outcome, again leading to upward biases in SG values.

Scale compatibility means that an individual assigns more weight to an attribute the higher its compatibility with the response scale used. In the TTO, the individual is asked how many years in full health are equivalent to a longer period of time in some intermediate state of health, and so the response scale is duration. If an individual exhibits scale compatibility in responding to TTO questions, this implies that they give more weight to duration than to health status. As a consequence, the individual will be less willing to give up life years for an improvement in health status, leading to an upward bias in TTO values. In SG, probability is used as the response scale. Therefore, scale compatibility predicts that an individual will focus upon probability in the evaluation of the SG question. Three probabilities are involved in the SG question, and so scale compatibility may lead to either downward or upward biases in the SG values, the overall effect being ambiguous. Table 4.1 summarizes the arguments made by Bleichrodt in relation to the biases in SG and TTO values (Bleichrodt 2002).

Doctor and colleagues (2010) undertook a systematic review and meta-analysis of health state values to establish the net effect of biases in VAS, SG, and TTO. A total of 2,206 VAS and TTO and 1,318 VAS and SG respondents in 27 studies of utilities were included in the meta-analysis. A data synthesis of computed VAS-TTO and VAS-SG differences was undertaken to reveal persistent dissimilarities in values. While no significant differences between VAS and TTO values were observed, it was found that

Table 4.1 Overview of the biases in SG and TTO values

Effect	Bias in SG values	Bias in TTO values
Utility curvature	None	Downward
Probability weighting	Generally upward	None
Loss aversion	Upward	Upward
Scale compatibility	Ambiguous	Upward

VAS values were significantly lower than SG values. In addition to analysis on raw standard gambles, Doctor *et al.* conducted two meta-analyses on corrected values. The first correction formula adjusted for the effects of bias associated with prospect theory (loss aversion, framing, and probability weighting) (Van Osch *et al.* 2004) and the second corrected only for probability weighting (Prelec 1998). The meta-analyses revealed that the probability weighting correction was effective in reducing SG and VAS differences, but left a very small measurable difference between SG and VAS values, while the correction adjusting for loss aversion, framing, and probability weighting eliminated these differences altogether.

In conclusion, there are theoretical concerns with all these techniques. The valuation of health is essentially subjective and there is no gold standard approach to employ in valuing health states. While the work conducted by Doctor and colleagues and others in the field has demonstrated that it is theoretically possible to apply correction formulate to reduce the differences between the values generated from the main health state valuation techniques, it is impossible to remove all of the problems and biases associated with the generation of health state values in practice. It is argued that unadjusted VAS values do not provide a valid basis for estimating preferences over health states, and satisfactory adjustments remain elusive. For trade-off-based valuations from an individual perspective, the current choice is between SG and TTO. Although TTO has been used more widely in recent years, the reasons outlined here indicate that the values generated by both SG and TTO are distorted by factors apart from preferences over health states, and currently there is no compelling basis on which to select one or the other. Thus, researchers in the field are increasingly opting to employ ordinal techniques such as ranking and discrete choice experiments, as we will discuss in Chapter 7. PTO continues to offer an interesting alternative for those wishing to adopt a social perspective to valuing health states, but there are other approaches to incorporating social concerns in QALYs (see Chapter 11).

4.5 The impact of different variants of health state valuation techniques—evidence for preference construction?

The debate around the appropriate technique for valuation has tended to be the focus of the academic literature; however, there are many variants of each technique and these too may have important implications. Techniques vary in terms of their mode of administration (interview or self-completion, online, digital computer, or paper administration), search procedures (e.g. iteration, titration, or open-ended), the use of props and diagrams, time allowed for reflection, and individual versus group interviews. There have been few publications in the health economics literature comparing these alternatives, but what evidence there is suggests that health state values vary considerably between variants of the same technique.

4.5.1 Format

Dolan and Sutton (1997) compared two variants of the SG and TTO, one using props and the other, no props. These two variants differed not only in terms of the materials used (props versus no props), but also their mode of administration (props is interviewer-administered and no props is designed for self-completion) and their procedure for finding the indifference value. The props variant used a 'ping–pong' search procedure and the no props used titration. Dolan and Sutton (1997) found that differences between variants were more pronounced than differences between techniques. In particular, they found that TTO props valuations tended to be higher than VAS responses for mild states and lower for more severe states. SG props valuations were broadly similar to VAS scores over a wide range, and titration method valuations were consistently higher than VAS valuations, especially for more severe states. In another study comparing titration versus ping–pong search procedures using a common mode of administration (a standardized computer programme), Lenert *et al.* (1998) found that health state values were between 0.10 and 0.15 higher with the titration search procedure than with the ping–pong search procedure for both SG and TTO methods. Differences due to search procedures were found to be similar in magnitude to the differences between SG and TTO methods using the same search procedure, with SG values being, on average, higher than TTO values for the same health state.

A study by Brazier and Dolan (2005) compared SG props (ping–pong with interviewer administration) to no props (titration with self-completion) and found that the mean titration values were significantly higher on average for the first four of the seven health states valued. Brazier and Dolan suggested that this result could be explained by anchoring, since titration typically starts eliciting preferences at the upper end of the scale, whereas the ping–pong iterates respondents between the upper and lower ends, thereby reducing any anchor point bias. Brazier and Dolan argue that this hypothesis is supported by the finding that a significantly lower proportion of respondents chose a probability of success of 1.0 with ping–pong compared with titration. A view expressed by some of the respondents in their study was that the ping–pong procedure actually confuses people and encourages them to take risks. This was a crossover study, and the last three states had values that were found to be contaminated by what went before.

A recent study by Luo and colleagues (2014) examined the impact of different formats for lead-time TTO. Specifically, this study investigated the effects on health state valuation of the length of lead time and the way in which the lead-time TTO task was displayed visually. It was found that health state values generated by TTO valuation tasks using a longer lead time were slightly lower than those generated by tasks using a shorter lead time. When lead time and unhealthy time were presented with visual aids highlighting the difference between the lead time and unhealthy time, respondents spent longer considering health states with a value close to 0. Luo *et al.* (2014) interpreted this result positively as an indicator of more thoughtful answers and recommend that future studies should investigate whether the special design in visual aids and a physical reminder at the value of 0 would generate more accurate values.

In a study to examine the effect that different specifications of the TTO had on values for the EQ-5D, Versteegh *et al.* (2013) compared lead-time and lag-time TTO with conventional TTO tasks. The study also investigated the impact of different health state durations and an online versus face-to-face mode of administration for each task. It was found that lag-time TTO produced lower values than lead-time TTO and this difference was larger for health states of longer durations. Conventional TTO values most closely resembled those of lag-time TTO in the longest (20-year) period in terms of mean absolute difference. It was also found that the relative importance of different domains of health was systematically related to the health state duration, with anxiety/depression having the largest negative impact in the 10-year time frame and pain/discomfort having the largest negative impact in the 5-year time frame. A lower level of task engagement was reported with the online mode of administration leading to lower data quality. Approximately two-thirds of the observations used a maximum of four iterations to reach a point of indifference leading to a bunching of health state values; a finding that was also noted earlier by Norman and colleagues (2010) in a randomized comparison of an online and face-to-face TTO task. Norman *et al.* recommended that the incorporation of a similar level of decision support for an online task as would be provided in a face-to-face interview may help alleviate this problem. Versteegh *et al.* commented that low levels of task engagement remained despite very careful design of the online TTO and the incorporation of both textual and graphical explanations similar to those presented in the face-to-face interview. The purported advantages of an online mode of administration for TTO include the ability to facilitate broad geographical coverage of a population at relatively low cost (Bansback *et al.* 2012). However, these advantages need to be balanced against the ongoing concerns relating to the quality of the responses achieved.

4.5.2 Chaining of health state values

It has been suggested in the literature that for valuing milder health states where respondents may be less willing to risk death, an alternative variant is to value such states (h_i) against an uncertain prospect of full health or another state worse than the one being valued (h_j) but not as bad as being dead (Drummond *et al.* 2005). This is essentially the approach suggested for valuing temporary states (Fig. 4.4). The lower state is then valued in an SG as the intermediate state against the gamble of full health or being dead. By a simple 'chaining' process, it is possible to transform the indifference probability value from the first gamble (P_x) using the indifference probability value from the second gamble (P_y) onto the full health–dead scale (i.e. $h_i = P_x + (1-P_y) \times P_x$). According to the axioms of EUT, the chained value for health state h_i should be the same as the value obtained from a single gamble involving full health and being dead as lower anchor (or the equivalent gamble for states worse than being dead).

A number of studies have found that values chained via the worst state are consistently higher than the values obtained directly (Llewellyn-Thomas *et al.* 1982; Jones-Lee *et al.* 1993; Rutten van Molken *et al.* 1995). As observed by Jones-Lee *et al.* (1993) in their studies of injury state valuation ' . . . Varying the severity of the consequence of failure in the risky treatment requires a conceptually more difficult adjustment than keeping the risky treatment the same and varying the severity of the injury description' (p. 62). There are a number of theoretical explanations of this phenomenon, including the existence of a gambling effect (Richardson 1994) and loss aversion due to a reference point effect (Oliver 2003). This would suggest that the process of chaining should be avoided where possible.

4.5.3 Implications

The evidence that results are majorly affected by the way people are questioned in preference elicitation techniques has a number of implications. Firstly, it demonstrates the importance of using a common variant to ensure comparability between studies. It is not enough to claim two studies used the same methods simply because they both claim to have used TTO or SG. It is necessary to demonstrate that the two studies used the same variant and the same technique (and respondents with the same characteristics). Secondly, there might be scope for correcting some of these differences if they prove to be systematic. This approach has been applied by Oliver (2003), Van Osch *et al.* (2004), and more recently by Doctor *et al.* (2010) with some success, but there has been little of such work to date. There is also a need to utilize cognitive techniques to better understand the reasons for the differences between variants.

More fundamentally, this evidence suggests that people do not have well-defined preferences over health prior to undertaking a valuation task, but rather their preferences are constructed during the task. This would account for the apparent willingness of respondents to be influenced by the precise framing of the question. This may be a consequence of the cognitive complexity of the task. With TTO and SG, respondents are typically asked to consider variations in up to eight health dimensions alongside a life and death scenario involving probabilities or survival. Evidence from the psychology literature suggests that respondents faced with such complex problems tend to adopt simple decision heuristic strategies (Lloyd 2003). This may be particularly true where the respondents have little time to consider their real underlying values. Also, much of the health state valuation work undertaken to date has used 'cold calling' techniques, that is, the respondents are members of the general public who have not been prepared in any way for the valuation task. A well conducted preference elicitation study should provide a full explanation of the task to the respondent and undertake a practice question, but typically respondents are then expected to generate health state values in one sitting with little time given for reflection.

These arguments suggest that respondents need to be given more time and support to reflect upon their values in order to process such complex information. There is a case for allowing respondents more time to learn the techniques, to ensure they understand them fully and to allow them more time to reflect on their health state valuations. It has been suggested that respondents could be re-interviewed after they have had time to reflect and deliberate on the health state in question, and that this process may be helpful in encouraging the development of 'well formed' preferences (Shiell *et al.* 2000; also see Box. 4.1). An implication may be to move away from the current large-scale surveys including members of the general public and involving one-off interviews or online surveys, to smaller scale studies including panels of members of the general public who are better trained and more experienced in the techniques, and who are given time to fully reflect on their valuations (Robinson and Bryan 2013; McTaggart-Cowan *et al.* 2011; Stein *et al.* 2006b).

Box 4.1 Preferences for health states: elicited or constructed?

In a study of health preferences in a sample of 62 members of staff and students from the Department of Community Medicine at the University of Sydney and Westmead Hospital (Shiell *et al.* 2000), participants were asked to value a set of states at three points in time (initial interview and repeat interviews one and eight weeks after the initial interview). A standard format was followed at each interview in which participants were asked to value two chronic health states: first using VAS and secondly using SG. At the end of the second and third interviews, all of the participants were asked whether they had given any thought to the issues raised in the previous interview and whether anything of significance had happened to them since the last interview which may have influenced their responses in the repeat interview. In order to control for unstable preferences, the analysis was repeated both with and without those respondents who reported a significant event between interviews. For the majority of participants, values were stable over repeat administrations. However, one-third of participants deliberately changed their answers and suggested that the interview process had forced them to think about their answers more deeply. The omission of those who experienced a significant event did not change the results. Despite being impossible to draw definitive conclusions from such a small sample, the key finding of this work is the suggestion that the assumption of completeness of preferences should not be taken for granted; a process of reflection and deliberation may be necessary before it is possible to elicit valid and reliable estimates of preference.

4.6 Aggregation of health state values

Once health state values have been obtained, individual responses must be aggregated in some way. The choice includes the mean, median, or modal response. Economists have generally advocated the mean average as representing the theoretically correct way to aggregate individual values, irrespective of the nature of the distribution. This is because the mean reflects people's intensity of preference and follows conventional welfare concerns by addressing whether the total benefits to those who gain are greater than the sum of the benefits to those who lose from a policy change. However, in the area of public policy it may be argued that group preferences should be expressed in terms of the median value. The median treats each person's valuations as equal in a voting context. A comparison of an EQ-5D population value set based upon mean values with a value set based upon median values revealed differences, in that the median-based value set exhibited higher values for less severe states and lower values for more severe states (Dolan 1997). Dolan suggests that the choice of population value set is a matter of judgement: 'without a gold standard by which to compare the two tariffs, this choice should ultimately be based upon a prior philosophical position on how preferences should be aggregated rather than on intuition about which set of valuations seem to produce better answers' (Dolan 1997).

The general consensus within health economics to date has been to adopt mean health state values as the most appropriate aggregation measure for informing decision making within the methodology of economic evaluation; while this would seem to follow from a conventional welfarist view, under the non-welfarist view there is scope to conceive and develop alternative value sets that reflect the population median or modal preference.

4.7 Who should value health?

Historically, it was recognized that values for health could be obtained from a number of different sources including patients, their carers, health professionals, and the community. Currently, health state values are usually obtained from members of the general public trying to imagine what the state would be like, but it has also been argued that values should be obtained from patients (Menzel *et al.* 2002; Ubel *et al.* 2003). This section concentrates on general population versus patients' values or, as it has been more recently characterized, the choice between using health state values based on hypothetical preferences versus experiences (Brazier *et al.* 2005; Dolan 2008; Burström *et al.* 2014).

4.7.1 Why does it matter?

The choice of whose values to elicit is important because it may influence the resulting values. A number of empirical studies have been conducted which indicate that patients with first-hand experience tend to place higher values on dysfunctional health states than members of the general population who do not have similar experience. The extent of this discrepancy tends to be much stronger when patients value their own health state (Tengs and Wallace 2000; Ratcliffe *et al.* 2007; Peeters and Stigglebout 2010). In relation to certain mental health conditions, in particular the case of dementia, there is some evidence that indicates a tendency for the opposite effect; patient and carer values for dementia health impairment states have been found to be lower than those elicited for identical states from the general population (Rowen *et al.* 2015).

There is also evidence to indicate that the extent of the differences in health state values between patient and general population may be influenced by the valuation method. A meta-analysis of published studies between 1970 and 2008 reporting patient and general population values for health states found that when elicitation methods were analysed separately, patient values were higher than general population values for the TTO and VAS, but no discernible differences were found for SG (Peeters and Stigglebout 2010).

Earlier empirical studies tended to use relatively small sample sizes and focus on differences in patient and general population values for a single medical condition or type of health problem. More recently, studies have attempted to use larger sample sizes and incorporate multiple patient samples. For example, Mann *et al.* (2009) compared EQ-5D profile and VAS data obtained from 3,376 patients covering eight different conditions, with general population data taken from the EQ-5D valuation set using regression modelling. Statistically significant differences were found between the coefficients for the EQ-5D health dimensions pain/discomfort, mobility and anxiety/depression. The decrements for anxiety/ depression were larger in the patient model but smaller for pain/discomfort and mobility relative to the general population model. The magnitude of disagreement between patient self-rated VAS model and the population VAS model was also found to vary depending upon the patients' condition. In a study to examine differences in the relative importance attributed to the EQ-5D dimensions between experienced health valuations from patients and hypothetical health valuations from the general population for EQ-5D states in the United States, Rand-Hendriksen *et al.* (2012) found considerable differences between stated preferences, particularly for self-care and usual activities. Self-care and pain/discomfort were found to be the most important dimensions for the hypothetical health valuations, whereas normal activity was the most important dimension for the experienced health valuations. Little *et al.* (2014) compared a European value set for the EQ-5D-3L based on hypothetical health valuations from the general population with a German value set for the same instrument based upon experienced health valuations. It was found that weightings of the EQ-5D-3L dimensions were systematically different. The experienced health value set gave significantly lower mean values for most, but not all, patient groups despite the hypothetical health value set generating lower values for 213 of the 243 EQ-5D-3L health states. Little *et al.* note that this apparently contradictory finding may be partly explained by the fact that most of the patient groups reported some problems in mobility, usual activities, and pain/discomfort and a relatively greater weight was assigned to 'some' problems in these dimensions when using the experienced health value set. Burström *et al.* (2014) estimated Swedish experience-based value sets for EQ-5D-3L health states using general population health survey data. A very large sample of N = 45,000 individuals was utilized in order to facilitate modelling of the association between the experience-based TTO and VAS values and the EQ-5D dimensions and severity levels. It was found that almost all dimensions and severity levels had less impact on TTO valuations compared with the UK study based on hypothetical general population values. The anxiety/depression dimension had the greatest impact on both TTO and VAS values, and both TTO and VAS values were consistently related to self-reported health.

In summary, although there are variations in the findings from these individual studies in terms of the relative impact of EQ-5D dimensions according to patient experience, the available evidence highlights the potential for systematic differences between hypothetical general population preferences and experienced patient preferences that in certain patient groups could drive the results of an economic evaluation. Therefore, the choice as to whose values are used may be critical when making resource allocation decisions.

4.7.2 Why do these discrepancies exist?

There are a number of possible contributing factors for observed differences between patient and general population values, including: poor descriptions of health states (for the general population), use of different internal standards, or response shift and adaptation (Ubel *et al.* 2003).

4.7.2.1 Poor descriptions of health states

An important potential source of discrepancy is found when descriptions provided to the general population may not accurately describe the health state. Most health state descriptive systems contain a limited number of attributes and tend to focus upon the negative aspects of a health state. As such, individuals tend to bring their own information to the valuation exercise by drawing upon their own personal experiences or stereotypes. Given that the personal experiences of patients and members of the general public are unlikely to be the same, it may mean that, in effect, they are evaluating different health states even when provided with identical descriptions of the health state to be valued. It has also been suggested that general population respondents focus too much on ill health and ignore the remaining positive aspects of a person's life (Ubel *et al.* 2003). It is possible that this problem could be reduced by more accurate health state descriptions.

4.7.2.2 Changing standards

A well-known phenomenon in the psychometric literature is 'response shift', which refers to the possibility that individuals will change their internal standards for evaluating their own health in response to changes in their health (Sprangers and Schwartz 1999). Response shift occurs due to changes in expectations. For example, an older person may rate his or her health according to their expectations of the best possible health for a person of their age rather than best possible health *per se*. Similarly, a patient may rate his or her health by comparing themselves with other patients rather than with healthy individuals. In either instance, response shift will contribute to discrepancies between patient and general population values for the same health states and, unlike the problem of incomplete or inaccurate health state descriptions, it is difficult to see how response shifts can be reduced or eliminated in practice. Indeed, it can be argued that response shift effects in health state valuation tasks conducted with patients should not be of concern, since these reflect the entirely laudable concepts of adaptation and coping.

4.7.3 **Adaptation to the state**

Someone in an ill health state is likely to adapt over time, both physically and emotionally. Physical changes include the acquisition of new skills to help cope with a disability, such as learning to use a walking stick. A person may also change the things they do in order to limit the impact of their disability or illness. For example, someone who once played football may take up a sport that has a lower impact on his or her knees. There are also psychological adaptations that include a shift in the weight people place on different aspects of health and quality of life and, more fundamentally, a change in their view of what matters in life. People may also lower their expectations of what they can achieve.

It is well established in the literature that people tend to underpredict their ability to adapt (Kahneman 2000; McTaggart-Cowan *et al.* 2011; Dolan 2011). When general population respondents read the description of a state, their valuation may reflect an initial response to say, going blind, rather than what it would be like for an extended period. In other words, they focus on the transition to the state rather than the longer-term consequences. This focus results in the general population giving lower values compared with patient self-reported values for chronic states of health.

4.7.4 **How do generic preference-based measures currently take patient views into account?**

The impact of response shift and adaptation on the size of the discrepancy between patient and general population valuations will depend on the descriptive system being used. A degree of adaptation to physical disability is already incorporated into those descriptive systems that have dimensions such as role and social functioning, for instance the SF-6D or usual activities in the EQ-5D (see Chapter 8 for a description of these preference-based measures). The developers of the HUI3, however, excluded these social dimensions of health in part to remove adaptation. Nonetheless, all the generic descriptive systems take some account of psychological adaptation through dimensions concerned with mood (such as anxiety, positive affect, and depression). Indeed, it could be argued that the wording of other dimensions, such as those concerned with physical functioning and pain, contain a significant element of self-evaluation and so also incorporate a degree of adaptation. For example, does a 90-year-old person reporting 'some problems with mobility' on the EQ-5D really mean the same as a 25-year-old reporting this level? Whether or not it is appropriate from a normative point of view to take any account of adaptation (as explored in the next section), it would seem that existing preference-based measures do take some account of adaptation.

4.7.5 Why use general population values?

The Washington Panel on the Cost-Effectiveness in Health and Medicine, a highly influential body who advocated the use of general population values, argued that ' . . . the best articulation of society's preferences for a particular state would be gathered from a representative sample of fully informed members of the community'. The Panel went on to use the notion of the 'veil of ignorance' to support the use of community values, where 'a rational public decides what is the best course of action when blind to its own self-interest, aggregating the utilities of persons who have no vested interest in particular health states seems most appropriate' (Gold *et al.* 1996). This reflects a concern that patients will only think of their own health state and not appreciate how it compares with those of other patients. They argue that the values of different patient groups are not comparable, whereas a general population sample provides a coherent set of values.

The main arguments for and against general population values are summarized in Box 4.2. A key argument is that the general population pays for the service. While members of the general population want to be involved in health care decision making, it is not clear that they want to be asked to value health states specifically (see Litva *et al.* 2002). At the very least, it does not necessarily imply the current practice of using relatively uninformed general population values.

4.7.6 Why use patient values?

While the recommendation for the use of general population values by the Washington Panel on Cost-Effectiveness in Health and Medicine in the United States has been influential in the guidelines for economic appraisal of new health care technologies in a number of countries including the United Kingdom and Canada (National Institute for Health and Care Excellence 2013; Canadian Agency for Drugs and Technologies in Health 2006), other regulatory authorities including Sweden and Germany recommend the use of experienced patient-based values (Burström *et al.* 2014; German Social Code 2013).

Box 4.2 Preferences versus experience

Using patient values based upon experience

For:

- Patients know their own health state better than anyone trying to imagine it.
- It is the well-being of the patient that we are interested in, since ultimately it is the patients who will be the losers and gainers from a public programme.

Against:

- It is possible that patients may behave strategically, for example, in overemphasizing the benefits of a new treatment in terms of the health improvement experienced in order to try to ensure that they will have access to it.
- Patients may be unable or unwilling to provide values (or indeed it may be unethical).
- Adaptation to a particular health state may work against the patient's best interests because it may result in them assigning higher health state values to a dysfunctional health state, thereby lessening the value of quality of life improvements due to new health care technologies, and some of this may be regarded as undesirable (e.g. low expectations).

Using general population values based upon preferences

For:

- The 'veil of ignorance' argument was advocated by the Washington Panel on Cost-Effectiveness in Health and Medicine to support the use of general population values where the utilities of individuals who have no vested interest in particular health states are aggregated to generate summary health state values.
- Public funding (in the form of taxation, for example) can essentially be seen as public insurance and so it is the *ex ante* public preferences that should be used to value health states.

Against:

- Members of the general population generally have little or no first-hand experience of the health states being valued.
- While members of the general population want to be involved in health care decision making, it is not clear that they want to be asked to value health states specifically (see for example Litva *et al.* 2002).

A common argument for using patient values is the fact that patients understand the impact of their health on their well-being better than someone trying to imagine it. As Buckingham has pointed out: 'To ask a person of 20 how s/he will value health at the age of 70 is to ask an enormous amount of their imagination. To ask a 70-year-old how important their health is to them is likely to result in far more valuable information' (Buckingham 1993). However, this fact does not imply that raw patient values should be used on their own to inform resource allocation decisions. This requires a value judgement that society wants to incorporate all the changes and adaptations that occur in patients who experience states of ill health over long periods of time. Some adaptation may be regarded as 'laudable', such as skill enhancement and activity adjustment, whereas cognitive denial of functional health, suppressed recognition of full health, and lowered expectations may be seen as less desirable (Menzel *et al.* 2002). Furthermore, there may be a concern that patient values are context-based, reflecting their recent experiences of ill health and the health of their immediate peers (Ubel *et al.* 2003).

Putting normative concerns to one side, asking patients to value their own health, and to do so sufficiently frequently, raises some major practical problems. Many patients by definition are quite unwell and may be unable or unwilling to undertake complex and quite intrusive valuation tasks. In addition, there may also be ethical concerns with asking patients in terminal conditions to imagine scenarios involving either the risk of death or shorter life expectancies.

The psychological work on 'experienced' utility mainly uses rating scales, which are criticized by health economists for lacking the choice context required to obtain a preference value, such as those achieved in SG, TTO, or WTP (willingness to pay). However, the use of choice-based methods presents a paradox. The accepted choice-based techniques for valuing health states, such as SG or TTO, require a patient to value their existing state by imagining what it would be like to be in full health, which they may not have experienced for many years. For patients who have lived in a chronic health state, for example chronic obstructive pulmonary disease or osteoarthritis, the task of imagining full health is as difficult as a healthy member of the general population trying to imagine a poor health state.

4.7.7 A middle way—further research

One conclusion from what we have explored here is that it seems difficult to justify the exclusive use of patient values or the currently widely adopted practice of using values from relatively uninformed members of the general population. It has already been argued that existing generic preference-based measures already take some account of adaptation and response shift, but whether this is sufficient is a normative judgement. If it is accepted that ultimately it is the values of the general population that are required to inform resource allocation in a public system, it might be argued that respondents should be provided with more information on what the states are like for patients experiencing them. This position has been proposed by a number of commentators on the subject (Menzel *et al.* 2002; Fryback 2003; Ubel *et al.* 2003; Dolan 2011; McTaggart-Cowan *et al.* 2011) and there are examples of some studies which have attempted to operationalize this in practice. A review examining all empirical studies published in 2009 and earlier identified a total of 14 studies reporting upon methods used to elicit informed general population values for health states (McTaggart-Cowan, 2011). Interventions used to inform the general population were categorized into the following: information to enrich the health state descriptions (n = 7); simulation to reproduce the symptoms of the health state (n = 2); opportunity to reflect and deliberate on the health state descriptions (n = 2); and exercises to evoke adaptation to the health state (n = 3).

The majority of the identified studies to date have attempted to generate informed general population values for health states by providing respondents with additional information through the use of audio recordings and videos. For example, a study by Clarke *et al.* (1997) examined the health state values for three Gaucher disease states by presenting information from patients currently living in the states through the use of multimedia equipment. The authors did not detect statistically significant differences in the utilities between the patients and the general population samples. In another study, descriptions of dentofacial deformities and photographs of dental patients corresponding to the health state descriptions were presented to both patient and general population respondents (Cunningham and Hunt 2000). Again, no statistically significant differences in the utilities between the patients and the general population samples were found.

A disadvantage of the provision of additional information is that respondents may still have difficulty imagining themselves living in the health state they are being asked to value. One method that has been utilized to overcome this limitation is the use of devices to enhance the effect of the health state. In a study to assess general population health state values for different visual impairment states, Aballéa and Tsuchiya used spectacles to simulate the symptoms of the health states being valued (Aballéa and Tsuchiya 2008). However, such simulation approaches are not applicable to all disease states. Deliberation and adaptation techniques explicitly encourage respondents to consider broader life aspects in relation to the health state. The deliberation approach may replicate the way in which 'real-life' decisions are made, whereas adaptation exercises inform the respondents about the possibility of adapting to an impaired health state over time.

In a study to assess the impact of discussion on preferences elicited in a group setting, Stein *et al.* (2006*b*) utilized the SG technique with a panel of 15 members of the general population who were asked to value 41 different health states five times over the course of six months. Following initial individual valuation, the group was given the opportunity to discuss the health states and after this discussion, individuals were given the opportunity to change their health state values. Although no statistically significant differences were detected before and after the discussion, respondents indicated that the group discussion brought reassurance and cohesion to their responses. In relation to accounting for adaptation, Damschroder *et al.* (2005) used a generic adaptation exercise whereby respondents were asked to think back to a previous different life event and assess the extent to which their emotions towards this event changed over time when valuing states pertaining to paraplegia, below-the-knee amputation, colostomy, and severe pain. A more recent study by McTaggart-Cowan *et al.* (2011) explored the extent to which members of the general population (n = 200) changed their initial values for three rheumatoid arthritis states following an adaptation exercise, where they listened to recordings of patients discussing how they adapted. After undergoing the adaptation exercise, the respondents increased their values for the rheumatoid arthritis states and it was found that younger and healthier individuals were more likely to increase their initial values after being informed.

Despite the evidence presented, in reality the vast majority of health state valuation exercises conducted to date have not attempted to incorporate methods to elicit informed general population values. Further research is needed to determine explicit methods for providing better ways of explaining hypothetical health states to general population respondents (Brazier *et al.* 2005; McTaggart-Cowan *et al.* 2011; Robinson and Bryan 2013).

4.8 Conclusions

This chapter has considered the issue of how to value the quality adjustment weight component of QALYs for use within the methodology of economic evaluation. The reader may feel somewhat overwhelmed by the large array of health state valuation techniques and variants on offer and the choice of sources of value. Indeed, there are further choices offered in the chapter on ordinal techniques (Chapter 6). Some of the decisions can be made on theoretical grounds (such as the use of a choice-based method for deriving preferences) or empirical grounds (some variants generate more consistent values than others), but often the analyst is left with either a trade-off between different types of distortion (e.g. the SG versus TTO), or a need to make normative choices (e.g. the extent to which adaptation should be incorporated).

The vastness of the array is not surprising. The mistake is to assume that there is a single set of 'true' values for health states or profiles. However, a decision maker needs a common and consistent set of methods for informing decisions and so choices need to be made about technique, variant, and source of values. Such choices are made for reasons of expediency for assisting decision making (e.g. National Institute for Health and Care Excellence 2013), but it is important to continue research into major outstanding issues; these include further developing our understanding of the theoretical basis of the different techniques, and the development of methods to improve their reliability and validity both in theory and in practice.

References

Aballéa S, Tsuchiya A (2007). Seeing for yourself: feasibility study towards valuing visual impairment using simulation spectacles. *Health Economics* **16**:537–43.

Attema AE, Brouwer WB (2008). Can we fix it? Yes we can! But what? A new test of procedural invariance in TTO-measurement. *Health Economics* **17**:877–85.

Attema AE, Versteegh MM (2013). Would you rather be ill now, or later? *Health Economics* **22**:1496–506.

Augestad LA, Rand-Hendriksen K, Stavem K, Kristiansen IS (2013). Time trade-off and attitudes toward euthanasia: implications of using 'death' as an anchor in health state valuation. *Quality of Life Research* **22**(4):705–14.

Augustovski F, Rey-Ares L, Irazola V, Oppe M, Devlin NJ (2013). Lead versus lag-time trade-off variants: does it make any difference? *European Journal of Health Economics* Jul;14 Suppl 1:S25–31.

Bansback N, Tsuchiya A, Brazier J, Anis A (2012). Canadian valuation of EQ-5D health states: preliminary value set and considerations for future valuation studies. PLoS One 7(2):e31115.

Bleichrodt H (2002). A new explanation for the difference between time trade off utilities and standard gamble utilities. *Health Economics* 11:447–56.

Bleichrodt H, Johannesson M (1997). An experimental test of a theoretical foundation for rating-scale valuations. *Medical Decision Making* 17:208–16.

Bleichrodt H, Pinto JL, Abellán-Perpiñán JM (2003). A consistency test of the time trade-off. *Journal of Health Economics* 22:1037–52.

Bombardier C, Wolfson A, Sinclair A, McGreer A (1982). Comparison of three measurement methodologies in the evaluation of functional status index. In: Deber R, Thompson G (eds). *Choices in health care: decision making and evaluation of effectiveness.* University of Toronto, Toronto, Canada, pp. 298–322.

Brazier J, Akehurst R, Brennan A, Dolan P, Claxton K, McCabe C, Sculpher M, Tsuchiya A (2005). Should patients have a greater role in valuing health states? *Applied Health Economics and Health Policy* 4:201–8.

Brazier J, Deverill M, Green C, Harper R, Booth A (1999). A review of the use of health status measures in economic evaluation. *Health Technology Assessment* 3(9):1–164.

Brazier J, Dolan P (2005). *Evidence of preference construction in a comparison of variants of the standard gamble method.* Health Economics and Decision Science Section Discussion Paper no 05/04, University of Sheffield, UK.

Brazier J, Roberts J, Deverill M (2002). The estimation of a preference-based single index measure for health from the SF-36. *Journal of Health Economics* 21:271–92.

Brooks R, Rabin RE, de Charro FTH (eds) (2003). The measurement and valuation of health status using EQ-5D: a European perspective. Kluwer Academic Press, Dordrecht, the Netherlands.

Broome J (1993). QALYs. *Journal of Public Economics* 50:149–67.

Bryce CL, Angus DC, Switala J, Roberts MS, Tsevat J (2004). Health status versus utilities of patients with end-stage liver disease. *Quality of Life Research* 13:773–82.

Buckingham K (1993). A note on HYE (healthy years equivalent). *Journal of Health Economics* 12:301–9.

Burström K, Sun S, Gerdtham UG, Henriksson M, Johannesson M, Levin LÅ, Zethraeus N (2014). Swedish experience-based value sets for EQ-5D health states. *Quality of Life Research* 23:431–42.

Cairns JA, Van der Pol MM (1997). Saving future lives: a comparison of three discounting models. *Health Economics* 6:341–50.

Canadian Agency for Drugs and Technologies in Health (2006). *Guidelines for Economic Evaluation of Health Technologies,* 3rd edn.

Chao LW, Szrek H, Pereira NS, Pauly MV (2009). Time preference and its relationship with age, health, and survival probability. *Judgement and Decision Making* 4:1–19.

Cher DJ, Miyamoto J, Lenert LA (1997). Incorporating risk attitude into Markov-process decision models: importance for individual decision making. *Medical Decision Making* 17:340–50.

Clarke AE, Goldstein MK, Michelson D (1997). The effect of assessment method and respondent population on utilities elicited for Gaucher disease. *Quality of Life Research* 6:169–84.

Craig BM, Busschbach JJ (2009). The episodic random utility model unifies time trade-off and discrete choice approaches in health state valuation. *Population Health Metrics* 13:7;3.

Craig BM, Oppe M (2010). From a different angle: a novel approach to health valuation. *Social Science and Medicine* 70:169–74.

Cunningham S, Hunt N (2000). A comparison of health state utilities for dentofacial deformity as derived from patients and members of the general population. *European Journal of Orthodontics* 22:335–42.

Damschroder LJ, Zikmund-Fisher BJ, Ubel PA (2005). The impact of considering adaptation in health state valuation. *Social Science and Medicine* 61:267–77.

Devlin NJ, Tsuchiya A, Buckingham K, Tilling C (2011). A uniform time trade off method for states better and worse than dead: feasibility study of the 'lead time' approach. *Health Economics* 20:348–61.

Devlin N, Shah K, Feng Y, Mulhern B, van Hout B (2015). An EQ-5D-5L value set for England. OHE Research Paper 15/03. Office of Health Economics, London, UK.

Doctor JN, Bleichrodt H, Lin HJ (2010). Health utility bias: a systematic review and meta-analytic evaluation. *Medical Decision Making* 30:58–67.

Dolan P (1996). Modelling valuations for health states: the effect of duration. *Health Policy* 38:189–203.

Dolan P (1997). Aggregating health state valuations. *Journal of Health Services Research and Policy* 2:160–7.

Dolan P (2008). Developing methods that really do value the 'Q' in the QALY. *Health Economics Policy and Law* 3:69–77.

Dolan P (2011). Thinking about it: thoughts about health and valuing QALYs. *Health Economics* 20:1407–16.

Dolan P, Gudex C (1995). Time preference, duration and health state valuations. *Health Economics* 4:289–99.

Dolan P, Gudex C, Kind P, Williams A (1996). Valuing health states: a comparison of methods. *Journal of Health Economics* 15:209–31.

Dolan P, Stalmeier P (2003). The validity of time trade-off values in calculating QALYs: constant proportional time trade-off versus the proportional heuristic. *Journal of Health Economics* 22:445–58.

Dolan P, Sutton M (1997). Mapping visual analogue scale health state valuations on to standard gamble and time trade-off values. *Social Science and Medicine* 44:1519–30.

Drummond MF, Sculpher MJ, Torrance GW, O'Brien BJ, Stoddart GL (2005). *Methods for the economic evaluation of health care programmes*, 3rd edn. Oxford University Press, Oxford, UK.

Dyer JS, Sarin RK (1982). Relative risk aversion. *Management Science* 28:875–86.

Evans M, Khunti K, Mamdani M, Galbo-Jørgensen CB, Gundgaard J, Bøgelund M, Harris S (2013). Health-related quality of life associated with daytime and nocturnal hypoglycaemic events: a time trade-off survey in five countries. *Health and Quality of Life Outcomes* 11:90.

Feeny D, Furlong W, Torrance G, Goldsmith C, Zenglong Z, DePauw S, Denton M, Boyle M (2002). Multiattribute and single attribute utility functions for the Health Utilities Index Mark 3 system. *Medical Care* 40:113–28.

Feng Y, Parkin D, Devlin NJ (2014). Assessing the performance of the EQ-VAS in the NHS PROMs programme. *Quality of Life Research* 23:977–89.

Froberg DG, Kane RL (1989). Methodology for measuring health-state preferences— II: Scaling methods. *Journal of Clinical Epidemiology* 42:459–71.

Fryback DG (2003). Whose quality of life? Or whose decision? *Quality of Life Research* **12**:609–10.

Gafni A (1996). HYEs: do we need them and can they fulfil their promise? (comment). *Medical Decision Making* **16**:215–6.

German Social Code (2013). (Sozialgesetzbuch) Book V (SGB V), Section 35, Paragraph 1b.

Gloth FM, 3rd, Scheve AA, Stober CV, Chow S, Prosser J (2001). The Functional Pain Scale: reliability, validity, and responsiveness in an elderly population. *Americal Medical Directors Association* **2**(3):110–4.

Gold MR, Siegel JE, Russell LB, Weinstein MC (1996). *Cost-effectiveness in health and medicine*. Oxford University Press, Oxford, UK.

Green C, Brazier J, Deverill M (2000). Valuing health-related quality of life. A review of health state valuation techniques. *Pharmacoeconomics* **17**:151–65.

Hawthorne G, Richardson J, Osbourne R (1999). The assessment of quality of life (AQoL) instrument: a psychometric measure of health related quality of life. *Quality of Life Research* **8**:209–24.

Hershey JC, Kunrather HG, Schoemaker PJH (1981). Sources of bias in assessment procedures for utility functions. *Management Science* **28**:936–54.

Horsman J, Furlong W, Feeny D, Torrance G (2003). The Health Utilities Index (HUI(R)): concepts, measurement properties and applications. *Health and Quality of Life Outcomes* **1**:54.

Jansen SJ, Stiggelbout AM, Nooij MA, Kievit J (2000). The effect of individually assessed preference weights on the relationship between holistic utilities and non preference-based assessment. *Quality of Life Research* **9**:541–57.

Jones-Lee M, Loomes G, O'Reilly D, Phillips P (1993). *The value of preventing non fatal road injuries: findings of a willingness to pay national sample survey*. Transport Research Laboratory, UK.

Joyce VR, Barnett PG, Chow A, Bayoumi AM, Griffin SC, Sun H, Holodniy M, Brown ST, Kyriakides TC, Cameron DW, Youle M, Sculpher M, Anis AH, Owens DK (2012). Effect of treatment interruption and intensification of antiretroviral therapy on health-related quality of life in patients with advanced HIV: a randomized, controlled trial. *Medical Decision Making* **32**:70–82.

Kahneman D (2000). Evaluation by moments: past and future. In: Kahneman D, Tversky AS (eds). *Choices, values and frames*. Cambridge University Press and the Russell Sage Foundation, New York, NY, pp. 693–708.

Kahneman D, Tversky A (1979). Prospect theory: an analysis of decision under risk. *Econometrica* **47**:263–91.

Kaplan RM, Anderson JP (1988). A general health policy model: update and applications. *Health Services Research* **23**:203–35.

Kaplan RM, Bush JW, Berry CC (1979). Health status indices: category rating versus magnitude estimation for measuring level of well being. *Medical Care* **17**:501–25.

Keeney RL, Raiffa H (1976). *Decisions with multiple objectives: preferences and value trade-offs*. John Wiley and Sons, New York, NY.

Kharroubi SA, Brazier JE, McGhee S (2013). Modeling SF-6D Hong Kong standard gamble health state preference data using a nonparametric Bayesian method. *Value in Health* **16**:1032–45.

Lenert LA, Cher DJ, Goldstein MK, Bergen MR, Garber A (1998). The effect of search procedures on utility elicitations. *Medical Decision Making* **18**:76–83.

Lenert LA, Sturley A, Watson ME (2002). iMPACT3: Internet based development and administration of utility elicitation protocols. *Medical Decision Making* **22**:522–5.

Little MH, Reitmeir P, Peters A, Leidl R (2014). The impact of differences between patient and general population EQ-5D-3L values on the mean tariff scores of different patient groups. *Value in Health* **17**:364–71.

Litva A, Coast J, Donovan J, Eyles J, Shepherd M, Tacchi J, Abelson J, Morgan K (2002). 'The public is too subjective': public involvement at different levels of health-care decision making. *Social Science and Medicine* **54**:1825–37.

Llewellyn-Thomas H, Sutherland HJ, Tibshirani R, Ciampi A, Till JE, Boyd NF (1982). The measurement of patients' values in medicine. *Medical Decision Making* **2**:449–62.

Lloyd AJ (2003). Threats to the estimation of benefit: are preference elicitation methods accurate? *Health Economics* **12**:393–402.

Loomes G (1993). Disparities between health state measures: is there a rational explanation? In: Gerrard W (ed). *The economics of rationality*. Routledge, London, UK, pp. 149–178.

Loomes G, McKenzie L (1989). The use of QALYs in health care decison making. *Social Science and Medicine* **28**:299–308.

Luo N, Wang P, Thumboo J, Lim YW, Vrijhoef HJ (2014). Valuation of EQ-5D-3L health states in Singapore: modeling of time trade-off values for 80 empirically observed health states. *Pharmacoeconomics* **32**:495–507.

Luo N, Wang Q, Feeny D, Chen G, Li SC, Thumboo J (2007). Measuring health preferences for Health Utilities Index Mark 3 health states: a study of feasibility and preference differences among ethnic groups in Singapore. *Medical Decision Making* **27**:61–70.

Mahboub-Ahari A, Pourreza A, Akbari Sari A, Rahimi Foroushani A, Heydari H (2014). Stated time preferences for health: a systematic review and meta-analysis of private and social discount rates. *Journal of Research in the Health Sciences* **14**:181–6.

Mann R, Brazier J, Tsuchiya A (2009). A comparison of patient and general population weightings of EQ-5D dimensions. *Health Economics* **18**:363–72.

Mannion AF, Junge A, Fairbank JC, Dvorak J, Grob D (2006). Development of a German version of the Oswestry Disability Index. Part 1: cross-cultural adaptation, reliability, and validity. *European Spine Journal* **15**:55–65.

McCabe C, Stevens K, Brazier J (2004). Utility values for the Health Utility Index Mark 2: an empirical assessment of alternative mapping functions. Health Economics and Decision Science Section Discussion Paper no 01/04, University of Sheffield, UK.

McTaggart-Cowan H (2011). Elicitation of informed general population health state utility values: a review of the literature. *Value in Health* **14**:1153–7.

McTaggart-Cowan H, Tsuchiya A, O'Cathain A, Brazier J (2011). Understanding the effect of disease adaptation information on general population values for hypothetical health states. *Social Science and Medicine* **72**:1904–12.

Measurement and Valuation of Health Group (1994). *Time trade-off user manual: props and self completion methods*. Centre for Health Economics, University of York. *Medical Decision Making* **24**:511–7.

Mehrez A, Gafni A (1991). The healthy-years equivalents: how to measure them using the standard gamble approach. *Medical Decision Making* **11**:140–6.

Mehrez A, Gafni A (1993). HYEs versus QALYs: in pursuit of progress. *Medical Decision Making* **13**:287–92.

Menzel P, Dolan P, Richardson J, Olsen A (2002). The role of adaptation to disability and disease in health state valuation: a preliminary normative analysis. *Social Science and Medicine* **55**:2149–58.

Murray CJ, Lopez AD (1997). Regional patterns of disability free life expectancy and disability adjusted life expectancy: Global Burden of Disease Study. *Lancet* **349**:1347–52.

National Institute for Health and Clinical Excellence (2013). *Guide to the methods of technology appraisal.* NICE, London, UK.

Nord E (1991). The validity of a visual analogue scale in determining social utility weights for health states. *International Journal of Health Planning and Management* **6**:234–42.

Nord E (1992). Methods for quality adjustment of life years. *Social Science and Medicine* **34**:559–64.

Nord E (1995). The person-trade-off approach to valuing health care programs *Medical Decision Making* **15**:201–8.

Nord E, Pinto JL, Richardson J, Menzel P, Ubel P (1999). Incorporating societal concerns for fairness in numerical valuations of health programmes. *Health Economics* **8**(1):25–39.

Norman R, King M, Clarke D, Viney R, Cronin P, Street D (2010). Does mode of administration matter? Comparison of online and face to face administration of a time trade off task. *Quality of Life Research***19**:499–508.

O'Brien B and Viramontes JL (1994). Willingness to pay: a valid and reliable measure of health state preference? *Medical Decision Making* **14**:289–97.

Oliver A (2003). The internal consistency of the standard gamble: tests after adjusting for prospect theory. *Journal of Health Economics* **22**:659–74.

Parducci A Wedell DH (1986). The category effect with rating scales: number of categories, number of stimuli and method of presentation. *Journal of Experimental Psychology* **12**:496–516.

Patrick DL, Bush JW, Chen MM (1973). Methods for measuring levels of well-being for a health status index. *Health Services Research* **8**:228–45.

Patrick DL, Erickson P (1973). *Health status and health policy. Quality of life in health care evaluation and resource allocation.* Oxford University Press, New York, NY.

Patrick DL, Starks HE, Cain KC, Uhlmann RF, Pearlman RA (1994). Measuring preferences for health states worse than death. *Medical Decision Making* **14**:9–18.

Peeters Y, Stiggelbout AM (2010). Health state valuations of patients and the general public analytically compared: a meta-analytical comparison of patient and population health state utilities. *Value in Health* **13**:306–9.

Petrou S, Kandala NB, Robinson A, Baker R (2013). A person trade-off study to estimate age-related weights for health gains in economic evaluation. *Pharmacoeconomics* **31**:893–907.

Pinto-Prades JL (1997). Is the person trade-off a valid method for allocating health care resources? *Health Economics* **6**:71–81.

Pinto-Prades JL, Abellán-Perpiñán JM (2005). Measuring the health of populations: the veil of ignorance approach. *Health Economics* **14**:69–82.

Pinto-Prades JL, Rodríguez-Míguez E (2015). The lead time tradeoff: the case of health states better than dead. *Medical Decision Making* **35**:305–15.

Prelec D (1998). The probability weighting function. *Econometrica* **66**:497–527.

Rand-Hendriksen K, Augestad LA, Kristiansen IS, Stavem K (2012). Comparison of hypothetical and experienced EQ-5D valuations: relative weights of the five dimensions. *Quality of Life Research* **21**:1005–12.

Rand-Hendriksen K, Augestad L, Ariane L (2014). MAT-study. Varied starting point and iteration sizes non-stopping TTO.

Ratcliffe J, Brazier J, Palfreyman S, Michaels J (2007). A comparison of patient and population values for health states in varicose veins patients. *Health Economics* **16**:395–405.

Ratcliffe J, Couzner L, Flynn T, Stevens K, Brazier J, Sawyer M (2011). Assessing the feasibility of applying best worst scaling discrete choice methods to value Child Health Utility 9D health states in a young adolescent sample. *Applied Health Economics and Health Policy* **9**:15–27.

Richardson J (1994). Cost utility analysis: what should be measured? *Social Science and Medicine* **39**:7–21.

Robberstad B, Cairns J (2007). Time preferences for health in northern Tanzania: an empirical analysis of alternative discounting models. *Pharmacoeconomics* **25**:73–88.

Robinson A, Dolan P, Williams A (1997). Valuing health states using VAS snd TTO: what lies behind the numbers? *Social Science and Medicine* **45**:1289–97.

Robinson A, Loomes G, Jones-Lee M (2001). Visual analogue scales, standard gambles and relative risk aversion. *Medical Decision Making* **21**:17–27.

Robinson A, Spencer A (2006). Exploring challenges to TTO utilities: valuing states worse than dead. *Health Economics* **15**:393–402.

Robinson S (2011). Test-retest reliability of health state valuation techniques: the time trade off and person trade off. *Health Economics* **20**:1379–91.

Robinson S, Bryan S (2013). Does the process of deliberation change individuals' health state valuations? An exploratory study using the person trade-off technique. *Value in Health* **16**:806–13.

Ross PC, Litterby B, Fearn P (2003). Paper standard gamble, a paper based measure of SG utility for current health. *International Journal of Technology Assessment in Health Care* **19**:135–47.

Rowen D, Brazier J (2011). Health utility measurement. In: Glied S, Smith PC (eds). *The Oxford handbook of health economics*. Oxford handbooks online 33.1–33.4.

Rowen D, Brazier J, Van Hout B (2015). A comparison of methods for converting DCE values onto the full health–dead QALY scale. *Medical Decision Making* **35**:328–40.

Rutten van Molken MP, Bakker CH, van Doorslaer EK, van der Linden S (1995). Methodological issues of patient utility measurement. Experience from two clinical trials. *Medical Care* **33**:922–37.

Schoemaker PJH (1982). The expected utility model: its variants, purposes, evidence and limitations. *Journal of Economic Literature* **20**:529–63.

Schwartz A (1998). Rating scales in context. *Medical Decision Making* **18**:236

Schwarzinger M, Lanoe J, Nord E, Durand-Zaleski I (2004). Lack of multiplicative transitivity in person trade-off responses. *Health Economics* **13**:171–81.

Shah K, Rand-Hendriksen K, Ramos-Goni JM, Prause AJ, Stolk E (2014). Improving the quality of data collected in EQ-5D-5L valuation studies: a summary of the EQ-VT research methodology programme. In: Proceedings of the 31st Scientific Plenary Meeting of the EuroQol Group; 2014. p. 1–18. Available at: http://www.euroqol.org/uploads/media/EQ14-CH01_Shah.pdf

Shaw JW, Johnson JA, Coons SJ (2005). US valuation of the EQ-5D health states: development and testing of the D1 valuation model. *Medical Care* **43**:203–20.

Shiell A, Seymour J, Hawe P, Cameron S (2000). Are preferences over health states complete? *Health Economics* **9**:47–55.

Sintonen H (1994). The 15D-measure of health-related quality of life. I. Reliability, validity and sensitivity of its health state descriptive system. National Centre for Health Program Evaluation, working paper 41, Melbourne, Australia.

Sonntag M, König HH, Konnopka A (2013). The estimation of utility weights in cost-utility analysis for mental disorders: a systematic review. *Pharmacoeconomics* **31**:1131–54.

Spencer A (2003). The TTO method and procedural invariance. *Health Economics* **12**:655–68.

Sprangers M, Schwartz C (1999). Integrating response shift into health-related quality of life research: a theoretical model. *Social Science and Medicine* **48**:1507–15.

Stavem K (1999). Reliabilty, validity and responsiveness of two multiattribute utility measures in patients with COPD. *Quality of Life Research* **8**:45–54.

Stein K, Dyer M, Crabb T, Milne R, Round A, Ratcliffe J, Brazier J (2006a). *An Internet 'Value of Health' Panel: recruitment, participation and compliance.* Health Economics and Decision Science Discussion Paper 08/06, ScHARR, University of Sheffield, UK. Available at: http://www.sheffield.ac.uk/scharr/sections/heds/discussion.html

Stein K, Ratcliffe J, Round A, Milne R, Brazier J (2006b). Impact of discussion on preferences elicited in a group setting. *Health and Quality of Life Outcomes* **4**:22.

Stevens K, McCabe C, Brazier J (2006). Mapping between visual analogue scale and standard gamble data; results from the UK Health Utilities Index 2 valuation survey. *Health Economics* **15**:527–33.

Stevens K, McCabe C, Brazier J (2007). Response to Shmueli. Mapping between visual analogue scale and standard gamble data; results from the UK Health Utilities Index 2 valuation survey. *Health Economics* **16**:759–61.

Stewart ST, Lenert L, Bhatnager V, Kaplan RM (2005). Utilities for prostate cancer health states in men aged 60 years and older. *Medical Care* **43**:347–55.

Stiggelbout AM, Kiebert GM, Kievit J, Leer JW, Stoter G, de Haes JC (1994). Utility assessment in cancer patients: adjustment of time trade off scores for the utility of life years and comparison with standard gamble scores. *Medical Decision Making* **14**:82–90.

Sutherland HJ, Llewellyn-Thomas H, Boyd D, Till JE (1982). Attitudes towards quality of survival: The concept of maximum endurable time. *Medical Decision Making* **2**:299–309.

Tengs TO, Wallace A (2000). One thousand health related quality of life estimates. *Medical Care* **38**:583–637.

Tilling C, Devlin N, Tsuchiya A, Buckingham K (2010). Protocols for TTO valuations of health states worse than dead: a literature review and framework for systematic analysis. Health Economics and Decision Science Section Discussion Paper no 08/09, University of Sheffield, UK.

Torrance G (1986). Measurement of health state utilities for economic appraisal. *Journal of Health Economics* **5**:1–30.

Torrance G, Feeny D, Furlong W, Barr R, Zhang Y, Wang Q (1996). Multiattribute utility function for a comprehensive health status classification system. Health Utilities Index Mark 2. *Medical Care* **34**:702–22.

Torrance GW (1976). Social preferences for health states: an empirical evaluation of three measurement techniques. *Socio-Economic Planning Science* **10**:129–36.

Torrance GW, Fenny D, Furlong W (2001). Visual analogue scales: do they have a role in the measurement of preferences for health states? *Medical Decision Making* **21**:329–34.

Ubel PA, Loewenstein G, Jepson C (2003). Whose quality of life? A commentary exploring discrepancies between health state evaluations of patients and the general public. *Quality of Life Research* **12**:599–607.

Van der Pol MM, Cairns JA (2000). The estimation of marginal time performance in a UK wide sample (TEMPUS) project. *Health Technology Assessment* **4**:i–iv, 1–83.

Van Osch SM, Wakker PP, Van der Hout WB, Stigglebout AM (2004). Correcting biases in standard gamble and time trade off utilities. *Medical Decision Making* **24**:511–17.

Versteegh MM, Attema AE, Oppe M, Devlin NJ, Stolk EA (2013). Time to tweak the TTO: results from a comparison of alternative specifications of the TTO. *European Journal of Health Economics* Suppl 1:S43–51.

Viney R, Norman R, King MT, Cronin P, Street DJ, Knox S, Ratcliffe J (2011). Time trade-off derived EQ-5D weights for Australia. *Value in Health* **14**:928–36.

Von Neumann J, Morgenstern O (1944). *Theory of games and economic behaviour.* Oxford University Press, New York, NY.

Wasserman J, Aday LA, Begley CE (2005). Measuring health state preferences for haemophilia, development of a disease specific utility instrument. *Haemophilia* **11**(1):49–57.

Wisløff T, Hagen G, Hamidi V, Movik E, Klemp M, Olsen JA (2014). Estimating QALY gains in applied studies: a review of cost-utility analyses published in 2010. *Pharmacoeconomics* **32**:367–75.

Appendix 4.1 Probability wheel for the standard gamble

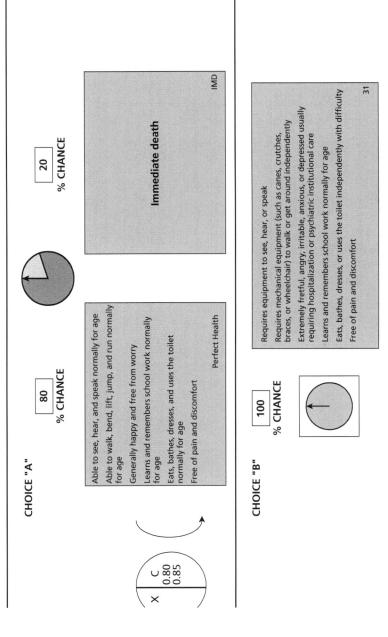

CHANCE BOARD

CHOICE "A"

| 80 | % CHANCE |

Able to see, hear, and speak normally for age
Able to walk, bend, lift, jump, and run normally for age
Generally happy and free from worry
Learns and remembers school work normally for age
Eats, bathes, dresses, and uses the toilet normally for age
Free of pain and discomfort

Perfect Health

| 20 | % CHANCE |

Immediate death

IMD

CHOICE "B"

| 100 | % CHANCE |

Requires equipment to see, hear, or speak
Requires mechanical equipment (such as canes, crutches, braces, or wheelchair) to walk or get around independently
Extremely fretful, angry, irritable, anxious, or depressed usually requiring hospitalization or psychiatric institutional care
Learns and remembers school work normally for age
Eats, bathes, dresses, or uses the toilet independently with difficulty
Free of pain and discomfort

31

X C 0.80 0.85

Appendix 4.2 Example extract from a script for eliciting health state valuations using the standard gamble probability wheel

In this part of the interview, we are interested in your views about different health states. However, the questions are going to be different from those using the feeling thermometer.

For the example, I will show you three different descriptions of health. I will describe two choices; one choice will involve taking a risk, the other choice will not. I want you to decide between the two choices. If you think the two choices are equal, tell me. The amount of risk will be changed until we find out how much risk you will take to avoid the certain choice. In order to make the task easier to understand we will use an aid similar to a game board.

Description of the 'chance board'

> Place the chance board on the table with the wheel set to 90/10. Open Standard Gamble Health State Description Card Envelope 1.

We call this a chance board because it indicates the chance or probability of a certain event occurring. As you can see, the top part of the board is labelled choice A and the bottom part of the board is labelled choice B.

You will be asked to choose between A

> (point to choice A)

and B

> (point to choice B)

Choice B, at the bottom of the board, will describe a state of health, here is an example:

> (place example card in pocket of choice B).

If you choose B, you are 100 per cent certain to be in that state of health for the *rest of your life*

> (point to example card).

Choice A is a little more complex as it is a treatment which does not always work. If the treatment DOES work, you will be in the health state shown on this pink card for the rest of your life

> (place the perfect health card in the left pocket of choice A).

However, if the treatment DOES NOT work, you will be in the health state shown on this blue card

(place the immediate death card in the right-hand pocket of choice A).

Therefore, if you choose A, there are *two* possible results.

The chances of each of these results occurring are shown by numbers appearing in the windows above each pocket

(point to the windows),

and by the amount of blue and pink inside the circle

(point to the circle).

Another way of explaining the chance aspect of choice A is that for every 100 patients who choose choice A, 90 will experience the health state on the left following treatment,

(point to 90),

but 10 will experience the health state on the right

(point to 10).

No one will know before choosing whether they will be one of the 90 or one of the 10. That is the chance they take.

During the interview, these chances will change and I will ask you to choose Choice A or Choice B each time I change the chances.

DEMONSTRATE BY TURNING THE WHEEL ON THE CHANCE BOARD TO 20/80

Now before we start looking at other health states, would you like me to explain how the chance board works again?

If the answer is yes, repeat the description of the chance board here. If the answer is no, go to instruction 2.

Instruction 2

Let's work through the first question carefully together. In choice A, the description will stay the same each time and is described by the pink card, Perfect Health, in the left-hand top pocket, and the blue card, Immediate Death, in the right-hand pocket. The health state of choice B is one described by a green card.

There are no right or wrong answers, only what *you* think.

Place the Perfect Health card in the left-hand pocket of choice A and the Immediate Death card in the right-hand pocket of choice A. Hand the green card to the respondent.

Please read over the description and when you are finished, I will put it in pocket B at the bottom of the board.

Place the green card in the choice B pocket and set wheel to 100/0.

C1.1. THE FIRST HEALTH STATE I WOULD LIKE YOU TO DECIDE ON IS THE ONE DESCRIBED BY THIS GREEN CARD.

You have already seen this card but could you please read over the description again.

SET THE WHEEL TO 100 ON THE LEFT AND 0 ON THE RIGHT. WHEN RESPONDENT HAS FINISHED READING, SAY

As you can see choice A is a 100 per cent chance of being in the health state described on the pink card, with zero chance of immediate death.

Choice B is a 100 per cent chance of being in the health state described on the green card.

Remember whichever choice you make you will be in the health state you end up in for the *rest of your life*. Would you prefer Choice A or Choice B now?

A	1 Go to C1.2
B	2 Go to C1.13
Can't decide	3 Go to instruction 3

C1.2. SET THE WHEEL TO 10 ON THE LEFT AND 90 ON THE RIGHT.

Choice A is now a 10 per cent chance of the health state described on the pink card, with a 90 per cent chance of immediate death. Choice B is still a 100 per cent chance of the health state described on the green card. Would you prefer Choice A or Choice B now?

A	1 Go to C1.3
B	2 Go to C1.4
Can't decide	3 Go to instruction 3

C1.3. PLACE COVER 1 OVER CHOICE A OF THE CHOICE BOARD.

Suppose now that choice A was a zero chance of the health state described on the pink card, with a 100 per cent chance of immediate death. Choice B is still a 100 per cent chance of the health state described on the green card.

Would you prefer Choice A or Choice B now?

A	1 Go to C1.14
B	2 Go to C1.4
Can't decide	3 Go to instruction 3

C1.4. SET THE WHEEL TO 90 ON THE LEFT AND 10 ON THE RIGHT

Choice A is now a 90 per cent chance of the health state described on the pink card, with a 10 per cent chance of immediate death. Choice B is still a 100 per cent chance of the health state described on the green card.

Would you prefer Choice A or Choice B now?

A	1 Go to C1.6
B	2 Go toC1.5
Can't decide	3 Go to instruction 3

C1.5. PLACE COVER 2 OVER CHOICE A OF THE CHOICE BOARD.

Suppose now that choice A was a 95 per cent chance of the health state described on the pink card, with a five per cent chance of immediate death. Choice B is still a 100 per cent chance of the health state described on the green card. Would you prefer Choice A or Choice B now?

A	1 Go to instruction 3
B	2 Go to instruction 3
Can't decide	3 Go to instruction 3

C1.6. SET THE WHEEL TO 20 ON THE LEFT AND 80 ON THE RIGHT

Choice A is now a 20 per cent chance of the health state described on the pink card, with an 80 per cent chance of immediate death.

Choice B is still a 100 per cent chance of the health state described on the green card.

Would you prefer Choice A or Choice B now?

A	1 Go to instruction 3
B	2 Go to C1.7
Can't decide	3 Go to instruction 3

C1.7. SET THE WHEEL TO 80 ON THE LEFT AND 20 ON THE RIGHT

Choice A is now an 80 per cent chance of the health state described on the pink card, with a 20 per cent chance of immediate death. Choice B is still a 100 per cent chance of the health state described on the green card.

Would you prefer Choice A or Choice B now?

A	1 Go to C1.8
B	2 Go to instruction 3
Can't decide	3 Go to instruction 3

C1.8. SET THE WHEEL TO 30 ON THE LEFT AND 70 ON THE RIGHT

Choice A is now a 30 per cent chance of the health state described on the pink card, with a 70 per cent chance of immediate death.

Choice B is still a 100 per cent chance of the health state described on the green card.

Would you prefer Choice A or Choice B now?

A	1 Go to instruction 3
B	2 Go to C1.9
Can't decide	3 Go to instruction 3

C1.9. SET THE WHEEL TO 70 ON THE LEFT AND 30 ON THE RIGHT

Choice A is now a 70 per cent chance of the health state described on the pink card, with a 30 per cent chance of immediate death.

Choice B is still a 100 per cent chance of the health state described on the green card.

Would you prefer Choice A or Choice B now?

A	1 Go to C1.10
B	2 Go to instruction 3
Can't decide	3 Go to instruction 3

C1.10. SET THE WHEEL TO 40 ON THE LEFT AND 60 ON THE RIGHT

Choice A is now a 40 per cent chance of the health state described on the pink card, with a 60 per cent chance of immediate death.

Choice B is still a 100 per cent chance of the health state described on the green card.

Would you prefer Choice A or Choice B now?

A	1 Go to instruction 3
B	2 Go to C1.11
Can't decide	3 Go to instruction 3

C1.11. SET THE WHEEL TO 60 ON THE LEFT AND 40 ON THE RIGHT

Choice A is now a 60 per cent chance of the health state described on the pink card, with a 40 per cent chance of immediate death.

Choice B is still a 100 per cent chance of the health state described on the green card.

Would you prefer Choice A or Choice B now?

A	1 Go to C1.12
B	2 Go to instruction 3
Can't decide	3 Go to instruction 3

C1.12. SET THE WHEEL TO 50 ON THE LEFT AND 50 ON THE RIGHT

Choice A is now a 50 per cent chance of the health state described on the pink card, with a 50 per cent chance of immediate death.

Choice B is still a 100 per cent chance of the health state described on the green card.

Would you prefer Choice A or Choice B now?

A	1 Go to instruction 3
B	2 Go to instruction 3
Can't decide	3 Go to instruction 3

C1.13.
Why did you choose a 100 per cent chance of the health state on the green card rather than a 100 per cent chance of the health state on the pink card?

RECORD VERBATIM RESPONSE

Go to instruction 3

C1.14.
Why did you choose a 100 per cent chance of immediate death rather than a 100 per cent chance of the health state on the green card?

RECORD VERBATIM RESPONSE

Appendix 4.3 Example of the titration method for the standard gamble

In the following exercises, the states of health in the upper boxes show the CERTAIN outcome of NOT having treatment (choice A), but differ in every exercise. The states of health in the lower two boxes show the UNCERTAIN outcomes of having treatment (choice B). One of these boxes shows the outcome for success, and the other shows the outcome for failure. These differ between exercises. For each choice there are a range of chances of a successful outcome and corresponding chances of failure (Table 4.A3.1). From now on, imagine that you yourself are in these states, and that they would last for the rest of your life without change.

N.B. Remember, there are no right or wrong answers—we are asking you to make value judgements.

Please put a ✓ against all cases where you are CONFIDENT that you would CHOOSE the risky treatment (choice B).

Please put an X against all cases where you are CONFIDENT that you would REJECT the treatment (choice B) and accept the certain health state (choice A).

Please put an = against all cases where you think it would be most difficult to choose between the treatment (choice B) and accept the certain health state (choice A).

Table 4.A3.1 Outcome of treatment

Chances of success	Chances of failure
100 in 100*	0 in 100*
95 in 100*	5 in 100
90 in 100	10 in 100
85 in 100	15 in 100
80 in 100	20 in 100
75 in 100	25 in 100
70 in 100	30 in 100
65 in 100	35 in 100
60 in 100	40 in 100
55 in 100	45 in 100
50 in 100	50 in 100
45 in 100	55 in 100
40 in 100	60 in 100
35 in 100	65 in 100
30 in 100	70 in 100
25 in 100	75 in 100
20 in 100	80 in 100
15 in 100	85 in 100
10 in 100	90 in 100
5 in 100	95 in 100
0 in 100	100 in 100

*You may be willing to accept the treatment but *only* if it has a chance of success of *higher* than 95 in 100 (i.e. a chance of failure which is less than 5 in 100). If so, at what level of success would you accept treatment?

Appendix 4.4 Example of a time trade-off board

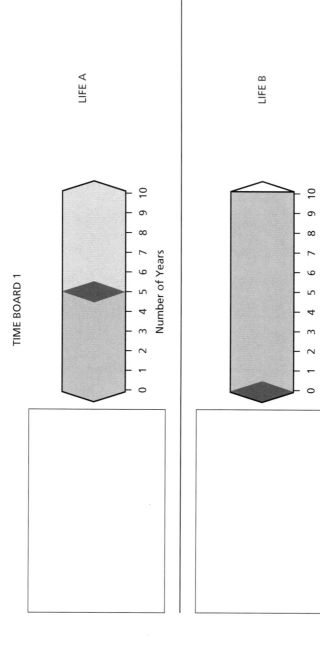

TIME BOARD 1

LIFE A

Number of Years
0 1 2 3 4 5 6 7 8 9 10

LIFE B

Number of Years
0 1 2 3 4 5 6 7 8 9 10

Appendix 4.5 Example extract from a script for eliciting health state valuations using the TTO board

PICK UP PINK AND BLUE CARD AND FIRST GREEN CARD
HAVE TTO BOARD SIDE '1' FACING UPWARDS
SET BOARD MARKER FOR LIFE A TO 10 YEARS

Now we are going to use a technique called the time trade-off to find out how good or bad you think living in some of the health states would be. The time trade-off asks you to compare living in two health states for a maximum period of 10 years. After this time period you must assume that you would die.

I am going to start with a practice using a health state that is similar to those which you have just ranked.

I am going to ask you to make a choice between living in this health state (Life B) and living in another health state (Life A). The pink scale and the green scale show the number of years you would be in each state for. Remember, I want you to imagine that *you* are in these states.

C2a. INTERVIEWER CHECK:
PICK OUT PRACTICE TTO CARD.
ENTER LETTERS ON TOP CORNER OF CARD: _____
PASS CARD TO THE RESPONDENT.

Please read this card carefully.

PLACE PRACTICE TTO CARD IN POCKET FOR LIFE B.
PLACE PINK CARD IN POCKET FOR LIFE A
MAKE SURE THAT BOARD MARKER FOR LIFE A IS AT 10 YEARS.

At the moment, each scale says 10 years. This means that you would either live in Life A for 10 years and then die, or you would live in Life B for 10 years and then die. Would you prefer Life A or Life B, or are they the same?

Life A	1. Go to C3
Life B	2.
The same	3. Ask c

c. IF 'LIFE B' AT b. Does this mean that you would rather live in Life B for 10 years than in Life A for 10 years?

IF 'THE SAME' AT b. Does this mean that living in Life B for 10 years would be the same as living in Life A for 10 years?

Yes	1. Go to C3
No (first time)	2. Repeat b
No (second time)	3. Go to C3

C3a. CONTINUE WORKING WITH CARD '**PRACTICE TTO**'.
ENTER LETTERS ON REVERSE OF CARD: _____
b. MOVE BOARD MARKER FOR LIFE A TO 0 YEARS.

Now you would either die immediately, or you would live in Life B for 10 years and then die. Would you prefer to die immediately or to have Life B, or are they the same?

Life A	1. Go to h. (state worse than death)
Life B	2. Go to c. (state better than death)
The same	3. Go to next health state

ASK IF 'LIFE B' (code 2) AT b.
c. STATE BETTER THAN DEATH
MARK 'X' UNDER 0 ON THE SCALE BELOW.

BETTER THAN DEATH SCALE	0	1	2	3	4	5	6	7	8	9	10

CONTINUE TO USE TIME BOARD WITH SIDE '1' UPWARDS
SET BOARD MARKER FOR LIFE A TO 5 YEARS ($t = 5$).

d. Now you would either live in Life A for 't' years and then die, or you would live in Life B for 10 years and then die. Would you prefer Life A or Life B, or are they the same?

CONTINUE TO WRITE ON SCALE *ABOVE ON THIS PAGE*.

IF A:	✓ UNDER 't' MOVE MARKER 1 YEAR TO THE LEFT.
	REPEAT d. WITH 't' 1 LESS THAN LAST TIME.
IF B:	X UNDER 't' MOVE MARKER 1 YEAR TO THE RIGHT.
	REPEAT d. WITH 't' 1 MORE THAN LAST TIME.
IF SAME:	= UNDER 't' GO TO next health state

REPEAT d. UNTIL:	
A) YOU ENTER ' = '	Go to next health state
B) 'X' AND '✓' APPEAR NEXT TO EACH OTHER	*OR* Go to e.

ASK IF d. ENDED WITH 'X' AND '✓' NEXT TO EACH OTHER
e. LET '*t*' NOW BE HALFWAY BETWEEN THE ADJACENT CROSS AND TICK,
I.E. 'SOMETHING AND 6 MONTHS'
   What if you would either live in Life A for '*t*' and then die, or you would live in Life
B for 10 years and then die. Would you prefer Life A or Life B, or are they the same?

Life A	1. Go to C4
Life B	2. Go to f
The same	3. Go to next health state

IF 'LIFE B' (code 2) AT e.

IF THERE IS A X UNDER 9	1. Go to g
IF THERE IS NOT A X UNDER 9	2. Go to next health state

f. INTERVIEWER CHECK:
ASK IF THERE IS 'X' UNDER 9 AND '✓' UNDER 10

Yes	1. Go to next
No	2. health state

g. Would you be prepared to sacrifice any time in order to avoid Life B?
IF YES: How many weeks?
ENTER WEEKS: _____
ASK IF 'LIFE A' (code 1) AT b.
h. STATE WORSE THAN DEATH
MARK '✓' UNDER 0 ON SCALE BELOW.

WORSE THAN DEATH SCALE	0	1	2	3	4	5	6	7	8	9	10

TURN TTO BOARD SIDE '2' UPWARDS.
MOVE GREEN CARD TO TOP LEFT POCKET ON SIDE '2'.
PLACE PINK CARD IN TOP RIGHT POCKET ON SIDE '2'.
PLACE BLUE CARD IN BOTTOM POCKET ON SIDE '2'.
SET BOARD MARKER FOR LIFE A TO 5 YEARS (t = 5).
Now here is a different choice.

i. Life A is now '*t*' years of this state (POINT TO THE GREEN CARD) followed by '10−*t*' years in this other state (POINT TO THE PINK CARD). Or instead of that you could choose to die immediately (POINT TO LIFE B). Would you prefer Life A, or to die immediately, or are they the same?
WRITE ON SCALE ABOVE ON THIS PAGE.

IF A:	✓ UNDER '*t*' MOVE MARKER 1 YEAR TO THE RIGHT.
	REPEAT i. WITH '*t*' 1 MORE THAN LAST TIME.
IF B:	X UNDER '*t*' MOVE MARKER 1 YEAR TO THE LEFT.
	REPEAT i. WITH '*t*' 1 LESS THAN LAST TIME.
IF SAME:	= UNDER '*t*' GO TO D4.

REPEAT i. UNTIL:	
A) YOU ENTER ' = '	GO TO next health state
B) "AND '✗' APPEAR NEXT TO EACH OTHER	*OR* Go to j.

ASK IF i. ENDED WITH '✓' AND 'X' NEXT TO EACH OTHER
j. LET '*t*' NOW BE HALFWAY BETWEEN THE ADJACENT TICK AND CROSS, I.E. 'SOMETHING AND 6 MONTHS'.
    What if Life A was '*t*' of this state (POINT TO THE GREEN CARD) followed by '10−*t*' in this other state (POINT TO THE PINK CARD). Or instead of that you could choose to die immediately (POINT TO LIFE B). Would you prefer Life A, or to die immediately, or are they the same?

Life A	1. Go to next health state
Life B	2.
The same	3.

Appendix 4.6 Example of titration method
for the time trade-off

Table 4.A6.1 Example of titration method of the time trade-off

Choice A	Choice B
25 years	25 years
25 years	24 years
25 years	23 years
25 years	22 years
25 years	21 years
25 years	20 years
25 years	19 years
25 years	18 years
25 years	17 years
25 years	16 years
25 years	15 years
25 years	14 years
25 years	13 years
25 years	12 years
25 years	11 years
25 years	10 years
25 years	9 years
25 years	8 years
25 years	7 years
25 years	6 years
25 years	5 years
25 years	4 years
25 years	3 years
25 years	2 years
25 years	1 years
25 years	0 years

Please put an 'A' against all cases where you are CONFIDENT that you would
choose choice A. Please put a 'B' against all cases where you are CONFIDENT
that you would choose choice B. Please put an '=' against *the case* where you
cannot choose between choice A and choice B.

Chapter 5

Modelling health state valuation data

5.1 Introduction to modelling health state valuation data

Preference-based measures of health have standardized, multidimensional descriptive systems that generate hundreds, and often thousands, of health states (Kaplan and Anderson 1988; Sintonen 1994; Dolan 1997; Brazier *et al.* 2002*a*; Feeny *et al.* 2002; Richardson *et al.* 2014). It is usually impractical to directly value all health states described by preference-based measures (PBMs) using techniques such as time trade-off (TTO) or standard gamble (SG). Hence, the solution adopted by most developers of preference-based measures is to value a subset of the health states described by the measure directly, and then to estimate a function for predicting the values of all the states defined.

Historically, there have been two approaches to estimating a function for valuing states for a health state descriptive system: the composite and decomposed approaches (Froberg and Kane 1989). The composite approach uses statistical modelling to estimate a function for predicting health state values defined by the classification. A sample of states for valuation are selected using a statistical design and a range of models fitted to the data. Health state values present a significant challenge for conventional statistical modelling procedures as the distribution is commonly skewed, truncated, non-continuous, and hierarchical (Brazier *et al.* 2002*b*). Attempts to model these data have met with some success for the generic Quality of Well-Being scale (QWB), EQ-5D, and SF-6D (Kaplan and Anderson 1988; Dolan 1997; Brazier *et al.* 2002*a*) as well as numerous condition-specific preference-based measures (Brazier *et al.* 2012). More advanced modelling methods have been applied, including a non-parametric approach using Bayesian methods (Kharroubi *et al.* 2007*a*) and a semi-parametric approach using inverse probability weighting techniques (Méndez *et al.* 2011).

The decomposed approach employs multiattribute utility theory (MAUT) to determine the functional form and the sample of states to be valued. MAUT reduces the valuation task by making simplified assumptions about the relationships between dimensions, with the most commonly used specifications being the additive and multiplicative functional forms. The application of MAUT decomposes the valuation task into four stages. Firstly, each dimension is valued separately to estimate single-attribute utility functions. Secondly, 'corner states' are valued; these are states in which one dimension is at one extreme (usually the worst level) and the rest are set at the other extreme (usually the best level). Thirdly, a set of multiattribute states determined by the model specification is valued. Finally, by applying MAUT it is possible to solve a system of equations using the mean values from the previous stages to calculate weights for each dimension and any parameter for preference interactions between dimensions as specified in the model. This approach has been used to value the various versions of the Health Utilities Index (HUI) (Torrance 1982; Torrance *et al.* 1996; Feeny *et al.* 2002), the assessment of quality of life (AQoL) (Richardson *et al.* 2014), and a condition-specific measure (Revicki *et al.* 1998).

This chapter describes the decomposed and composite approaches to analysing cardinal valuation data, followed by how they have been applied and how to assess their performance. The debate concerning which approach provides the best way to predict health state values is also addressed. The chapter aims to provide the reader with sufficient knowledge to undertake this type of modelling and to understand some of the controversies in the field. It provides an outline of the more recent developments in statistical modelling of health state preference data. Chapter 6 considers the modelling of ordinal preference data.

5.2 Statistical modelling

This section draws on the paper by Brazier *et al.* (2002*a*) on modelling the UK SF-6D data and subsequent experience with the SF-6D and condition-specific instruments (e.g. Yang *et al.* 2011; Rowen *et al.* 2012). Consequently, this work built upon the pioneering research to value the QWB (Kaplan and Andersen 1988) and EQ-5D (Dolan 1997; Busschbach *et al.* 1999).

5.2.1 Selection of health states

In order to describe the problem, consider the example of the health state classification of the SF-6D. (The other main preference-based measures, including the EQ-5D and HUI3, are similar in construction.) SF-6D is composed of six multilevel dimensions of health: *physical functioning, role limitation, social functioning, bodily pain, mental health*, and *vitality* (Table 5.1). An SF-6D health state is defined by selecting a level from each dimension, starting with *physical functioning* and ending with *vitality*. Level 1 in each dimension represents no loss of health or functioning in that dimension, so that state 111111 denotes the best state. The worst possible state is 645655, known as 'the pits'. A total of 18,000 health states can be defined in this way.

There is little guidance on how to select health states for valuation from a multidimensional descriptive system such as the SF-6D to value for statistical modelling. One approach has been to use an orthogonal array to select the states required to estimate an additive model (e.g. by applying the Orthoplan procedure of SPSSwin). This was supplemented in the SF-6D UK valuation study by randomly selecting additional states to enable the estimation of more sophisticated models (e.g. including additional terms for capturing interaction between dimensions) and to provide states to test the predictive properties of the model. Other approaches have included balanced design, which ensures that any dimension level has an equal chance of being combined with

Table 5.1 The SF-6D

Level		Level	
	Physical functioning		**Pain**
1	Your health does not limit you in *vigorous activities*	1	You have *no* pain
2	Your health limits you a little in *vigorous activities*	2	You have pain but it does not interfere with your normal work (both outside the home and housework)
3	Your health limits you a little in *moderate activities*	3	You have pain that interferes with your normal work (both outside the home and housework) *a little bit*
4	Your health limits you a lot in *moderate activities*	4	You have pain that interferes with your normal work (both outside the home and housework) *moderately*
5	Your health limits you *a little in bathing and dressing*	5	You have pain that interferes with your normal work (both outside the home and housework) *quite a bit*
6	Your health limits you *a lot in bathing and dressing*	6	You have pain that interferes with your normal work (both outside the home and housework) *extremely*
	Role limitations		**Mental health**
1	You have *no* problems with your work or other regular daily activities as a result of your physical health or any emotional problems	1	You feel tense or downhearted and low *none of the time*
2	You are limited in the kind of work or other activities as a result of your physical health	2	You feel tense or downhearted and low *a little of the time*
3	You accomplish less than you would like as a result of emotional problems	3	You feel tense or downhearted and low *some of the time*
4	You are limited in the kind of work or other activities as a result of your physical health and accomplish less than you would like as a result of emotional problems	4	You feel tense or downhearted and low *most of the time*
		5	You feel tense or downhearted and low *all of the time*

(*continued*)

Table 5.1 Continued

Level		Level	
	Social functioning		**Vitality**
1	Your health limits your social activities *none of the time*	1	You have a lot of energy *all of the time*
2	Your health limits your social activities *a little of the time*	2	You have a lot of energy *most of the time*
3	Your health limits your social activities *some of the time*	3	You have a lot of energy *some of the time*
4	Your health limits your social activities *most of the time*	4	You have a lot of energy *a little of the time*
5	Your health limits your social activities *all of the time*	5	You have a lot of energy *none of the time*

The SF-36 items used to construct the SF-6D are as follows: physical functioning, items 1, 2, and 10; role limitation due to physical problems, item 3; role limitation due to emotional problems, item 2; social functioning, item 2; both bodily pain items; mental health items, 1 (alternative version) and 4; and vitality, item 2.

[1]Most severe is defined as levels 4–6 for physical functioning, levels 3 and 4 for role limitation, 4 and 5 for social functioning, mental health and vitality, and 5 and 6 for pain.

the levels of other dimensions (see the example in Yang *et al.* 2011) and random samples drawn from different severity groups.

There is some evidence that the method for sampling states has implications for the performance of the mode. Lamers and colleagues (2006) compared different samples of states and numbers of respondents from the original Measurement and Valuation of Health (MVH) valuation of EQ-5D conducted in the United Kingdom. Unsurprisingly they showed a negative relationship between the mean absolute error (MAE) (i.e. the absolute difference between observed and predicted mean values) and both the numbers of states and respondents. Norman and colleagues (2009) argued for a more balanced design than that used in the UK MVH study.

The samples of states selected for valuation are usually too large for a respondent to value at a single sitting. Therefore, previous surveys have further divided the sample of states into smaller blocks for each respondent to value. These blocks have been chosen to ensure that respondents face a balance of severe, moderate, and mild health states in order to minimize the risk of bias. The optimal number of states per respondents is unknown, with some studies opting to present as few as six. However, there is evidence that respondents can value substantially more in one sitting; a study in Poland conducted by Golicki and colleagues (2013) using TTO showed no significant impact on the coefficients from models estimated on observation 18 to 23 compared with one to five.

The design of studies using cardinal techniques like TTO and SG have tended to be less sophisticated than those using ordinal techniques like discrete choice experiment (DCE) (see Chapter 6). There are important choices to be made in the design of a valuation survey, including the selection of states, the blocking of those states for completion by respondents, and the numbers of respondents that have been shown to have implications for model performance. This is an area requiring more systematic research.

5.2.2 **Data preparation**

The preparation of data from valuation surveys for statistical modelling has involved the exclusion of certain types of respondents and transformations.

5.2.2.1 Exclusions

Previous studies have 'cleaned' health state valuation data by eliminating respondents who were thought to have been confused by the valuation task or had not paid it sufficient attention (Kaplan and Anderson 1988; Torrance *et al.* 1996; Brazier *et al.* 2002*a*). Participants have been excluded who valued all states as the same (e.g. Brazier *et al.* 2002*a*; Devlin *et al.* 2015), or exhibited some degree of logical inconsistency with the health state classification (i.e. where one state is better than another on at least one dimension but no worse on any other and yet given a lower value). The number of participants or values excluded varies between surveys and is subject to research judgement. The advantage of excluding participants who do not seem to understand or engage with the task is that this usually reduces the variability. However, it also reduces the sample size and representativeness of the sample; the latter can be important when the measure is being used to inform political decisions.

5.2.2.2 Adjustments to data

Adjustments may need to be made to the raw responses to preference elicitation, including those that generate data that is treated as cardinal, such as TTO and SG. One is the treatment of values for states worse than dead. States regarded as worse than dead by participants are usually valued using a different task (see Chapter 4). The TTO and SG tasks used in the valuation of EQ-5D, SF-6D, and HUI3, for example, used a task for states worse than dead that results in values ranging from + 1 to very low negative values. The MVH protocol for valuing EQ-5D results in values as low as −39. It has been argued that this gives greater weight to negative values in the calculation of mean scores (Dolan 1997). One solution has been to transform the value in various ways; for the MVH survey, this was calculated by the negative of the number of years in full health at indifference divided by 10 (Patrick *et al.* 1994; Dolan 1997), which has the effect of bounding negative values at minus one. However, this has no theoretical basis and other transformations have been used (e.g. Shaw *et al.* 2005 for the US valuation of the EQ-5D). Chapter 4 considers other variants of TTO that eliminate this problem by introducing additional time to trade (e.g. lead-time TTO), although this has a different problem as the additional time can be exhausted. Below is a brief review of an alternative proposed solution using econometric methods.

Another transformation of data that is sometimes required is chaining. For example, the SF-6D valuation survey asked respondents to value states against full health and the worst state (i.e. the 'pits') defined by the descriptive system. In order to estimate health state values on the conventional full health–dead scale, these values had to be transformed using the valuation of the 'pits' state on the full health–dead scale obtained from each respondent. The health state values used in the modelling for the SF-6D were therefore computed as: $U_x = P + (I - P) (U_y)$, where P is the unadjusted SG value for each state and U_y is the value of the 'pits' state against full health and dead. Similar types of transformations are sometimes required for temporary states.

5.2.3 Features of health state valuation data

Two hundred and forty-nine health states defined by the SF-6D were valued by a representative sample of the UK general population using the SG valuation technique. From the 611 respondents in the sample, there were 148 missing values from 117 individuals, resulting in 3,518 observed SG valuations across 249 health states. Each health state was valued an average of 15 times. Mean health state values ranged from 0.10 to 0.99 and generally had large standard deviations (up to 0.5). A histogram and descriptive statistics for the 3,518 individual adjusted health state valuations are presented in Figure 5.1. Median health state values usually exceeded mean values, reflecting the negative skewness of the data. Negative observations (suggesting states worse than dead) were comparatively rare (245/3518) and over 23 per cent of observations lay between 0.9 and 1.0.

The distribution of observed health state values usually diverges substantially from normality (e.g. Fig. 5.1). Left skew and bimodality are common, depending on the

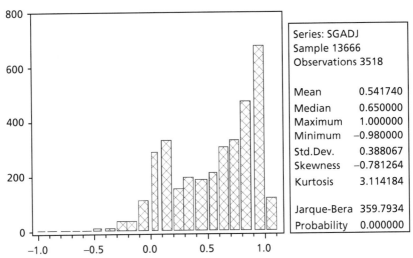

Fig. 5.1 Histogram and descriptive statistics for SG values of SF-6D health states. Reprinted from *Journal of Health Economics*, Volume 21, Issue 2, Brazier JE and Deverill M, 'The estimation of a preference-based measure of health from the SF-6D', pp. 271–92, Copyright © 2002 Elsevier, with permission from Elsevier, http://www.sciencedirect.com/science/journal/01676296

valuation technique employed. The TTO valuation of the EQ-5D generated data that were skewed and multimodal (Dolan 1997). The recent TTO valuation of the EQ-5D-5L produced pronounced spikes in the distribution at key points including 1.0, 0.5, 0.0, –0.5, and –1.0 (Devlin *et al.* 2015). The presence of spikes raises questions about the validity of the data (see Chapter 4 for a discussion of this problem), in addition to statistical challenges. It also seems to be the product of the valuation procedure for finding the point of indifference used by the EuroQol group's method for valuation (Oppe *et al.* 2014).

Skewness in the data also raises questions about the appropriate measure of central tendency, which essentially determines whose values are given greatest weight. In the case of highly skewed distributions, the mean takes into account the values of the extreme responses, whereas the median ignores the extremeness of the values. In welfare economics, the mean should be used as it reflects strength of preference, whereas a more democratic solution is arguably to use the median (Williams 1995). Published algorithms for the preference-based measures are based on predicting mean health state values. A further complexity is that the distribution of health state values is generally truncated and non-continuous. For example, SG scores are truncated at an upper limit, as the chance of treatment success cannot be greater than one. Additionally, the design of most surveys means that respondents can only answer in discrete values.

These features of health state valuation data pose major challenges to statistical modelling.

5.2.4 Specifying the model

The aim of statistical modelling is to estimate health state values for all states defined by descriptive systems such as the SF-6D. The value associated with a health state is assumed to be a function of that state; hence, by estimating a relationship between the descriptive system and the observed values, we can infer values for all states. Any model specification should deal with the complexities described here and the fact that the data are likely to be clustered by respondents. Respondents do not value the same set of states, and although allocation of states to respondents should be stratified in such a way as to remove systematic differences, the data will be clustered around the individual.

A number of alternative models have been proposed for estimating functions from health state valuation data (Busschbach *et al.* 1999; Brazier *et al.* 2002*a*). The general model defined in Brazier *et al.* (2002*a*) is as follows:

$$y_{ij} = g(\beta'\mathbf{x}_i + \theta'\mathbf{r}_{ij} + \delta'\mathbf{z}_j) + \varepsilon_{ij}$$

where $i = 1, 2, \ldots, n$ individual health states and $j = 1, 2, \ldots, m$ represents respondents. The dependent variable, y_{ij}, is the value for health state i valued by respondent j. $\mathbf{X}$ is a vector of binary dummy variables ($X_{\Omega\lambda}$) for each level λ of dimension Ω of the classification. Level $\lambda = 1$ acts as a baseline for each dimension, so in a simple linear model the intercept represents state 1111111, and summing the coefficients of the 'on' dummies (which are expected to be negative) derives the value of all other states. The **r** term is a vector of terms to account for interactions between the levels of different dimensions. $\mathbf{z}$ is a vector of the respondent's personal characteristics that may also affect the value an individual gives to a health state, for example age, sex, and education. g is a function specifying the appropriate functional form. ε_{ij} is an error term whose autocorrelation structure and distributional properties depend on the assumptions underlying the particular model used.

5.2.4.1 The constant term

The constant term has an expected value of 1, but the estimate has been found to be significantly lower than 1 in a number of empirical studies (e.g. Dolan 1997; Brazier *et al.* 2002*a*). There are several responses to this problem. The developers of the UK value set for the three-level version of EQ-5D regarded 1 as full health (i.e. 11111), and the value of any ill health state is calculated to be the decrement associated with dimension levels (where different from 1) and a term representing the divergence of the constant term from 1.00. This results in the state of 11211 having a value of 0.883 (i.e. the decrement of 0.036 for level 2 of usual activities and a constant decrement of −0.81; see Table 7.8 for the full scoring algorithm), which causes a large gap between full health and the most mild ill health state defined by EQ-5D.

There are arguments for restricting the intercept to unity, where the best state defined by the health classification (i.e. 111111 in the SF-6D, or 11111 for EQ-5D) is the upper anchor in the SG or TTO task, since by definition this should be 1. There are studies where the upper anchor is not defined by the health state classification, but by states such as full or perfect health. In this case, it is possible for the intercept to be smaller than unity. This was the approach in modelling the SF-6D and it resulted in the magnitude of β coefficients being larger. A third solution would be to treat the constant term as though it provides an estimate of the instrument-specific full health state, and transform the scale by dividing it through by the value of the full health state obtained in a separate exercise, where the upper anchor is a generic state of full health (rather like the chaining transformation described above).

It has been suggested that the estimate for the constant term may be an artefact of bounding at 1.0 in the TTO and SG tasks (Devlin *et al.* 2015). Participants can give a value for states of less than 1 but not more than 1, which has the effect of biasing the value of the mildest states downward. The constant term is simply picking up this effect. The solution proposed to deal with such asymmetry in the modelling of the English EQ-5D-5L valuation was to consider the values to be censored at 1.0 (Devlin *et al.* 2015).

5.2.4.2 Interactions

A simple additive model of the $X_{\Omega\lambda}$ dummies does not impose an interval scale between the levels of each dimension, nor does it insist on a particular ordering of levels (indeed for the SF-6D the expected ordering of states was contradicted by the model results). However, it does not permit interaction between dimensions. The $\mathbf{r}$ term is a vector of terms to account for interactions between the levels of different dimensions. To analyse first order interactions alone is problematic, since the large number of possible interactions means there is the potential for collinearity and a risk of finding that some are significant purely by chance. To overcome these problems there would need to be a larger number of states valued and participants to value them. The approach adopted for a number of preference-based measures has been to use simple composite terms for describing interactions (Dolan 1997; Brazier *et al.* 2002*a*). The model used to value the SF-6D had one example of this called MOST, which takes a value of 1 if any dimension in the health state is at one of the most severe levels, and 0 if not. There is a similar term in the modelling of the UK EQ-5D TTO valuation survey called the N3, which is a dummy that takes a value of 1 when at least one dimension is at the worst level (i.e. level 3). This means that the second and subsequent level 3 terms have a much smaller impact.

5.2.5 **Estimation**

An ordinary least squares (OLS) model would ignore the clustering in the data, as it assumes that each individual health state value is an independent observation, regardless of whether or not it was valued by the same respondent. A more valid specification, which takes account of variation both within and between respondents, is the one-way error components random effects (RE) model. This model divides the error between respondent-specific variation (assumed to be random across individuals) and an error term for the health state being valued by the respondent. Estimations are calculated via generalized least squares or maximum likelihood (MLE). A fixed effects model could also deal with clustering, but the RE model has been found to be more appropriate using the Hausman test in analyses of SF-6D and HUI2 valuation data (Brazier *et al.* 2002*a*; McCabe *et al.* 2005*a*).

Another way to handle the clustering of data is to aggregate the data prior to analysis. This was undertaken in the analysis of the SF-6D data, where an OLS model was estimated using mean health state values. RE models use individual level data (i.e. y_{ij} in equation 1), which has the advantage of greatly increasing the number of degrees of freedom available for the analysis (for the SF-6D model by increasing the number of observations to model from 249 mean health state values to over 3,500 individual level observations) and enabling the analysis of respondent background characteristics on health state valuations. Despite these apparent advantages, it is not clear whether it is necessarily superior for the purposes of predicting mean health state values (Gravelle 1995). Indeed, mean models were found to perform better at predicting mean health state values in the SF-6D valuation (Brazier *et al.* 2002*a*).

The literature has examined a number of alternative functional forms to account for the skewed distribution of health state valuations. These have included a logit transformation and two complementary log–log transformations suggested by Abdalla and Russell (1995). These are chosen to map the data from the range (−1,1) to the range (−∞,∞). Secondly, left skew in these data, whereby 25 per cent of the values lie between 0.9 and 1, can be accounted for in a Tobit model with upper censoring which treats the data as if they arise from a censored observation mechanism through which observations with true values greater than 1 are observed as 1. However, these transformations have not been found to improve the fit of models (Brazier *et al.* 2002*a, b*), and new methods have been proposed for modelling preference data.

5.2.5.1 **New approaches to estimation**

More recently alternative techniques for analysing preference data have been explored. These include Bayesian non-parametric and semi-parametric approaches, and a hybrid approach that combines cardinal preference data with the results of paired data from a discrete choice experiment. These approaches are briefly described in the next section. This is an active area of research and other methods are likely to be explored and compared in the near future.

5.2.5.2 Bayesian 'non-parametric' approach

A Bayesian 'non-parametric' approach has been applied to offer a more flexible solution to some of the problems with modelling health state valuation data. It has been applied to valuation data from the SF-6D (Kharroubi *et al.* 2007*a*), HUI-2 (Kharroubi and McCabe 2008), EQ-5D (Kharroubi *et al.* 2010), and a number of condition-specific measures (e.g. Kharroubi *et al.* 2014). It has been shown to more effectively represent the nature of individual respondent effects, using the repeated measurements from each individual and the skew in the distribution of their values in all applications to date. The non-parametric model achieved better performances in an 'out of sample' validation in terms of root mean square error (RMSE) (5.2.6) and standardized predictive errors. Although the improvements have been modest, the values tend to be more consistent with the health state classification and better reflected the lower health state values in the SF-6D. It has the potential to utilize prior information and reduce the scale of surveys, such as in cross-country valuation work. It also offers a flexible way to incorporate background characteristics (the results of this are reported later in this chapter). However, the extra flexibility comes at a price in terms of complexity and needing specialist software, though the programme can be adapted to other measures (the software is available from Dr Samer Kharoubi at *samer.kharroubi@york.ac.uk*).

5.2.5.3 Semi-parametric approach

An alternative semi-parametric method has been developed that uses inverse probability weighting techniques (Méndez *et al.* 2011). This approach makes no assumptions about the distribution of health state values, allows for heterogeneity in the variablity in the health state valuations, and is also able to accommodate covariates in a flexible way. Méndez *et al.* (2011) claim it is easier to implement and interpret than the non-parametric method described here. The authors make use of SF-6D valuation data, but there have not been other applications of this approach, nor any direct comparison with the results of the non-parametric model of Kharroubi and colleagues to date.

5.2.5.4 Hybrid models

Another innovation in the analyses of health state preference data has been to combine the cardinal data from a technique like TTO with ordinal data from DCE. The use of ordinal data to value health states is described in Chapter 6 and this 'hybrid' approach can be seen as a means of anchoring DCE data onto the quality-adjusted life year (QALY) full health to dead scale (Rowen *et al.* 2015). In terms of analysing cardinal data, it has been used in the UK valuation of the EQ-5D-5L. The 'hybrid' approach has been adopted for this purpose due to the problems found in the models generated from the TTO data, particularly for the mild levels where all level 2s were non-significant (3 had the wrong sign) and three out of five level 3s were insignificant. Furthermore, the coefficients on severe and extreme for anxiety and depression were in reverse order. DCE data are more consistent with the classification system and provide coefficients that are more sensitive at the upper end of the scale. It could be argued that the solution is to obtain better quality TTO data, since these problems were not found with the models of the MVH TTO data, nor other uses of TTO (e.g. Yang *et al.* 2011), but this 'hybrid' approach offers a practical solution to the problems with these data obtained using EQ-VT.

The basis for this hybrid approach is that, while the two elicitation methods use different techniques to elicit utility values, they do so for the same underlying preference function. The generalized linear regression on the TTO data and the Probit regression on the DCE data contain a similar linear component $\beta' x_i$ underlying the TTO values and pairwise choices. It estimates the parameters by using a single likelihood function that is the product of the likelihood of the TTO data and the likelihood of the DCE data. There is a single parameter relating both linear functions with each other by assuming different variances for the heterogeneity (or errors) in the TTO data and the DCE data. This hybrid model has been implemented using a likelihood model and a Bayesian method, where the former was found to perform better (Rowen *et al.* 2015) and has been adopted by the EQ Group in the valuation of the EQ-5D-5L (Devlin *et al.* 2015).

5.2.6 **Model performance**

Model performance has been assessed in a number of ways in the literature. It is common to report a model's explanatory power in terms of its adjusted R-squared, but this has limited value for comparing models that are estimated using different specifications, such as RE and OLS, and has no meaning for models without a constant term. Models have also been assessed in terms of the sign, significance, and consistency of the estimated coefficients of the dimension levels with any prior assumptions about the ordinality of the descriptive system. On the natural scale for valuations, with higher values indicating preferred health states, coefficients should be negative and the more severe the health problem, the larger the magnitude of the negative coefficient should be. However, for some descriptive systems, there might be some ambiguity regarding the ordering of statements (e.g. between 'your health limits you a little in bathing and dressing' versus 'your health limits you a lot in moderate activities' in the SF-6D). Furthermore, interaction terms would interfere with these orderings.

Ultimately, the purpose of modelling these data is to predict mean health state values. Thus, another way to evaluate models has been to examine the average absolute difference between predicted and observed mean health state values. This has been done by calculating the mean absolute error and the root mean squared error. Models are sometimes also compared in terms of the numbers of errors greater than 0.05 and 0.10 in absolute value. Bias in predictions has been assessed using a t-test and the normality of prediction errors (e.g. the Jarque–Bera test). It is important to examine the pattern of error by health state severity, such as by plotting observed against predicted mean health state values. For example, models have been estimated for the SF-6D that were found to underpredict values at the top end of the scale (see Fig. 5.2). This problem has also been found for TTO data. It was suggested earlier that it was an

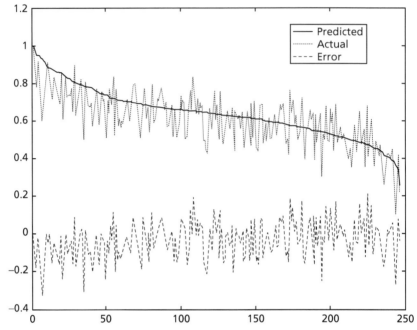

Fig. 5.2 Comparison of observed and predicted SF-6D health state values.
Reprinted from *Journal of Health Economics*, Volume 21, Issue 2, Brazier JE and Deverill M, 'The estimation of a preference-based measure of health from the SF-6D', pp. 271–92, Copyright © 2002 Elsevier, with permission from Elsevier, http://www.sciencedirect.com/science/journal/01676296

artefact of the bounding at 1.0, which tends to create a downward bias in the estimate. One solution suggested for the EQ-5D-5L TTO data is to consider the values to be censored at 1.0 (Devlin *et al.* 2015).

5.3 **Multiattribute utility theory**

5.3.1 **Specification of functional form**

The decomposed approach uses MAUT to specify a functional form in advance of undertaking the valuation survey. It is based on decision theory and is consistent with expected utility theory (Keeney and Raiffa 1976). MAUT reduces the valuation task by making simplifying assumptions about the relationship between dimensions. These simplifying assumptions place stringent restrictions on the way in which dimensions and dimension levels can interact with each other.

There are three functional forms used in practice: additive, multiplicative, and multilinear (Box 5.1). The most restrictive is the additive functional form which assumes that dimensions are independent. It permits no interactions and simply adds up the decrements associated with each dimension. The multiplicative function permits a very limited form of interaction between dimensions as it assumes the preference dependence to be the same between all dimensions. The multilinear form is the least restrictive as it allows pairs of states, and indeed higher order interactions, to be estimated separately so as to not impose a limitation on the direction of the preference dependence. It is far more demanding in terms of the amount of valuation work required to parameterize such a model. Interactions can result in either more or less than the sum of the individual effects of the two dimensions. For multilinear models, the degree of complementarity or substitutability can vary across pairs of dimensions, but for the multiplicative case it is fixed to be the same.

Evidence from work on the HUI (Torrance 1982; Torrance *et al.* 1996; Feeny *et al.* 2002) shows that the assumptions of additivity did not hold (i.e. the k_js in equation 2 in Box 5.1 do not sum to unity). They found that dimensions were complements in preference terms, and this has been confirmed for the EQ-5D and SF-6D (Dolan 1997; Brazier *et al.* 2002*a*). The developers of the HUI3 have examined a limited form of the multilinear equation. Health states were selected for valuation in an independent sample in order to estimate 26 of the 28 first order interactions and four of the 56 second order interactions (Feeny 2002). Some of these were found to be potentially important (i.e. >0.025) and the direction was always the same (i.e. preference complements). Feeny (2002) concludes that although the multilinear form is less restrictive, the multiplicative form seems to capture the important interactions, and indeed it outperformed their version of the multilinear model. The estimation of a full multilinear equation for a descriptive system such as the HUI3 would require too many states to be valued within the resources usually at the disposal of researchers in this field.

5.3.2 Design of valuation survey

The application of MAUT decomposes the valuation task into three parts: valuing single dimension states; 'corner' states; and other multidimensional states. Next, the procedure used for the HUI3 (Feeny *et al.* 2002) is described.

5.3.2.1 Single dimension states

The aim is to estimate single dimension utility functions. A single dimensional state is defined as a level of functioning on one dimension of the descriptive system, such as being 'Able to walk around the neighbourhood with walking equipment, but without the help of another person' (a single dimensional health state on the ambulation dimension). Firstly, the respondent is asked to assume that all other dimensions are at level 1, the highest level of functioning. For the HUI3, a visual analogue scale (VAS) is used in the valuations, though TTO or SG could have been used. The VAS is anchored by the highest level of functioning, for example 'Able to walk around the neighbourhood without difficulty and without walking equipment' and the lowest level of functioning, for example 'cannot walk', which are set to one and zero, respectively. The descriptive system of the HUI3 has 37 such single dimension health states to value.

5.3.2.2 Corner states

Secondly, 'corner states' are valued; these are multidimensional states where one dimension is at one extreme (usually the worst level of functioning), and the rest are set at the other extreme (usually the highest level of functioning). This requires the

Box 5.1 Types of multiattribute utility theory models

Additive

$$u(x) = \sum_{j=1}^{n} k_j u_j(x_j)$$

where $\sum_{j=1}^{n} k_j = 1$.

Multiplicative

$$u(x) = (1/k)\left[\prod_{j=1}^{n}(1+kk_j u_j(x_j)) - 1\right]$$

where $(1+k) = \prod_{j=1}^{n}(1+kk_j)$.

Multilinear

$$u(x) = k_1 u_1(x_1) + k_2 u_2(x_2) + \cdots$$
$$+ k_{12} u_1(x_1) u_2(x_2) + k_{13} u_1(x_1) u_3(x_3) + \cdots$$
$$+ k_{123} u_1(x_1) u_2(x_2) u_3(x_3) + \cdots$$
$$+ \cdots$$

where the sum of all ks equals 1.

Hybrid

Various hybrid models are possible, based on hierarchically nested subsets of attributes.

Notation: $u_j(x_j)$ is the single-attribute utility function for attribute j.

$u(x)$ is the utility for health state x, represented by an n-element vector. k and k_j are model parameters. Σ is the summation sign. Π is the multiplication sign.

The multiplicative model contains the additive model as a special case. In fitting the multiplicative model, if the measured k_j sum to 1, then $k = 0$ and the additive model holds.

Reproduced from *PharmacoEconomics*, 'Multi-attribute preference functions. Health Utilities Index', Volume 7, Issue 6, 1995, pp. 503–20, Torrance GW *et al.*, Copyright © 1995 Adis International Limited. With permission from Springer.

dimensions to be structurally independent, which implies that they are not correlated, otherwise the respondent may have difficulty imagining the state. For example, it may be difficult to imagine a state with very severe pain but with no impact on social or role activities. This problem occurred for the HUI2 and so the developers used states 'backed off' from the corner, whereby the extreme levels are replaced with the next extreme ones and then additional calculations performed to extrapolate for the missing values (Torrance *et al.* 1996).

5.3.2.3 Multiattribute utility states

Thirdly, a set of multiattribute states are valued. These are determined by the exact specification of the multiattribute utility function (MAUF). A simple additive model only needs two multidimensional states to be valued, whereas multiplicative models require an extra state in order to calculate a value for the k parameter in equation 3 (Box 5.1).

5.3.3 **Analysis of data**

Using the chosen functional form, it is possible to solve a system of equations to calculate weights for each dimension and any parameter for preference interactions specified in the model.

The MAUFs for the HUI2 and HUI3 have been constructed in a number of stages (Torrance *et al.* 1996; Feeny *et al.* 2002; McCabe *et al.* 2005a). The first stage is to estimate the mean VAS value for each single and multidimensional state. (The MAUFs are often constructed to predict the disutility of a health state, i.e. one minus the utility, to make the valuation task easier for respondents.)

A VAS-SG mapping function is then estimated in order to convert the VAS into SG. This is done by asking respondents to value three states by SG as well as VAS, followed by estimating a power function between the two and applying this to all the other states they valued (details of this procedure and a critique are provided in Chapter 4 and Stevens *et al.* 2006). The final stage in the construction of the valuation tariff is to solve one of the MAUFs presented in Box 5.1. Past work in health has tended to use the multiplicative form.

As for statistical modelling, there is a choice in the level of analysis. MAUFs can be calculated for each individual (provided each respondent undertook all the necessary valuations) or at an aggregate level. Individual MAUFs can be aggregated to give population mean estimates, but an aggregate analysis means it is not possible to estimate respondent-specific effects. Whether or not it is important to explore the impact of covariates on health state values depends upon the policy context. For economic evaluation, it can be argued that it is the population that is important and, since the developers of the HUI2 found that the two approaches yield virtually identical results, there seems little reason to pursue the more laborious process of estimating individual level functions (Torrance 1986). For some policy makers, however, it may be relevant to understand how values vary by key background characteristics.

5.4 **Comparison of statistical modelling and MAUT**

There is a choice between using statistical modelling and MAUT to predict health state values, and there have been arguments on both sides (Dolan 2002; Feeny 2002; McCabe *et al.* 2005a). This section will summarize the debate.

MAUT provides a stronger and more explicit theoretical foundation for the design of valuation studies based on decision theory. However, it could be argued that this theoretical advantage counts for little unless it is able to predict health state values more effectively. Furthermore, the statistical approach draws upon a theoretical framework, but is one based on statistical rather than economic theory.

MAUT seems to require direct valuation of a smaller set of states than the number that must be valued directly for estimating a statistical model. The HUI2 valuation function was estimated on the direct valuation of just 29 states and HUI3 used 40 states, compared with 249 for the SF-6D. The EQ-5D was valued using 43 states in the UK valuation and just 17 in a number of other countries, but this is a much smaller descriptive system. This advantage of MAUT has been exploited by the AQoL, which has a 35-item descriptive system that would define many billions of states (Richardson *et al.* 2014). The extent of this advantage is difficult to gauge as little is known about the optimal number of states for statistical modelling. Using a simple additive design, the SPSS 'orthoplan procedure' selected 49 states for the SF-6D, but this was felt to be inadequate to model possible interactions and so a further 200 were selected at random. More recently, valuation of condition-specific descriptive systems with five dimensions each with five levels has been undertaken successfully with 100 states using a balanced statistical design (Yang *et al.* 2011). Further work is required to determine the optimal statistical design, but current evidence suggests that MAUT requires fewer states to be valued and that this advantage is likely to increase with larger descriptive systems.

There is a question surrounding the plausibility of some of the MAUT valuation tasks, particularly the valuation of corner states. The developers had to undertake a 'backing off' procedure to reduce this problem with the HUI2, but avoided the problem for the HUI3 by designing the descriptive system to be orthogonal. However, this may cause a problem with descriptive systems involving dimensions that are more correlated. This is also a potential problem with the statistical approach, since some of the states selected to achieve an orthogonal array or balanced design may be implausible, though these states are usually less extreme in nature than the corner states required for MAUT.

Predictive validity for these two approaches can be compared. The EQ-5D was able to achieve mean absolute error of around 0.04 and SF-6D 0.08, compared to 0.09 for the HUI3 in an 'out of sample' set of states. These types of comparisons are contaminated by other differences in the descriptive systems, valuation technique, and the source of values. A more rigorous test would be to compare the predictive abilities of these estimation methods using the same descriptive system, valuation technique, and sample of respondents in an 'out of sample' set of states. This has been done by Stevens *et al.* (2007) in a comparison of the predictions of a multiplicative MAUF and a statistical method estimated on an independent random sample of the general population who valued 14 HUI2 health states. The statistically estimated additive model was found to outperform the MAUF in terms of MAE, root mean square error, and the proportion of predictions plus or minus three per cent from the actual mean value. A similar result was found by Currim and Sarin (1984) in a study of job choice in 100 MBA graduates in the United States using a self-administered questionnaire.

The superior performance of the statistical model may reflect the problems with using the MAUT methodology, which relies heavily on the valuation of corner states that rarely exist in practice, rather than the more mixed sets of states used by the statistical approach. However, this is far from being conclusive evidence on the relative performance of these approaches. The Stevens *et al.* (2007) study used the HUI methodology, so health state valuations were elicited using VAS and then mapped onto SG. There are numerous criticisms of using VAS to derive preference data, and the specific mapping function they employed could confound the result. There need to be more studies comparing these two approaches that use the same descriptive system and the same valuation method (preferably using a choice-based technique throughout) on independent samples.

It has also been argued that the relative advantages of each approach depend on the descriptive system (Dolan 2002). MAUT requires a greater degree of structural independence than statistical modelling as it depends on being able to value extreme corner states, whereas statistical modelling is more flexible in this regard. At the same time, Dolan (2002) has argued that '*Ceteris paribus*, as the total number of states (generated by the descriptive systems) increases, the robustness of the parameter estimates from the composite approach decreases, and so the axiomatic basis of the decomposed approach might become more attractive' (parentheses added). It is interesting to note that the developers of the larger systems, including the AQoL and 15D, have chosen to use MAUT (Richardson *et al.* 2014; Sintonen 1994). However, the developers of AQoL did not only use MAUT, but combined it with statistical inference to correct systematic errors found as a result of using MAUT (to be discussed in the following chapter).

5.5 The role of background variables

This section examines the extent of variation in health state values between subgroups of the population. Early research in this field suggested that there was little or no relationship between the background characteristics of respondents and health state values, but these tended to be either small-scale studies with fewer than 200 respondents (Llewellyn-Thomas *et al.* 1984; Balaban *et al.* 1986; Froberg and Kane 1989), or studies using rating scales and simple pairwise choices (Badia *et al.* 1995; Hadorn and Uebersax 1995) rather than one of the established cardinal preference-based methods for valuing health states, such as TTO or SG. Furthermore, they were mainly univariate studies, examining one characteristic at a time.

It is better to explore the impact of covariates using a multivariate approach with a comparatively large valuation data set over many health states. One such study analysed a UK EQ-5D TTO valuation data set and found some evidence for a systematic variation of TTO values by age, sex, and marital status (Dolan and Roberts 2002). The most important of these was age, but this finding may have been partly the result of an artefact of the TTO variant used for states worse than dead. Robinson and colleagues (1997) found that approximately 50 per cent of respondents over 60 years of age regarded the scenario as implausible because it involves a full recovery from a state worse than dead to full health. Another study examined the SG health state valuations produced from the UK SF-6D survey (as described earlier in this chapter) using a non-parametric Bayesian approach (Kharroubi *et al.* 2007b). It found that 11 covariates had a reasonable probability of effecting the values given to health states. Age was found to have the strongest association, with a quadratic relationship where health state values initially increase from 18 to around 60 years, and then fall slowly until around 70, followed by a more rapid decline. The largest difference was between those under 40 and the over 65s for the worst state of 0.14, other things being equal, but this difference shrank as states became milder. Own physical functioning was found to have a strong relationship, with poorer own physical functioning being associated with higher health state values (with a posterior probability (PP) of more than 0.95). A weaker relationship in the same direction was found with social functioning (PP 0.9). Non-manual employment was associated with higher values than manual workers, as was being male (PP >0.95). Weaker relationships (PP >0.9 or <0.1) were also found for having a degree (lower for those with a degree), being in employment (lower for those employed), being a student (lower), and understanding of the SG task. The size of the impact depended on the mean utility value.

There are a number of explanations for these relationships. The findings regarding own physical and social functioning support the arguments reviewed in Chapter 4 that people learn to adapt or cope to some extent with disability (Menzel *et al.* 2002; Ubel *et al.* 2003). As a consequence, they would regard the states described to them as having less of an impact than those not currently experiencing ill health. Interestingly, evidence reviewed in Chapter 4 suggests that adaptation is more likely with physical and functioning aspects of health than pain or mental health, and indeed this was the case in the SF-6D SG data.

The findings regarding age may reflect an adaptation effect or at least the consequences of experiencing many of the states in the past, or it could be the context of mixing with older, (on average) less healthy individuals. It may be to do with a person's change in living circumstances, with respondents in middle age being less willing to risk their life due to having greater responsibilities than both the young and elderly. However, the underlying reasons for these findings are not fully understood (Robinson *et al.* 1997). The reasons for sex, class, education, and employment are also unclear.

While these background variables are significant, their impact on the mean health state values tends to be quite modest (usually 0.05 or less). Only age had an impact of more than 0.1 (for the more severe states). These can be used to adjust health state values for the unrepresentativeness of a valuation sample, although this was found to have very little impact on the results from the UK SF-6D SG valuation survey (Kharroubi *et al.* 2007b). Another response could be to argue for using health state values that are more specific to the population they are being applied to. The debate surrounding whose values should be used to estimate health state values has been reviewed in Chapter 4. However, one limitation with age-specific QALYs, for example, is the difficulty of making the cross-age group comparisons necessary to inform resource allocation in the context of a cash limited health system.

5.6 Conclusion

Modelling health state values is an important task in the valuation of health state descriptive systems. It has become a highly technical area, using a range of different mathematical and statistical techniques. This chapter has described in some detail the different techniques that can be used, along with their pros and cons. Research in this field is likely to continue developing better methods for estimating models and comparing the performance of different methods.

References

Abdalla M, Russell I (1995). Tariffs for the Euroqol health states based on modelling individual VAS and TTO data of the York Survey In: **MVH Group** (eds). *Final report on the modelling of valuation tariffs*. Centre for Health Economics, University of York, UK. pp. 3–21.

Badia X, Fernandez E, Segura A (1995). Influence of socio-demograpjhic and health status variables on evaluation of health states in a Spanish population. *European Journal of Public Health* 5:87–93.

Balaban DJ, Sagi PC, Goldfarb NI, Nettler S (1986). Weights for scoring the quality of well-being instrument among rheumatoid arthritics: a comparison to the general population. *Medical Care* 24:973–80.

Brazier JE, Roberts J, Deverill M (2002a). The estimation of a preference-based measure of health from the SF-36. *Journal of Health Economics* 21:271–92.

Brazier JE, Rice N, Roberts J (2002b). Modelling health state valuation data. In: Murray C, Salomon J, Mathers C, Lopez A, Lozano R (eds). *Summary measures of population health: concepts, ethics, measurement and applications*. World Health Organization, Geneva, Switzerland. pp. 529–48.

Brazier J, Rowen D, Mavranezouli I, Tsuchiya A, Young T, Yang Y (2012) Developing and testing methods for deriving preference-based measures of health from condition specific measures (and other patient based measures of outcome). *Health Technology Assessment* 16:1–114.

Busschbach JV, McDonnell J, Essink-Bot M-L, van Hout BA (1999). Estimating parametric relationships between health state description and health valuation with an application to the EuroQol EQ-5D. *Journal of Health Economics* 18:551–71.

Currim IS, Sarin RK (1984). A comparative evaluation of multi-attribute consumer preference models. *Management Science* 30:543–61.

Devlin N, Shah K, Feng Y, Mulhern B, van Hout B (2015). An EQ-5D-5L value set for England. OHE Research Paper 15/03. Office of Health Economics, London, UK.

Dolan P (1997). Modeling valuation for Euroqol health states. *Medical Care* 35:351–63.

Dolan P (2002). Modelling the relationship between the description and valuation of health states. In: Murray C, Salomon J, Mathers C, Lopez A (eds). *Summary measures of population health: concepts, ethics, measurment and applications*. World Health Organization, Geneva, Switzerland. pp. 501–14.

Dolan P, Roberts J (2002). To what extent can we explain time trade-off values from other information about respondents? *Social Science and Medicine* 54:919–29.

Feeny D (2002). The utility approach to assessing population health. In: Murray C, Salomon J, Mathers C, Lopez A (eds). *Summary measures of population health: concepts, ethics, measurment and applications*. World Health Organization, Geneva, Switzerland.

Feeny DH, Furlong WJ, Torrance GW, Goldsmith CH, Zenglong Z, Depauw S, Denton M, Boyle M (2002). Multi-attribute and single-attribute utility function for the Health Utility Index Mark 3 system. *Medical Care* 40:113–28.

Froberg DG, Kane RL (1989). Methodology for measuring health-state preferences— I: measurement strategies. *Journal of Clinical Epidemiology* 42:345–54.

Golicki D, Jakubezyk M, Niewada M, Wrona W (2013). Extending of a TTO experiment to 23 states per respondent justifiable? An empirical answer from Polish EQ-5D valuation study. *Journal of Health Policy and Outcomes Research* **1**:18–23.

Gravelle H (1995). Valuations of Euroqol health states: comments and suggestions. Paper presented at the ESRC/SHHD Workshop on Quality of Life, Edinburgh, UK (unpublished).

Hadorn DC, Uebersax J (1995). Large-scale health outcomes evaluation: how should quality of life be measured? 1—Calibration of a brief questionnaire and search for preference subgroups. *Journal of Clinical Epidemiology* **48**:607–18.

Kaplan RM, Anderson JP (1988). A general health policy model: update and application. *Health Services Research* **23**:203–35.

Keeney RL, Raiffa H (1976). *Decisions with multiple objectives: preferences and value trade-offs.* John Wiley and Sons, New York, NY.

Kharroubi SA, O'Hagan A, Brazier JE (2010). A comparison of United States and United Kingdom EQ-5D health states valuations using a nonparametric Bayesian method. Published online in *Statistics in Medicine* **29**:1622–34.

Kharroubi SA, McCabe C (2008). Modelling HUI 2 health state preference data using a nonparametric Bayesian method. *Medical Decision Making* **28**:875–87.

Kharroubi SA, Brazier JE, Roberts J, O'Hagan A (2007*a*). Modelling SF-6D health state preference data using a nonparametric Bayesian method. *Journal of Health Economics* **26**:597–612.

Kharroubi SA, Brazier JE, O'Hagan A (2007*b*). Modelling covariates for the SF-6D standard gamble health state preference data using a nonparametric Bayesian method. *Social Science and Medicine* **64**:1242–52.

Kharroubi SA, Brazier JE, Yang Y (2014). Modelling a Preference-Based Index for two condition specific measures (asthma and overactive bladder) using a nonparametric Bayesian method. *Value in Health* **17**:406–15.

Lamers LM, McDonnell J, Stalmeier PF, Krabbe PF, Busschbach JJ (2006). The Dutch tariff: results and arguments for an effective design for national EQ-5D valuation studies. *Health Economics* **15**:1121–32.

Llewellyn-Thomas H, Sutherland HJ, Tibshirani R, Ciampi A, Till JE, Boyd NF (1984). Describing health states: methodological issues in obtaining values for health states. *Medical Care* **22**:543–52.

McCabe C, Stevens K, Roberts J, Brazier JE (2005*a*). Health state values from the HUI-2 descriptive system: results from a UK survey. *Health Economics* **14**:231–44.

Menzel P, Dolan O, Richardson J, Olsen JA (2002). The role of adaptation to disability and disease in health state valuation: a preliminary normative analysis. *Social Science and Medicine* **55**:2149–58.

Norman R, Cronin P, Viney R, King M, Street D, Ratcliffe J (2009). International comparisons in valuing EQ-5D health states: a review and analysis. *Value in Health* **12**:1194–200.

Méndez I, Abellán-Perpiñán JM, Sánchez FI, Martínez JE (2011). Inverse probability weighted estimation of social tariffs: an illustration using SF-6D value sets. *Journal of Health Economics* **30**:1280–92.

Oppe M, Devlin NJ, van Hout B, Krabbe P, de Charro F (2014). A programme of methodological research to arrive at the new international EQ-5D-5L valuation protocol. *Value in Health* **17**:445–53.

Patrick DL, Starks HE, Cain KC, Uhlmann RF, Pearlman RA (1994). Measuring preferences for health states worse than death. *Medical Decision Making* **14**:9–18.

Revicki DA, Leidy NK, Kline N, Brennen-Diema F, Sorensen S, Togian A (1998). Integrating patient preferences into health outcomes assessment: the multi-attribute Asthma Symptom Utility Index. *Chest* **114**:998–1007.

Richardson J, Sinha K, Iezzi A, Khan MA (2014). Modelling utility weights for the Assessment of Quality of Life (AQoL)-8D. *Quality of Life Research* **23**(8):2395–404.

Robinson A, Dolan P, Williams A (1997). Valuing health status using VAS and TTO: what lies behind the numbers? *Social Science and Medicine* **45**:1289–97.

Rowen D, Brazier J, Young T, Gaugris S, Craig BM, King MT, Velikova G (2011). Deriving a preference-based measure for cancer using the EORTC QLQ-C30. *Value in Health* **14**:721–31.

Rowen D, Brazier J, Van Hout B (2015). A comparison of methods for converting DCE values onto the full health-dead QALY scale. *Medical Decision Making* **35**:328–40.

Shaw JK, Johnson JA, Coons SJ (2005). US valuation of the EQ-5D health states: development and testing of the D1 model. *Medical Care* **43**:203–20.

Sintonen H (1994). The 15D-measure of health-related quality of life. I. Reliability, validity and sensitivity of its health state descriptive system. National Centre for Health Program Evaluation, Working Paper 41, Melbourne, Australia.

Stevens KJ, McCabe CJ, Brazier JE (2006). Mapping between visual analogue and standard gamble data; results from the UK Health Utilities Index 2 valuation. *Health Economics* **15**:527–34.

Stevens KJ, McCabe CJ, Brazier JE (2007). Multi-attribute utility function or statistical inference models: a comparison of health state valuation models using the HUI2 health state classification system. *Journal of Health Economics.* **26**(5):992–1002.

Torrance GW (1982). Multi attribute utility theory as a method of measuring social preferences for health states in long-term care. In: Kane RL, Kane RA (eds). *Values in long-term care.* Lovington Books, DC Heath & Co., MA, pp. 127–56.

Torrance GW (1986). Measurement of health state utilities for economic appraisal: a review. *Journal of Health Economics* **5**:1–30.

Torrance GW, Furlong W, Feeny D, Boyle M (1995). Multi-attribute preference functions. Health Utilities Index. *Pharmaco Economics* **7**:503–20.

Torrance GW, Feeny DH, Furlong WJ, Barr RD, Zhang Y, Wang Q (1996). Multi-attribute utility function for a comprehensive health status classification system: Health Utility Index mark 2. *Medical Care* **34**:702–22.

Ubel PA, Loewenstein G, Jepson C (2003). Whose quality of life? A commentary exploring discrepancies between health state evaluations of patients and the general public. *Quality of Life Research* **12**:599–607.

Williams A (1995). *The measurement and valuation of health: a chronicle.* Centre for Health Economics, Discussion Paper, University of York, UK.

Yang Y, Brazier J, Tsuchiya A, Young T (2011). Estimating a preference-based index for a 5-dimensional health state classification for asthma (AQL-5D) derived from the Asthma Quality of Life Questionnaire (AQLQ). *Medical Decision Making* **31**:281–91.

Chapter 6

Using ordinal response data to estimate cardinal values for health states

6.1 Introduction to ordinal response data for estimating cardinal values for health states

In Chapter 4, we reviewed the range of different methods that are most commonly used to elicit cardinal valuations of health states. Chapter 5 introduced approaches to modelling health state values using scoring functions estimated for health state classification systems. In this chapter, we consider the potential role of ordinal data collection techniques as an alternative to the more widely used valuation techniques highlighted in Chapter 4. We review the variety of techniques for eliciting ordinal information on health state values, with an emphasis on discrete choice, ranking, and best–worst scaling methods, and we describe the methods used for modelling these ordinal data in a way that produces health state utility values analogous to the valuation models estimated from cardinal responses.

6.2 Why consider ordinal valuation methods?

Although many of the major pioneering health state valuation studies included ordinal ranking tasks (e.g. Fryback *et al.* 1993; Dolan *et al.* 1996; Brazier *et al.* 2002), the ranking exercise in these studies was typically intended as a 'warm-up' task rather than as a basis for deriving cardinal valuations. There exists a strong methodological foundation, however, for estimating cardinal values from ordinal information, originating in psychology but commonly applied in areas as diverse as consumer marketing (Louviere *et al.* 2000), political science (Koop and Poirier 1994), transportation research (Beggs *et al.* 1981), and environmental economics (Adamowicz *et al.* 1994). Over recent years, there has been a steady rise in the use of these approaches to estimate health state values.

Potential advantages claimed for ordinal data collection approaches include relative ease of comprehension and administration, and greater reliability corresponding to reduced measurement error. Particularly in settings or subpopulations in which educational attainment and numeracy are limited, an ordinal measurement strategy may have practical advantages over more commonly applied techniques such as the

SG and time trade-off (TTO), which may place a greater cognitive burden on respondents and can demand a higher degree of abstract reasoning. However, the existence and extent of these advantages depend on the specific design of the study; some ordinal tasks, such as pairwise choices in which the two options are described in multiple dimensions, require a respondent to process more information than in an SG or TTO for a single state.

Another advantage of some types of ordinal data collection methods is that the preferences or judgements they elicit are not contaminated by risk aversion (as in the standard gamble) or by time preference (as in the TTO). An exception in the latter case is discrete choice methods that explicitly include duration as a dimension of the choice, as some recent studies have done (e.g. Bansback *et al.* 2012). As discussed in Chapter 4, the methods that have been favoured in the traditional health economics literature all elicit responses that reflect both valuations of the health levels associated with different states as well as other values, considerations, or biases (see also Bleichrodt 2002; Salomon and Murray 2004). With ordinal methods, questions posed to respondents may be framed strictly in terms of choices over health states, without the need for 'calibrators' such as time or risk that can confound interpretation of responses as 'pure' valuations of health states. Additionally, ordinal elicitation techniques may avoid ordering biases inherent to conventional, iterative valuation techniques, wherein responses may be sensitive to the sequence of questions that are used to arrive at an indifference point for a particular trade-off (Ternent and Tsuchiya 2013).

6.3 Types of ordinal information

There are a variety of different types of ordinal information, corresponding to different modes of data collection. In this chapter we focus on discrete choice, ranking, and best–worst scaling.

6.3.1 Discrete choice

Discrete choice data are elicited by asking respondents to choose between two or more alternatives, typically described by their levels along several dimensions. In the context of health valuations, these choices are *stated choices* by which respondents indicate their selection from among a set of alternatives. The framing of the choice may be in terms of which state the respondent would choose to live in for some defined amount of time, or in terms of a judgement as to which state is associated with the best health level overall. Discrete choices may take the form of paired comparisons, in which respondents indicate the preferred option between two alternatives (see Box 6.1 for an example), or they may be presented as choices of the most preferred alternative among a choice set including more than two alternatives. A special case and variant of the latter type of question is best–worst scaling, described separately in section 6.3.3.

6.3.2 Ranking

Respondents may be asked to produce a complete ranking of a set of health states from the best to the worst (or vice versa). This information may be elicited either through an open-ended ranking task, or through a more structured interview protocol.

Box 6.1 Examples of discrete choice and best–worst scaling questions, with states described using EQ-5D-3L

Discrete choice example

Consider the following two health states.

Health state A	Health state B
No problems in walking about	Some problems in walking about
No problems with self-care	No problems with self-care
Some problems with performing usual activities	No problems with performing usual activities
No pain or discomfort	Moderate pain or discomfort
Moderately anxious or depressed	Not anxious or depressed

Which health state do you think is better? (please check one)

	Health state A
	Health state B

Best–worst scaling example (profile case)

Imagine you were living in the following health state. Check which aspect of this state would be best to live with and which would be worst to live with.

Best		Worst
	Some problems in walking about	
✓	No problems with self-care	
	Some problems with performing usual activities	
	Extreme pain or discomfort	✓
	Moderately anxious or depressed	

An example of the latter procedure, respondents may first be asked to identify the best health state out of some set of states, followed by the next best state, and so on, until the complete ordering is obtained. Alternatively, they may be asked to identify the best state, followed by the worst state, followed by a state in the middle, and so on. The more structured mode of eliciting rankings bears a greater resemblance to the discrete choice methods described here, and also shares features with best–worst scaling.

6.3.3 **Best–worst scaling**

Best–worst scaling, as noted above, resembles both discrete choice and ranking methods in certain aspects. Three types of best–worst scaling have been proposed (Flynn 2010). In two of the types, respondents are asked to indicate the best and worst alternatives among a choice set containing at least three options; in one case, the alternatives are presented as profiles consisting of levels on multiple attributes (a familiar scheme in health state valuation), whereas in the other case, the alternatives are presented without this classification structure. The third type of best–worst scaling, perhaps most familiar to researchers in health measurement, presents respondents with a single profile at a time and elicits choices regarding which attribute is the best (most attractive) and which is the worst (least attractive) based on the attribute levels in the profile (see Box 6.1 for an example).

6.4 **How can ordinal data be used to derive cardinal information?**

We begin with an overview of the conceptual basis for deriving cardinal values from ordinal responses. Later we will elaborate on the statistical models that are used to formalize these intuitive notions. We first describe the concepts in terms of a discrete choice model, then consider how rankings over a choice set may be conceptualized in a discrete choice framework.

The starting point for imputing cardinal valuations from ordinal information is an assumption that choices over sets of alternatives are related to latent cardinal values that are distributed around the population mean value for each alternative. Under this framework, a person may choose an alternative with a lower mean value than another alternative due to individual variability or random error. The frequency of these reversals is related to the proximity of the mean values for different alternatives on the latent scale. Mean values that are far apart, in other words, will produce greater agreement in choices than mean values that are close together.

A similar logic applies to a complete ordering of states if we regard this ordering as resulting from a series of discrete choices. For example, the ordering of three alternatives A, B, and C may be regarded as a sequence of discrete choices, either through paired comparisons (A over B, A over C, and B over C) or choices within subsets (A from the set {A,B,C}, then B from the set {B,C}). The key assumption that allows this translation is called Luce's choice axiom, or *independence from irrelevant alternatives* (see Section 6.6.2).

6.5 **Historical foundations for ordinal approaches: Thurstone and beyond**

The notion of inferring cardinal values from ordinal choices has its origins in the pioneering work of Thurstone (1927). Thurstone first proposed the *law of comparative judgement* as a measurement model representing 'discriminal processes' by which perceptions or judgements arise along some dimension of interest. Initially proposed in reference to physical stimuli such as weights, Thurstone later extended the law to describe non-physical entities such as attitudes (Thurstone 1928).

Thurstone's logic is as follows: a given stimulus, presented to a respondent, evokes a 'discriminal' process, which is subject to some random error, such that the same stimulus presented to the same respondent over multiple occasions will produce a distribution of 'discriminal processes', assumed to be normal. The distributions of discriminal processes cannot be observed directly, but can be inferred from comparisons between different stimuli. The *law of comparative judgement* comprises a set of mathematical relationships that imputes relative values (along some dimension of measurement) for two stimuli, based on the frequency with which one stimulus is regarded as greater on that dimension than the other stimulus. Thurstone distinguished five 'cases' of his law, corresponding to different simplifying assumptions that would enable solution of the mathematical equations defining the law. The most commonly invoked assumption (representing Thurstone's 'case V') is that all stimuli are associated with distributions that are uncorrelated and have the same variance.

The estimation of relative scale values based on the law of comparative judgement involves matrix operations undertaken on data reporting the proportion of times a particular stimulus is judged as greater than each other stimulus. A requirement of the procedure is that comparisons between stimuli are replicated a large number of times, based either on repeated observations from a single individual, observations from multiple individuals, or some combination of the two. In the standard approach to collecting data for Thurstone models, responses are elicited through paired comparisons, by which respondents consider two stimuli and indicate which one is greater on the measurement dimension of interest.

Following Thurstone's original approach, there have been several modifications proposed by later contributors. Two directions of advancement in the approach include its generalization to accommodate other probability models besides the normal density function suggested by Thurstone, and its incorporation in a statistical estimation model formalized as a 'random utility' framework. The best-known development in the first category is probably the Bradley–Terry–Luce model (sometimes referred to as the Bradley–Terry model), which uses a logistic function in place of the normal density function (Bradley and Terry 1952; Luce 1959). The Bradley–Terry–Luce model also provided the initial basis for the second category of developments, which have produced regression-based approaches to estimating valuation functions from ordinal data, as we will describe in the following section.

6.6 **Statistical models for ordinal response data**

The logic of Thurstone's law of comparative judgement provides the basic foundation for estimating cardinal values from ordinal information. The key premise is that choices between two or more objects derive from comparisons that include both a systematic component and a random error term. For our purposes, the 'objects' of analysis are health states, so we will present the following explication in reference to health state comparisons. Formally, statistical models in a random utility framework assume that a respondent i has a latent value for state j, U_{ij}, that includes a systematic component (the mean health state value μ_j) and a random error term:

$$U_{ij} = \mu_j + \varepsilon_{ij}. \tag{6.1}$$

The probabilistic interpretation of the random error term has evolved in the translation of choice models from psychology to economics, from a model of repeated choice by an individual, to one of choices made by a population of individuals, with the latter perspective solidified by McFadden (1974) and typifying the modern application of the method in health state valuation.

In the formulation described by equation 6.1, the latent values for a given health state are characterized by the mean value across all respondents; a more general specification of the model would allow for systematic variation in latent values that depends on the characteristics of the respondent as well. Given a choice between two states, a respondent will select state j over state k if $U_{ij} > U_{ik}$. Allowing for the stochastic element in the model, the probability of this ordering is given by:

$$P(U_{ij} > U_{ik}) = P(\varepsilon_{ij} - \varepsilon_{ik} < \mu_j - \mu_k). \tag{6.2}$$

Different statistical models arise from different assumptions about the distributions of the random errors, with prominent alternatives including logit and probit models and their variants, relating to logistic and normal distributions, respectively.

6.6.1 Incorporating valuation functions

The framework for modelling ordinal response data as just described may be elaborated to capture the relationships between choices and the attributes of the alternatives in the choice set. For the purposes of health state valuation, what this implies is that ordinal data may be used as the basis for models of valuation functions, allowing for discrete choice, ranking, or best–worst scaling data to extend the empirical basis for estimating the types of models described in Chapter 5.

Building from equation 6.1, in which μ_j represents the average valuation of a particular health state in a population of respondents, we may express μ_j as a function of the multiple domain levels in the descriptive system, i.e. to specify the form of a valuation function. A range of different specifications is possible for the valuation function that relates the utility of a given health state to levels on different domains of health (see Chapter 5). The general specification may be represented as:

$$\mu_j = x_j'\beta, \tag{6.3}$$

with x_j a vector of indicator variables referring to levels on the relevant domains comprising the descriptive system and β a vector of unknown parameters.

6.6.2 Models for multinomial choice

In equation 6.2, we describe a choice between two alternatives. Many (though not all) discrete choice experiments are formulated in terms of this type of paired comparison. Alternatively, choices may be framed in terms of comparisons involving three or more alternatives. Such a multinomial choice may be elicited in a discrete choice experiment, as part of best–worst scaling, or in a ranking exercise. To accommodate multinomial choice data, the simple probabilistic model in equation 6.2 must be extended. A popular choice for the statistical modelling of multinomial choice data is logit regression, which assumes that the error terms in equation 6.1 are described by an extreme value distribution. In this case, the probability that individual i will choose alternative j out of all K alternatives in the choice set is given by:

$$P_{ij} = \frac{exp(\mu_j)}{\sum_{k=1}^{K} exp(\mu_k)}. \tag{6.4}$$

A key assumption that is common to models of multinomial choice is *independence from irrelevant alternatives* (IIA), which states that the probability of choosing one alternative over another does not depend on other alternatives that are available (Luce 1959).

The extreme value distribution is a convenient option for the joint distribution of the error terms, because it offers a simple closed-form expression for the choice probabilities. Given two variables X and Y with extreme value distributions, the difference $X–Y$ has a logistic distribution, hence the logit regression model. While other alternatives are possible, options such as the multinomial probit (which assumes normal distributions, as in Thurstone's original law of comparative judgement) require evaluation of complex integrals (Chapman and Staelin 1982; Allison and Christakis 1994).

The basic logic of multinomial choice can be extended from a data set comprised of discrete choice responses (as in the aforementioned example, in which a respondent chooses one alternative from a set) to a data set comprised of rankings of a set of alternatives. In a ranking dataset, each respondent is observed to rank K states, with Y_{ij} denoting the rank given to state j by respondent i (following the convention that 1 is the 'highest' ranking). Rank responses are often analysed using conditional logit regression, a modelling approach that has also been referred to as the rank-ordered logit (Koop and Poirier 1994) or exploded logit model (Chapman and Staelin 1982). The name *exploded logit* derives from the fact that an observed rank ordering of K alternatives may be regarded as an 'explosion' into $K - 1$ independent observations, each of them a discrete choice of one option from among a set. Based on this premise, the ranking $U_{i1} > U_{i2} > \cdot > U_{ij}$ is treated as equivalent to the following sequences of choices: $(U_{i1} > U_{ij}, j = 2, ..., K), (U_{i2} > U_{ij}, j = 3, ..., K), ..., (U_{i(K-1)} > U_{iK})$ (Chapman and Staelin 1982). In other words, ranking data are treated as equivalent to one state being chosen over all other alternatives, a second state chosen over all except the first, and so on.

6.6.3 Normalizing scale values estimated from statistical models for ordinal response data

Probabilistic choice models, as described here, produce estimated valuations on an interval scale, such that meaningful comparisons of differences are possible (Stevens 1946). However, the origin and units of the scale are defined arbitrarily by the identifying assumptions in the model. In other words, the probability that a person chooses a particular alternative over one or more other alternatives in a set will be the same under any positive affine transformation of the latent values for all of the alternatives, which implies the following more general specification of equation 6.1 (cf. Chapman and Staelin 1982):

$$U_{ij} = \gamma_1 \left(\mu_j + \varepsilon_{ij} \right) + \gamma_2. \qquad (6.5)$$

Substituting from equation 6.3, the predicted utility for a given health state, conditional on the parameter values estimated in the model, would be $\gamma_1 x'_j \beta + \gamma_2$. In the context of health state valuations, there are certain conceptual constraints on the possible values for the parameters γ_1 and γ_2, that lead to a limited number of logical alternatives. As applied here, γ_2 represents the value assigned to a state characterized by the best possible levels on all of the health dimensions in the relevant classification system. Intuitively, $\gamma_2 = 1$ is a reasonable choice which implies that a person with no difficulties on any dimension will have an expected health state valuation of 1.

For the value of γ_1, which defines a normalizing constant for the model coefficients, there is a somewhat larger number of possibilities. In two of the earliest studies analysing ranking data for health state valuations, Salomon (2003) and McCabe *et al.* (2006) described three different possible choices.

♦ Normalization using the exogenously defined value for at least one state. For example, the observed mean value (using TTO, VAS, or SG values, for instance) for the state consisting of the worst levels on all dimensions, or the so-called 'pits' state, could anchor the lower end of the scale.

♦ Normalization to produce a utility of 0 for the 'pits' state.

♦ Normalization to produce a utility of 0 for dead. The scale may be defined with 'dead' at 0 if respondents have ranked 'dead' among the health states in the study. By including an indicator for 'dead' in the regression model alongside the indicator variables for the domain levels, the modelled utility for dead on the untransformed scale of the regression coefficients may be used to rescale the results with dead located at 0.

More recently, Rowen *et al.* (2015) compared different rescaling methods, including those used in the earlier ranking studies, as well as a hybrid approach that combines ordinal data with limited information from TTO data. The study suggested that methods for measurement and scaling based on a combination of ordinal and cardinal valuation information may present a promising direction for further development in the effort to identify valid, reliable, and efficient techniques for estimating health valuations (see Chapter 7 for an application to the valuation of EQ-5D-5L).

6.7 Applications

Application of Thurstone's paired comparison approach to estimate health valuations was first proposed by Fanshel and Bush (1970) in one of the earliest examples of a time-based health index model. Kind (1982) offered another early precedent in a comparison of Thurstone and Bradley–Terry models for scaling the sleep dimension of the Nottingham Health Profile. More recently, Thurstone scaling has been used by Kind

(2005) and Krabbe (2008) to analyse data from valuation studies for the EQ-5D instrument in the United Kingdom and the Netherlands, respectively.

Salomon (2003) proposed the use of a random utility approach to modelling health state valuations from ordinal data and presented a first application using data on rankings of EQ-5D states from the UK Measurement and Valuation of Health study. Several subsequent studies have adopted the same approach to analyse ranking data from various populations (McCabe *et al.* 2006; Craig *et al.* 2009a; Craig *et al.* 2009b, Hernández Alava *et al.* 2013).

Hakim and Pathak (1999) presented an early example of a discrete choice experiment used to estimate values for EQ-5D health states. Studies that followed have examined discrete choice responses relating to both condition-specific and generic valuation instruments (Ratcliffe *et al.* 2009; Stolk *et al.* 2010; Brazier *et al.* 2012; Oppe *et al.* 2014; Krabbe *et al.* 2014). The literature using discrete choice techniques for health state valuation has grown substantially in recent years as the approach has gained considerable currency. A variant of the general approach has been introduced to incorporate duration as a dimension of the choices in order to use the results to calculate quality of life years (QALYs) (Bansback *et al.* 2012; Bansback *et al.* 2014).

An early example of best–worst scaling applied in health valuation was a 1999 study among patients with multiple myeloma, who rated EQ-5D health states using best–worst scaling and other techniques (Szeinbach *et al.* 1999). More recently, studies have also applied the method to the ICECAP-O (Coast *et al.* 2008) and Child Health Utility 9D (Ratcliffe *et al.* 2011; Ratcliffe *et al.* 2012) instruments.

In the following section, we review highlights from selected studies in this area; readers seeking more information are referred to the original studies, and those seeking an overview of the array of different probabilistic choice models for ordinal data are referred to a recent review by Arons and Krabbe (2013).

6.7.1 Examples of applications using ranking data

One of the studies that helped trigger the recent revival of interest in ordinal measurement methods was the study by Salomon (2003), which explicated the random utility framework for health valuation based on ordinal response data. It presented a first application of conditional logit modelling for ranking data from the Measurement and Valuation of Health study in the United Kingdom (Dolan *et al.* 1996; Kind *et al.* 1998). Health states in the survey were described using the EQ-5D descriptive system, and respondents provided rankings of 13 different hypothetical states described by EQ-5D profiles, plus outcomes labelled as 'immediate death' and 'unconscious', as well as valuations of the same states using a visual analogue scale and time trade-offs.

The conditional logit model was specified to be analogous to Dolan's widely cited model of the TTO values from the same study (Dolan 1997). Three alternative rescalings of the model results were considered: matching to the mean TTO value for the 'pits' state; setting the valuation of the 'pits' state to 0; or setting the valuation of dead to 0 based on an extended model with a coefficient for dead estimated from the empirical rankings of dead in relation to the hypothetical states. After fitting the model and using it to generate predicted valuations for the 42 EQ-5D states included in the

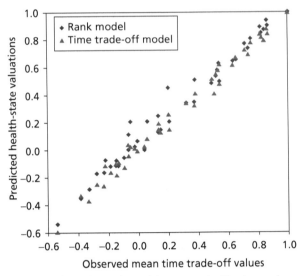

Fig. 6.1 Predicted values from the rank model compared with observed mean time trade-off values in the UK Measurement and Valuation of Health study.

Reproduced with permission from Salomon JA, 'Reconsidering the use of rankings in the valuation of health states: a model for estimating cardinal values from ordinal data', *Population Health Metrics*, Volume 1, Article 12, Copyright © 2003 Salomon; licensee BioMed Central Ltd. This is an Open Access article: verbatim copying and redistribution of this article are permitted in all media for any purpose, available from http://www.pophealthmetrics.com/content/1/1/12.

study, these predictions (under the three alternative rescaling options) were compared with observed mean TTO values. The rank-based predictions were strongly correlated with observed TTO values: of the three rescaling alternatives, the rescaling to the lowest observed TTO was the best-fitting alternative (Fig. 6.1), with a fit that was only marginally lower than the fit for predictions based on the directly estimated TTO tariff function reported previously by Dolan (1997).

McCabe and colleagues (2006) fitted a similar conditional logit model to data from two other valuation surveys in the United Kingdom, which used the HUI2 and the SF-6D. In both surveys, respondents ranked health states, and then valued the same states using the SG. Conditional logit models were estimated with indicator variables for each level on each domain. The models included an indicator variable for the state dead, and predictions from the model were rescaled based on setting the valuation of dead to 0. Models were assessed in terms of the logical consistency of the coefficients (i.e. that lower levels of functioning are associated with greater decrements in health valuations), and model predictions were compared with observed mean SG values. In the HUI2 data set, the rank-based model was very similar to a model estimated directly from the SG values. For the SF-6D data set, the rank-based and SG-based models were different, with fewer logical inconsistencies in the rank model, but slightly lower validity for the rank model compared with the SG model in predicting observed SG values (Fig. 6.2).

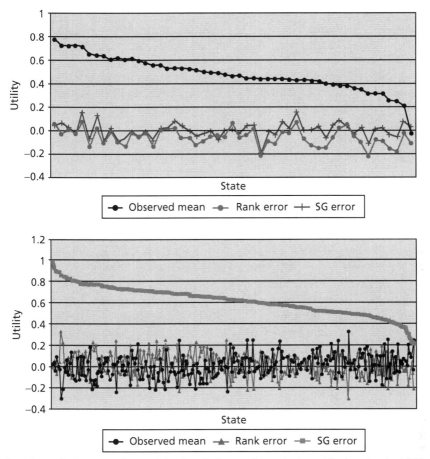

Fig. 6.2 Prediction errors for models of rank data and standard gamble data for the HUI2 (top panel) and SF-6D (bottom panel). The top line in each graph shows the observed mean standard gamble values, while the two lower lines show the average deviations from these for model predictions.

These early studies on ranking data together offered encouraging evidence that models of health state values based on ordinal data can provide results that are similar to those obtained from more widely analysed valuation techniques, such as the TTO or SG.

6.7.2 Examples of applications using discrete choice data

Studies using discrete choice data have focused on both condition-specific and generic measurement instruments. Ratcliffe *et al.* (2009) used a discrete choice experiment

(DCE) to estimate a value function for health states defined by the Sexual Quality of Life Questionnaire and compared the results with those obtained from ranking and TTO. A representative sample of the UK general population was interviewed and asked to rank a series of health states from best to worst. Following this exercise, the TTO technique was used to elicit utilities for each health state. Four weeks following the interview, consenting individuals received a postal self-completion questionnaire containing a DCE. Rank data were analysed using a conditional logit model (normalized around zero for 'immediate death') and DCE data by a random effects probit model (normalized on the TTO value for pits). The rank and DCE models produced significant coefficients that were consistent with the health state descriptive system, but with larger mean absolute errors compared with TTO in predicting actual TTO values.

In another discrete choice modelling study, focusing on an asthma quality of life questionnaire and a similar classification system relating to overactive bladder, Brazier *et al.* (2012) surveyed representative samples of the UK general population, who were asked to rank a series of health states from the two classification systems (each included in a separate sample) and being dead from best to worst, followed by a TTO elicitation exercise. Consenting respondents in the sample subsequently received a postal self-completion questionnaire containing a DCE. A separate general population sample was sent the same postal questionnaire without having completed the interview. Rank data were analysed using a conditional logit model, and DCE data were analysed using a random effects probit model, normalized either using the TTO value for pits, or using the pairwise comparisons with the 'dead' state. The rank model was found to predict actual TTO values very closely; DCE predictions varied from the TTO values in different ways depending on the normalization approach, with normalization using the TTO value for the pits state tending to produce values higher than observed TTO values, and normalization using dead tending to produce values lower than observed TTO.

Recently, discrete choice modelling has been used in the estimation of valuation functions for the five-level version of the EQ-5D (i.e. the EQ-5D-5L) (Stolk *et al.* 2010; Oppe *et al.* 2014; Krabbe *et al.* 2014). The findings, based on data collected in several countries (including the Netherlands, Canada, England, and the United States) support the feasibility of using DCEs for valuing EQ-5D states, and confirm earlier findings on the strong potential for ordinal data collection and modelling approaches to health state valuation.

6.7.3 Examples of applications using discrete choice experiments including duration

Several recent studies have incorporated duration as an attribute of a DCE, which creates a discrete choice task resembling the conventional TTO (Bansback *et al.* 2012; Bansback *et al.* 2014). An advantage noted by the authors of these studies is that a single task may be used for all health states regardless of whether they are considered better than or worse than being dead. A potential disadvantage of the approach is the need to collect data on a relatively large number of different combinations of health state levels and duration in order to identify duration effects with reasonable certainty, though this has been successfully done with online panels at comparatively low cost (e.g. Bansback *et al.* 2012). Overall, the studies indicate that a discrete choice question with duration as an attribute appears to be feasible for data collection in general population samples. This technique has been applied recently in the estimation of EQ-5D and SF-6D population values in Australia (Viney *et al.* 2014; Norman *et al.* 2014).

6.7.4 Examples of applications using best–worst scaling

Recent work has used variants of best–worst scaling to estimate values for health measurement instruments and other similar measures. Coast *et al.* (2008) used a best–worst scaling exercise to estimate values for the ICECAP index of capability for older people. While somewhat broader in concept than health, this example nevertheless provides a template for scaling profile measures based on the so-called 'attribute' or 'profile' case of best–worst scaling. In the study, a sample of respondents aged 65 years and older who had previously participated in the Health Survey for England were surveyed. Respondents considered a series of profiles consisting of combinations of the four levels on five attributes of ICECAP, and were asked to indicate which of the attribute levels was most and least attractive. Data were analysed using conditional logit regression, and scale values were normalized so that the combination of worst levels on all attributes had a scale value of 0, and the combination of best levels on all attributes had a scale value of 1. The study found that most of the older adult sample was able to complete the best–worst scaling task without difficulty.

Best–worst scaling has been used more recently in establishing values for the Child Health Utility 9D (CHU9D). A feasibility study conducted among young adolescents (Ratcliffe *et al.* 2011) suggested that best–worst scaling methods may be more easily understood and completed in this population group than conventional TTO or SG questions. A subsequent study (Ratcliffe *et al.* 2012) applied this method in a larger web-based survey of adolescents and used conditional logit regression to estimate values for each level of the nine attributes in the CHU9D. Comparing the results in this study to those obtained in prior studies among adults pointed to certain significant differences in values for the same health states.

6.8 Conclusions

The application of ordinal data collection methods for purposes of measuring and valuing health states is an area of rising interest, and a growing array of examples, including those selected in this chapter, confirm a number of advantageous features that make ordinal measurement strategies an attractive option for health state valuation. Overall, the findings from studies to date have suggested that the information content in aggregate-level ordinal data can be surprisingly similar to that in aggregated data collected using more commonly recommended techniques in health economics such as the TTO or SG, although a number of studies have pointed to important differences between the results from ordinal and cardinal elicitation techniques. An important limitation in ordinal techniques is the need to normalize values to the scale needed for QALYs, and the approach taken to normalization will critically affect the degree of correspondence between different measurement approaches. Comparisons of discrete choice and rank-based results provide mixed results on the relationship between alternative modes of eliciting ordinal information, and so conclusions about the optimal approach to ordinal data collection in health valuation awaits further empirical study. A potential advantage of discrete choice methods, particularly those involving paired comparisons, is the simplification of the measurement task, which has—among other benefits—facilitated the incorporation of these methods in online surveys. The recent attention to best–worst scaling methods reflects a similar interest in seeking relatively simple tasks that allow efficient elicitation of the information need to estimate health state values.

A range of additional methodological issues warrant further research, including testing the assumption of IIA in ranking exercises and relaxing this assumption in models if needed. As discussed in Chapter 4 in reference to methods such as the SG or TTO, ordinal valuation techniques may also be susceptible to framing effects that produce significant differences in responses based on subtle variants in question wording, context, and mode of administration. Important procedural aspects of how responses are elicited, for example, via face-to-face or online surveys, discussed in Chapter 4 with regard to cardinal measurement methods, pertain as well to ordinal methods where online methods are becoming widespread.

Part of the appeal of ordinal data collection methods is their apparent ease of administration, particularly among populations in which other techniques may be difficult to implement because of their complexity or abstract nature. As described in Chapter 11, this feature has been exploited in a large-scale empirical effort to measure health state values from diverse populations around the world for the global burden of disease study, which has relied heavily on discrete choice measurement methods (Salomon *et al.* 2012). With their relative simplicity, we may postulate that ordinal methods will reduce survey administration times and simplify data collection efforts, but this issue should be evaluated more thoroughly via direct comparison of methods within the same population groups. On balance, the combination of potential advantages of ordinal data collection methods with the encouraging results shown in a growing number of applications of these approaches justify the increased recognition of their importance as tools for health state valuation.

References

Adamowicz W, Louviere J, Swait J (1994). Combining stated and revealed preference methods for valuing environmental amenities. *Journal of Environmental Economics and Management* **26**:65–84.

Allison PD, Christakis NA (1994). Logit models for sets of ranked items. *Sociological Methodology* **24**:199–228.

Arons AM, Krabbe PF (2013). Probabilistic choice models in health-state valuation research: background, theories, assumptions and applications. *Expert Review of Pharmacoeconomics & Outcomes Research* **13**:93–108.

Bansback N, Brazier J, Tsuchiya A, Anis A (2012). Using a discrete choice experiment to estimate health state utility values. *Journal of Health Economics* **31**:306–18.

Bansback N, Hole AR, Mulhern B, Tsuchiya A (2014). Testing a discrete choice experiment including duration to value health states for large descriptive systems: addressing design and sampling issues. *Social Science & Medicine* **114**:38–48.

Beggs S, Cardell S, Hausman J (1981). Assessing the potential demand for electric cars. *Journal of Econometrics* **161**:1–19.

Bleichrodt H (2002). A new explanation for the difference between time trade-off utilities and standard gamble utilities. *Health Economics* **11**:447–56.

Bradley RA, Terry ME (1952). Rank analysis of incomplete block designs, I. The method of paired comparisons. *Biometrika* **39**:324–45.

Brazier J, Roberts J, Deverill M (2002). The estimation of a preference-based measure of health from the SF-36. *Journal of Health Economics* **21**:271–92.

Brazier J, Rowen D, Yang Y, Tsuchiya A (2012). Comparison of health state utility values derived using time trade-off, rank and discrete choice data anchored on the full health-dead scale. *European Journal of Health Economics* **13**:575–87.

Chapman RG, Staelin R (1982). Exploiting rank ordered choice set data within the stochastic utility model. *Journal of Marketing Research* **19**:288–301.

Coast J, Flynn TN, Natarajan L, Sproston K, Lewis J, Louviere JJ, Peters TJ (2008). Valuing the ICECAP capability index for older people. *Social Science and Medicine* **67**:874–82.

Craig BM, Busschbach JJ, Salomon JA (2009a). Modeling ranking, time trade-off, and visual analog scale values for EQ-5D health states: a review and comparison of methods. *Medical Care* **47**:634–41.

Craig BM, Busschbach JJ, Salomon JA (2009b). Keep it simple: ranking health states yields values similar to cardinal measurement approaches. *Journal of Clinical Epidemiology* **62**:296–305.

Dolan P (1997). Modeling valuations for EuroQol health states. *Medical Care* **35**:1095–108.

Dolan P, Gudex C, Kind P, Williams A (1996). The time trade-off method: results from a general population study. *Health Economics* **5**:141–54.

Fanshel S, Bush JW (1970). A health status index and its application to health services outcomes. *Operations Research* **18**:1021–66.

Flynn TN (2010). Valuing citizen and patient preferences in health: recent developments in three types of best-worst scaling. *Expert Review of Pharmacoeconomics & Outcomes Research* **10**:259–67.

Fryback DG, Dasbach EJ, Klein R, Klein BE, Dorn N, Peterson K, Martin PA (1993). The Beaver Dam Health Outcomes Study: initial catalog of health-state quality factors. *Medical Decision Making* **13**:89–102.

Hakim Z, Pathak DS (1999). Modelling the EuroQol data: a comparison of discrete choice conjoint and conditional preference modelling. *Health Economics* **82**:103–16.

Hernández Alava M, Brazier J, Rowen D, Tsuchiya A (2013). Common scale valuation across different preference-based measures: Estimation using rank data. *Medical Decision Making* **33**:839–52.

Kind P (1982). A comparison of two models for scaling health indicators. *International Journal of Epidemiology* **11**:271–5.

Kind P, Dolan P, Gudex C, Williams A (1998). Variations in population health status: results from a United Kingdom national questionnaire survey. *British Medical Journal* **316**:736–41.

Kind P (2005). Applying paired comparisons models to EQ-5D valuations—deriving TTO utilities from ordinal preferences data. In: Kind P, Brooks R, Rabin R (eds). *EQ-5D concepts and methods: a developmental history*. Springer, Dordrech, the Netherlands, pp. 201–20.

Koop G, Poirier DJ (1994). Rank-ordered logit models: an empirical analysis of Ontario voter preferences. *Journal of Applied Econometrics* **9**:369–88.

Krabbe PFM (2008). Thurstone scaling as a measurement method to quantify subjective health outcomes. *Medical Care* **46**:357–65.

Krabbe PFM, Devlin NJ, Stolk EA, Shah KK, Oppe M, Van Hout B, Quik EH, Pickard AS, Xie F (2014). Multinational evidence of the applicability and robustness of discrete choice modeling for deriving EQ-5D-5L health-state values. *Medical Care* **52**:935–43.

Louviere JJ, Hensher DA, Swait JD (2000). *Stated choice methods: analysis and application.* Cambridge University Press, Cambridge, UK.

Luce RD (1959). *Individual choice behavior: a theoretical analysis.* John Wiley & Sons, Inc., New York. NY.

McCabe C, Brazier J, Gilks P, Tsuchiya A, Roberts J, O'Hagan A, Stevens K (2006). Using rank data to estimate health state utility models. *Journal of Health Economics* **25**:418–31.

McFadden D (1974). Conditional logit analysis of qualitative choice behavior. In: Zarembka P (ed.). *Frontiers in econometrics.* Academic Press, New York, NY, pp. 105–42.

Norman R, Viney R, Brazier J, Cronin P, King MT, Ratcliffe J, Street D (2014). Valuing SF-6D health states using a Discrete Choice Experiment. *Medical Decision Making* **34**(6):773–86.

Oppe M, Devlin NJ, Van Hout B, Krabbe PFM, De Charro F (2014). A program of methodological research to arrive at the new international EQ-5D-5L valuation protocol. *Value in Health* **17**:445–53.

Ratcliffe J, Brazier J, Tsuchiya A, Symonds T, Brown M (2009). Using DCE and ranking data to estimate cardinal values for health states for deriving a preference-based single index from the sexual quality of life questionnaire. *Health Economics* **18**:1261–76.

Ratcliffe J, Flynn T, Terlich F, Stevens K, Brazier J, Sawyer M (2012). Developing adolescent-specific health state values for economic evaluation: an application of profile case best-worst scaling to the Child Health Utility 9D. *Pharmacoeconomics* **30**:713–27.

Ratcliffe J, Couzner L, Flynn T, Sawyer M, Stevens K, Brazier J, Burgess L (2011). Valuing Child Health Utility 9D health states with a young adolescent sample: a feasibility study to compare best-worst scaling discrete-choice experiment, standard gamble and time trade-off methods. *Applied Health Economics and Health Policy* **9**:15–27.

Rowen D, Brazier J, Van Hout B (2015). A comparison of methods for converting DCE values onto the full health-dead QALY scale. *Medical Decision Making* **35**:328–40.

Salomon JA (2003). Reconsidering the use of rankings in the valuation of health states: a model for estimating cardinal values from ordinal data. *Population Health Metrics* **1**:12. Available at: http://www.pophealthmetrics.com/content/1/1/12

Salomon JA, Murray CJ (2004). A multi-method approach to measuring health-state valuations. *Health Economics* **13**:281–90.

Salomon JA, Vos T, Hogan DR, Gagnon M, Naghavi M, Mokdad A, *et al.* (2012). Common values in assessing health outcomes from disease and injury: disability weights measurement study for the Global Burden of Disease Study 2010. *The Lancet* **380**:2129–43.

Stevens SS (1946). On the theory of scales of measurement. *Science* **103**:677–80.

Stolk EA, Oppe M, Scalone L, Krabbe PFM (2010). Discrete choice modeling for the quantification of health states: the case of the EQ-5D. *Value in Health* **13**: 1005–13.

Szeinbach SL, Barnes JH, McGhan WF, Murawski MM, Corey R (1999). Using conjoint analysis to evaluate health state preferences. *Drug Information Journal* **33**:849–58.

Ternent L, Tsuchiya A (2013). A note on the expected biases in conventional iterative health state valuation protocols. *Medical Decision Making* **33**:544–46.

Thurstone LL (1927). A law of comparative judgement. *Psychological Review* **34**:273–86.

Thurstone LL (1928). Attitudes can be measured. *American Journal of Sociology* **33**:529–54.

Viney R, Norman R, Brazier J, Cronin P, King MT, Ratcliffe J, Street D (2014). An Australian discrete choice experiment to value EQ-5D health states. *Health Economics* **23**: 729–42.

Chapter 7

Methods for obtaining health state utility values: generic preference-based measures of health

7.1 Introduction to generic preference-based measures of health

The generic preference-based measures of health (also known as multiattribute utility scales) are becoming the most widely used method for obtaining health state utility values on the utility scale (where zero is for states as bad as being dead and one for full health). They are relatively simple to use and widely accepted by policy makers concerned with using economic assessments of cost-effectiveness around the world (Chapter 12). There are numerous generic preference-based measures (GPBMs) and they all have a description of health status and a set of values to assign to each health state defined by the descriptive system. GPBMs vary enormously in the way they describe health and in the methods used to value health.

Each measure has a health state classification with multilevel dimensions that together describe a large quantity of health states. The original EQ-5D, for example, has five dimensions each with three levels that together describe 243 states (see Table 2.5 in Chapter 2). An individual is assigned to a state within the descriptive system by completing a questionnaire that takes less than 10 minutes to complete, and less than 5 minutes for most patients. A proxy could also complete the questionnaire on behalf of the patient. These questionnaires can be readily incorporated into most clinical trials and routine data collection systems with little additional burden for respondents. A preference-based single index score is generated by an off-the-shelf scoring algorithm, which is estimated from a survey of the general population who were asked to provide values for a set of states defined by the instrument. These measures are generic and designed to be relevant to all (or most) patient groups (including the general population) and provide a means of making comparisons across different disease areas.

This chapter describes the leading six GPBMs of health used in adult populations. These measures are then compared in terms of the generated scores and the possible reasons for any differences found. Their performance is compared using published evidence across different conditions and the implications for use in policy making is discussed. The chapter then briefly reviews the generic measures available for children and adolescents.

7.2 Generic preference-based measures of health

The number of GPBMs have increased over the past four decades, and include the following: Quality of Well-Being (QWB) scale (Kaplan and Anderson 1988); Health Utility Index one, two, and three (HUI1, HUI2, and HUI3) (Torrance 1982; Torrance *et al.* 1996; Feeny *et al.* 2002); EQ-5D (Dolan 1997; Shaw *et al.* 2005); 15D (Sintonen and Pekurin 1993); SF-6D—a derivative of the SF-36 and SF-12 (Brazier *et al.* 2002; Brazier and Roberts 2004); and various versions of the assessment of quality of life (AQoL) (Hawthorne *et al.* 1997; Richardson *et al.* 2014*a*). This list is not exhaustive and does not account for some of the variants of these instruments, but it includes the vast majority of those that have been used. While these measures all claim to be generic, they differ considerably in terms of the content and size of their descriptive system, the methods of valuation and the populations used to value the health states (although most aim for a general population sample). They also differ in terms of their relative use, with EQ-5D being by far the most widely used measure, followed by SF-6D and HUI3 before the other measures.

Section 7.3 describes in detail six leading GPBMs for use in adults—these will be reviewed in the sections that follow.

7.3 Description of scales

A summary of the main characteristics of these six GPBMs of health (and some of their variants) is presented in Tables 7.1 and 7.2. Table 7.1 summarizes the descriptive content of these measures, including their dimensions, dimension levels, and number of states they define, which are presented in full throughout this chapter. Each instrument has a questionnaire to be completed by the patient (or proxy) or to be administered by interview, and is used to assign the patient a health state from the instrument's descriptive system. These questions are mainly designed for adults, typically aged 16 or above. Table 7.2 summarizes the valuation methods used in terms of the valuation technique, the country (or countries) of the populations providing the values, the method of modelling the preference data, and the health state value of the worst state of the most widely used algorithms.

7.3.1 Quality of Well-Being scale

The QWB scale was developed from the Index of Well-Being and is the oldest of the GPBMs (though its developers initially preferred the term 'well-year'). It was developed as part of a general health policy model to inform resource allocation in health services (Fanshel and Bush 1970; Patrick *et al.* 1973). This earlier version had two components: three multilevel dimensions relating to function (mobility, physical activity, and social activity) that produce a total of 46 functional levels (including 'death') and a list of 27 symptom and problem complexes (e.g. 'general tiredness, weakness, or weight loss'; 'wore eyeglasses or contact lenses'). It takes between one and two weeks

Table 7.1 Descriptive systems of generic preference-based measures (GPBMs)

Instrument	Dimension	Levels	Health states
QWB-SA	Mobility, physical activity, social functioning	2	945
	68 symptoms/problems	2	
HUI3	Vision, hearing, speech, ambulation, dexterity, emotion, cognition, pain	5–6	972,000
EQ-5D	Mobility, self-care, usual activities, pain/discomfort, anxiety/depression	3 or 5	243 or 3,125
15D	Mobility, vision, hearing, breathing, sleeping, eating, speech, elimination, usual activities, mental function, discomfort/symptoms, depression, distress, vitality, sexual activity	4–5	31 billion
SF-6D	Physical functioning, role limitation, social functioning, pain, energy, mental health	4–6	18,000 (36), 7,500 (12), and 18,750 (V2)
AQoL-8D	Independent living (n = 4 items), pain (3), senses (3), mental health (8), happiness (4), coping (3), relationship (7), self-worth (3) (sleep, anxiety and depression, pain)	4-6	$2.37*10^{23}$

Table 7.2 Valuation methods of GPBMs

	Country	Valuation technique	Type of model	Minimum
QWB-SA	USA (San Diego)	VAS	Statistical additive, except for symptom/problem complexes	0.08
HUI3	Canada (Hamilton), France	VAS transformed into SG	MAUT multiplicative	−0.36
EQ-5D	3L: UK, US, and 16 others 5L: UK plus others	3L: TTO, VAS, ranking; 5L: Hybrid of TTO and DCE	Statistical—3L additive, with interaction term and 5L additive	3L UK: −0.59 5L UK: −0.208
15D	Finland	VAS	MAUT additive	0.11
SF-6D	UK and 5 others	SG, ranking V2: DCE with duration	Statistical additive with interaction term	0.301
AQoL-8D	Australia	VAS transformed into TTO	MAUT multiplicative and statistical	−0.04

to train interviewers to administer the questionnaire (Read *et al.* 1987) and between 7 and 15 minutes to conduct an interview (Kaplan 1994), although the range reported in published studies has reached up to 20 minutes (Bombardier and Ramboud 1991). For ease of use, a self-completed version called the QWB-SA has been developed, and is described in the next section (Kaplan *et al.* 1997).

7.3.1.1 Descriptive system

The newer version was developed for completion by the patient and the developers state that it takes less than 10 minutes to complete. The recall period is three days. The descriptive system is still largely dominated by dichotomous symptom lists with 19 chronic symptoms or problems (e.g. hearing loss, eczema), 25 acute symptoms (e.g. headache, toothache), and 14 mental health symptoms or behaviours (e.g. excessive worry or anxiety, a loss of appetite or overeating) (see Table 7.3). The symptoms lists were based on focus groups with clinicians. There are 17 items to cover three functional dimensions of mobility, physical activity, and social activity, that ask about number of days effected. These 68 items define 945 states in all.

7.3.1.2 Valuation

Weights for the descriptive system were obtained from a community sample of 330 who were recruited in primary care and two college campuses in San Diego. The age and gender distribution approximated the US population according to the authors (Seiber *et al.* 2008). Each respondent valued 12 states in all, including single symptom states and states with symptoms combined with impairments in mobility, physical activity, and social activity. The states were valued using a rating scale from 0 (worst or dead) to 100 (optimum). The weights (see Table 7.3) were calculated using an additive approach: the individual symptom weights were calculated first, and then the weights for the three functional dimensions by the state score minus the symptom weights. This resulted in a lower minimum score of 0.09, compared to 0.33 for the original QWB.

The QWB questionnaire (including the self-administered version) and its scoring algorithm are available from the developers (for more information see https://hoap.ucsd.edu/qwb-info/).

7.3.2 Health Utilities Index

The HUI has evolved over time into three different versions. Torrance and colleagues developed the first version (HUI1) in the late 1970s for use in an economic evaluation of neonatal intensive care (Torrance 1982). This version has been succeeded by the HUI2 and HUI3. The HUI2 was originally developed for use in studies of childhood cancer (Torrance *et al.* 1996) and is now used as a GPBM for children—this is reviewed later in the chapter. The HUI3 is designed for adults and is the most widely used of the three (Feeny *et al.* 2002).

7.3.2.1 Descriptive system

HUI3 was developed from HUI2, for which six dimensions were derived from a literature review and a survey of patients who were asked to rank the importance of 15 symptoms. The changes were partly made to increase the degree of independence between the

Table 7.3 Quality of well-being preference weights

Symptoms (CPX)

Blindness or severely impaired vision in both eyes	0.523
Blindness or severely impaired vision in only one eye	0.358
Speech problems such as stuttering, or being unable to speak clearly	0.358
Missing or paralysed hands, feet, arms, or legs	0.423
Missing or paralysed fingers or toes	0.297
Any deformity of the face, fingers, hand/arm, foot/leg or back	0.408
General fatigue, tiredness, or weakness	0.256
A problem with unwanted weight gain or weight loss	0.233
A problem with being under or overweight	0.225
Problems chewing your food adequately	0.204
Any hearing loss or deafness	0.274
Any noticeable skin problems (i.e. bad acne, large burns, or scars)	0.187
Eczema or burning/itching rash	0.187

Health aides used:

Dentures	0.153
Eye glasses or contact lenses	0.066
Hearing aide	0.148
Any problems with your vision not corrected with glasses or contact lenses	0.293
Any eye pain, irritation, discharge, or excessive sensitivity to light	0.389
A headache	0.189
Dizziness, earache, or ringing in your ears	0.299
Difficulty hearing or discharge or bleeding from an ear	0.35
Stuffy or runny nose or bleeding from the nose	0.178
A sore throat, difficulty swallowing, or hoarse voice	0.204
Toothache or jaw pain	0.298
Sore or bleeding lips, tongue, or gums	0.271
Coughing or wheezing	0.386
Shortness of breath or difficulty breathing	0.208
Chest pain, pressure, palpitations, fast or skipped heart beat, or other discomfort in the chest	0.343
An upset stomach, abdominal pain, nausea, heart burn, or vomiting	0.260
Difficulty with bowel movements, diarrhoea, constipation, rectal bleeding, black tar-like stools, or any pain or discomfort in the rectal area	0.278

(continued)

Table 7.3 Continued

Pain, burning, or blood in urine	0.424
Loss of bladder control, frequent night-time urination of difficulty with urination	0.259
Genital pain, itching, burning, or abnormal discharge or pelvic cramping or abnormal bleeding (does not include menstruation)	0.369
Broken arm, wrist, foot, leg, or other broken bone (other than in back)	0.365
Pain, stiffness, cramps, weakness or numbness in the neck or back	0.318
Pain, stiffness, cramps, weakness or numbness in the hips or sides	0.365
Pain, stiffness, cramps, weakness or numbness in any of the joints or muscles of the hand, feet, arms, or legs	0.318
Swelling of ankles, hands, feet, or abdomen	0.306
Fever, chills, or sweats	0.320
Loss of consciousness, fainting, or seizures	0.517
Difficulty with your balance, standing, or walking	0.377
Trouble falling asleep or staying asleep	0.296
Spells of feeling nervous or shaky	0.286
Spells of feeling upset, downhearted, or blue	0.327
Excessive worry or anxiety	0.324
Feelings that you had little or no control over events in your life	0.430
Feelings of being lonely or isolated	0.311
Feelings of frustration, irritation, or close to losing your temper	0.378
A hangover	0.297
Any decrease of sexual interest or performance	0.307
Confusion, difficulty understanding the written or spoken word or significant memory loss	0.559
Thoughts or images you could not get out of your mind	0.255
Take any medication including over-the-counter remedies (aspirin, Tylenol, allergy medications, insulin, hormone, oestrogen, thyroid, predisone)	0.160
To stay on a medically prescribed diet for health reasons	0.201
A loss of appetite or overeating	0.223

Mobility

Spend any part of the day or night as a patient in a hospital, nursing home, or rehabilitation centre	0.089
Either not drive a motor vehicle or not use public transportation because of your health or need help from another person to use	0.031

Table 7.3 Continued

Physical activity	
Have trouble climbing stairs or inclines, or walking off the kerb	0.072
Avoid or have trouble walking, or walk more slowly than other people your age	0.072
Limp, use a cane, crutches, or walker	0.072
Avoid or have trouble bending over, stooping, or kneeling	0.072
Have any trouble lifting or carrying everyday objects such as books, a briefcase, or groceries	0.072
Have any other limitations in physical movements	0.072
Spend all or most of the day in a bed, chair, or couch	0.163
Spend all or most of the day in a wheelchair	0.102
If in wheelchair, someone else controlled its movement	0.163

Social and self-care activity	
Need help with your personal needs such as eating, dressing, bathing, or getting around your home	0.096
Avoid, need help with, or were limited in doing some of your usual activities such as work, school, or housekeeping	0.054

Reproduced with permission from Seiber WJ, Groessl EJ, Kristen MD, Ganiats TG, and Kaplan RM, *Quality of Wellbeing self-administered (QWB-SA) scale: User's Manual*, Health Services Research Center, University of California, San Diego, Copyright © 2008 William J. Sieber *et al.* available from https://hoap.ucsd.edu/qwb-info/QWB-Manual.pdf

dimensions and to increase sensitivity. The number of dimensions was increased from six to eight, and include *vision* and *hearing* as separate dimensions, along with *speech, ambulation, dexterity, emotion, cognition*, and *pain*. The number of levels is between five and six, and the classification defines 972,000 health states (Table 7.4). Patients can be assigned to HUI3 using a 15-item self-completed questionnaire or from an interview-administered version (by face-to-face or telephone), or by asking a proxy to complete it on their behalf.

7.3.2.2 Valuation

HUI3 has been valued by a representative sample of 256 respondents who provided data for the modelling, and a further 248 respondents who provided a validation sample. The total sample of 504 adults were recruited from Hamilton, Ontario, obtained using a probability sample and made up 65 per cent of eligible respondents who could be contacted. The function for estimating health state values calculated using multiattribute utility theory (MAUT) is described in Chapter 5. In brief, respondents were first asked to value single dimensional states to derive the single dimension utility functions. Then they were asked to value a set of 'corner' states, where one dimension is presented at its worst level while all other dimensions are set to best. Finally, respondents are asked to value multiattribute utility states. These valuation

Table 7.4 Health Utilities Index Mark 3 (HUI3)

Attribute	Level	Description
Vision	1	Able to see well enough to read ordinary newsprint and recognize a friend on the other side of the street, without glasses or contact lenses
	2	Able to see well enough to read ordinary newsprint and recognize a friend on the other side of the street, but with glasses or contact lenses
	3	Able to read ordinary newsprint with or without glasses but unable to recognize a friend on the other side of the street, even with glasses or contact lenses
	4	Able to recognize a friend on the other side of the street with or without glasses but unable to read ordinary newsprint, even with glasses or contact lenses
	5	Unable to read ordinary newsprint and unable to recognize a friend on the other side of the street, even with glasses or contact lenses
	6	Unable to see at all
Hearing	1	Able to hear what is said in a group conversation with at least three other people, without a hearing aid
	2	Able to hear what is said in a conversation with one other person in a quiet room without a hearing aid, but requires a hearing aid to hear what is said in a group conversation with at least three other people
	3	Able to hear what is said in a conversation with one other person in a quiet room with a hearing aid, and able to hear what is said in a group conversation with at least three other people, with a hearing aid
	4	Able to hear what is said in a conversation with one other person in a quiet room without a hearing aid, but unable to hear what is said in a group conversation with at least three other people even with a hearing aid
	5	Able to hear what is said in a conversation with one other person in a quiet room with a hearing aid, but unable to hear what is said in a group conversation with at least three other people even with a hearing aid
	6	Unable to hear at all
Speech	1	Able to be understood completely when speaking with strangers or people who know me well
	2	Able to be understood partially when speaking with strangers but able to be understood completely when speaking with people who know me well
	3	Able to be understood partially when speaking with strangers or people who know me well

Table 7.4 Continued

Attribute	Level	Description
	4	Unable to be understood when speaking with strangers but able to be understood partially by people who know me well
	5	Unable to be understood when speaking to other people (or unable to speak at all)
Ambulation	1	Able to walk around the neighbourhood without difficulty, and without walking equipment
	2	Able to walk around the neighbourhood with difficulty, but does not require walking equipment or the help of another person
	3	Able to walk around the neighbourhood with walking equipment, but without the help of another person
	4	Able to walk only short distances with walking equipment, and requires a wheelchair to get around the neighbourhood
	5	Unable to walk alone, even with walking equipment. Able to walk short distances with the help of another person and requires a wheelchair to get around the neighbourhood
	6	Cannot walk at all
Dexterity	1	Full use of two hands and 10 fingers
	2	Limitations in the use of hands or fingers, but does not require special tools or help of another person
	3	Limitations in the use of hands or fingers, is independent with use of special tools and does not require the help of another person
	4	Limitations in the use of hands or fingers, requires the help of another person for some tasks (not independent even with use of special tools)
	5	Limitations in the use of hands or fingers, requires the help of another person for most tasks (not independent even with use of special tools)
	6	Limitations in use of hands or fingers, requires the help of another person for all tasks (not independent even with use of special tools)
Emotion	1	Happy and interested in life
	2	Somewhat happy
	3	Somewhat unhappy
	4	Very unhappy
	5	So unhappy that life is not worthwhile

(continued)

Table 7.4 Continued

Attribute	Level	Description
Cognition	1	Able to remember most things, think clearly, and solve day-to-day problems
	2	Able to remember most things, but has little difficulty when trying to think and solve day-to-day problems
	3	Somewhat forgetful but able to think clearly and solve day-to-day problems
	4	Somewhat forgetful, and has a little difficulty when trying to think or solve day-to-day problems
	5	Very forgetful, and has great difficulty when trying to think or solve day-to-day problems
	6	Unable to remember anything at all, and unable to think, or solve day-to-day problems
Pain	1	Free of pain and discomfort
	2	Mild to moderate pain that prevents no activities
	3	Moderate pain that prevents a few activities
	4	Moderate to severe pain that prevents some activities
	5	Severe pain that prevents most activities

tasks were undertaken with a version of the visual analogue scale (VAS) that uses a visual aid known as the feeling thermometer. Another three states were valued using VAS and standard gamble (SG) in order to estimate a power function to transform the VAS values into SG values. MAUT enabled the developers to estimate a multiplicative functional form that permits a limited degree of interaction between dimensions (Table 7.5). This function was found to predict the values for 73 out of sample health states with a mean difference of 0.008 and a mean absolute difference of 0.087. It generates a score range from 1.00 down to −0.36.

HUI3 has been valued in France using the original methods on a sample of 365 members of the general population aged 20–65 (Le Gales *et al.* 2002). The authors found that the French results were similar to those obtained in Canada.

The HUI3 is available in at least 15 languages and can be obtained from the developers for a survey administration fee. Further information can be found at http://www.healthutilities.com.

7.3.3 **The 15D**

This measure originally had 12 dimensions but was revised upwards to 15 dimensions (Sintonen and Pekurinen 1993). The dimensions were developed in part from a review of Finnish policy documents. Further revisions in response to feedback have resulted in the 15D.2, which is the recommended version for future applications (Sintonen 1994).

Table 7.5 HUI3 Canadian scoring algorithms

HUI3 single attribute utility functions

Level	Vision	Hearing	Speech	Ambulation	Dexterity	Emotion	Cognition	Pain
1	1.00	1.00	1.00	1.00	1.00	1.00	1.00	1.00
2	0.95	0.86	0.82	0.83	0.88	0.91	0.86	0.92
3	0.73	0.71	0.67	0.67	0.73	0.73	0.92	0.77
4	0.59	0.48	0.41	0.36	0.45	0.33	0.70	0.48
5	0.38	0.32	0.00	0.16	0.20	0.00	0.32	0.00
6	0.00	0.00		0.00	0.00		0.00	

HUI3 multiattribute utility function on dead–healthy scale

Vision		Hearing		Speech		Ambulation		Dexterity		Emotion		Cognition		Pain	
x_1	b_1	x_1	b_1	x_1	b_1	x_1	b_1	x_1	b_1	x_1	b_1	x_1	b_1	x_1	b_1
1	1.00	1	1.00	1	1.00	1	1.00	1	1.00	1	1.00	1	1.00	1	1.00
2	0.98	2	0.95	2	0.94	2	0.93	2	0.95	2	0.95	2	0.92	2	0.96
3	0.89	3	0.89	3	0.89	3	0.86	3	0.88	3	0.85	3	0.95	3	0.90
4	0.84	4	0.80	4	0.81	4	0.73	4	0.76	4	0.64	4	0.83	4	0.77
5	0.75	5	0.74	5	0.68	5	0.65	5	0.65	5	0.46	5	0.60	5	0.55
6	0.61	6	0.61	6		6	0.58	6	0.56			6	0.42		

Where x_n is the attribute level and b_n is the attribute utility score

Formula (dead–perfect health scale) $u^* = 1.371(b_1 \times b_2 \times b_3 \times b_4 \times b_5 \times b_6 \times b_6 \times b_7 \times b_8) - 0.371$

Where u^* is the utility of a chronic health state[1] on a utility scale where dead[2] has a utility of 0.00 and healthy has a utility of 1.00.

[1] Chronic states and healthy states are defined as lasting for a lifetime.

[2] Dead is defined as intermediate.

7.3.3.1 Descriptive system

The 15 dimensions are *mobility, vision, hearing, breathing, sleeping, eating, speech, elimination, usual activities, mental function, discomfort and symptoms, depression, distress, vitality,* and *sexual activity* (see Table 7.6). Each dimension has either four or five levels; therefore, the classification is able to define billions of health states. Patients are classified by a self-completed questionnaire, which asks them to indicate their level of health on each of the 15 dimensions.

7.3.3.2 Valuation

Health state values are estimated from a simple additive formula, where a value is assigned to each dimension level, multiplied by a weight representing the relative importance of that dimension, and summed to derive a single index. The valuation of the 15D.2 has been based on the survey of five random samples of the Finnish general population of 500 each (from response rates of 43, 46, 45, 52, and 72 per cent) (Sintonen 1994). The valuation method was a variant of a VAS where respondents are asked to regard the scale as having ratio properties. MAUT was used to estimate an additive function. It produces a score range of 1.0 down to 0.11. Permission to use the 15D.2 and its scoring algorithm must be obtained from Professor Sintonen (see http://www.15d-instruments.net/15d).

7.3.4 **EQ-5D**

This instrument was developed by a multidisciplinary group of researchers from seven research centres across five European countries (EuroQol group 1990). The original version of the instrument had six dimensions and was developed from a review of existing health status measures at the time. Kind (1996) has described the process as one where '. . . researchers principally drew on their own expertise and the evidence available from the literature in order to determine the dimensions of interest'. The aim was to develop an instrument that addressed a 'core' of domains common to other GPBMs and which reflected the most important concerns of patients themselves. The first version had six dimensions, but the energy dimension was dropped following empirical work to suggest that it did not have a significant impact on health state valuation (Brooks 1996). It is the simplest of the six GPBMs reviewed here and was originally intended to be used alongside more specific instruments. It has been translated into 169 languages. A five-level version (EQ-5D-5L) has recently been developed and is starting to be adopted by researchers around the world (Herdman *et al.* 2011). The following section describes both versions.

7.3.5 **EQ-5D-3L**

7.3.5.1 Descriptive system

The five dimensions of the EQ-5D are *mobility, self-care, usual activities, pain/discomfort*, and *anxiety/depression* (Table 7.7). They each have three levels and together define 243 health states. Patients are classified onto the EQ-5D by a simple one-page questionnaire that can be administered by post, via telephone, or by face-to-face interviews. It takes about a minute to complete for the average responder, though older

Table 7.6 Child generic preference-based measures

	HUI 2	16D	17D	AQoL-6D Adolescent	EQ-5D-Y	CHU9D
Country of origin	Canada	Finland	Finland	Australia	UK	UK
Age range (year)	≥5, aged 5–8 use proxy	12–15	8–11, younger than 8 years old use proxy	Adolescents	8–15, aged 4–7 use proxy	7–17
Respondent	Self-assess/interviewer-administered/proxy-assess	Self-assess/interviewer-administered/proxy-assess	Interviewer-administered/proxy-assess	Self-assess	Self-assess/proxy-assess	Self-assess/proxy-assess
Dimensions	7	16	17	6 (20 items)	5	9
Response levels	3–5	5	5	4–6	3	5
Health states defined	24,000	1.5×10^{11}	7.6×10^{11}	7.8×10^{13}	243	1,953,125
Physical						
Physical ability/vitality/coping/control		1	1	3		1
Body function/self-care	1	1	1	1	1	1
Dexterity						
Pain/discomfort	1	1	1	3	1	1
Senses	1	2	2	2		
Usual activities/school/hobbies	1	1	1	2	1	2
Mobility/walking	1	1	1	1	1	

(continued)

Table 7.6 Continued

	HUI 2	16D	17D	AQoL-6D Adolescent	EQ-5D-Y	CHU9D
Communication	1	1	1	1		
Breathing		1	1			
Elimination		1	1			
Self-image (physical appearance)		1	1			
Concentration			1			
Fertility	1					
Dimension of Psychosocial						
Sleeping		1	1			1
Psychological	1	2	2	4	1	3
Cognition	1	1	1			
Social, friends, or family function/relationships		1	1	3		

Note: Values in the tables are number of items. Adapted from from Chen G and Ratcliffe J, 'A Review of the Development and Application of Generic Multi-Attribute Utility Instruments for Paediatric Populations', *PharmacoEconomics*, Volume 33, Issue 10, pp. 1013–28, Copyright © 2015 Springer International Publishing Switzerland, with permission from Springer.

Table 7.7 EQ-5D classification

Dimension	Level	Description
Mobility	1	I have no problems walking about
	2	I have some problems walking about
	3	I am confined to bed
Self-Care	1	I have no problems with self-care
	2	I have some problems washing or dressing myself
	3	I am unable to wash or dress myself
Usual activities	1	I have no problems with performing usual activities (e.g. work, study, housework, family, or leisure activities)
	2	I have some problems with performing usual activities
	3	I am unable to perform usual activities
Pain/discomfort	1	I have no pain or discomfort
	2	I have moderate pain or discomfort
	3	I have extreme pain or discomfort
Anxiety/depression	1	I am not anxious or depressed
	2	I am moderately anxious or depressed
	3	I am extremely anxious or depressed

people may take longer. The EQ-5D is sometimes presented as having a sixth question, the EQ-VAS, but this is not a preference-based measure and tends to be used rather less than the preference-based index estimated from the five items (Chapter 4).

7.3.5.2 Valuation

The most widely used scoring algorithm has been estimated from a valuation survey that was undertaken by the UK Measurement and Valuation of Health (MVH) group at York. They developed a variant of the time trade-off (TTO) to be used in an interview survey of 3,395 members of the UK general population (a response rate of 56 per cent). Respondents were interviewed in their own home to value 13 hypothetical EQ-5D states using VAS followed by TTO. Across respondents, a total of 43 EQ-5D states were valued in this way. Regression techniques were used to model these data to estimate additive functions, with decrements for the moderate and severe dysfunctional categories of the five dimensions, a constant term for any kind of dysfunction, and the dummy term 'N3' for whenever any of the dimensions are at the worst sever-ity level (Table 7.8) (Dolan 1997). Separate UK TTO algorithms are available for the whole population and by age and sex groups, though these are rarely used. The UK TTO algorithm results in nearly one-third of states having a negative value, with a lowest value of −0.59.

There are value sets available in 18 countries (including USA, Spain, Japan, Netherlands, Singapore, and many others), which were obtained using either a VAS rating scale (e.g. van Agt *et al.* 1994; Badia *et al.* 1995; Selai and Rosser 1995) or TTO (Tsuchiya *et al.* 2002; Badia *et al.* 2001; Shaw *et al.* 2005). The US survey was the larg-est of these, with over 3,773 respondents (a response rate of 59 per cent). The TTO valuations have been shown to differ between many of the countries, which suggests that country-specific values should be used, where possible, for national applications.

There has also been a valuation using rankings based on an analysis of existing data from the UK and US valuation surveys (Salomon 2003; Craig *et al.* 2009). More recently, discrete choice experiments (DCEs) with duration have been successfully used to value the EQ-5D in Canada (Bansback *et al.* 2012), Australia, (Viney *et al.* 2014) and the United Kingdom (Mulhern *et al.* 2014) (see Chapter 6 for description of the method).

The EuroQol group has placed the EQ-5D in the public domain, though it is neces-sary to obtain permission to use it by going to http://www.euroqol.org.

7.3.6 **EQ-5D-5L**

7.3.6.1 **Descriptive system**

As a response to concerns with the insensitivity of the three-level version, the EuroQol group has developed a five-level version (Table 7.9). It has the same dimensions but with minor changes in wording to *mobility* ('confined to bed' replaced by 'unable to walk') and *usual activities* (from 'performing' to 'doing'). Five levels were achieved by incorporating 'slightly' between 'no problem' and 'moderately', and 'severe' between 'moderate' and 'unable' or 'extreme'. This version generates 3,125 states in total. Initial evidence suggests that the EQ-5D-5L reduces to some extent the proportion of re-sponses reporting no problems (i.e. level 1 for all dimensions).

7.3.6.2 **Valuation**

An interim tariff was estimated from mapping the EQ-5D-5L onto the three-level ver-sion, in order to be able to use it while a value set was being developed (van Hout *et al.* 2012). This mapping function will continue to have relevance for researchers after an EQ-5D-5L value set is available for those wishing to achieve consistency with previous studies using the EQ-5D-3L. The EuroQol group has been developing a valu-ation protocol for valuing the EQ-5D-5L based on an extensive programme of work. To overcome the concerns with the valuation of states worse than dead described in Chapter 4, a new composite variant has been adopted that uses conventional TTO for states better than dead and lead-time TTO for states worse than dead. Initial at-tempts to collect TTO data online failed to produce data of sufficient quality (Oppe *et al.* 2013), and so a computer-assisted version called the EQ-VT has been developed (which at the time of writing continues to be modified).

Table 7.8 EQ-5D scoring algorithm

Full health	1.00
Constant	−0.081
Mobility	
Level 2	0.069
Level 3	0.314
Self-care	
Level 2	0.104
Level 3	0.214
Usual activity	
Level 2	0.036
Level 3	0.094
Pain/discomfort	
Level 2	0.123
Level 3	0.386
Anxiety/depression	
Level 2	0.071
Level 3	0.236
N3	0.269

EuroQol time trade-off scores are calculated by subtracting the relevant coefficients from 1.00. The constant term is used if there is any dysfunction at all. The N3 term is used if any dimension is at level 3. The term for each dimension is selected based on the level of that dimension. The algorithm for computing scores is quite straightforward. For example, for state 12123:

Full health	1.000
Constant term (for any dysfunctional health state)	−0.081
Mobility (level 1)	−0
Self-care (level 2)	−0.104
Usual activities (level 1)	−0
Pain or discomfort (level 2)	−0.123
Anxiety or depression (level 3)	−0.236
N3 (level 3 occurs within at least one dimension)	−0.269
Therefore the estimated value for 12123 is	0.187

Contact developers for application details and use registration.

Table 7.9 EQ-5D-5L classification

Dimension	Level	Description
Mobility	1	I have no problems walking about
	2	I have slight problems walking about
	3	I have moderate problems walking about
	4	I have severe problems walking about
	5	I am unable to walk about
Self-Care	1	I have no problems with washing or dressing myself
	2	I have slight problems washing or dressing myself
	3	I have moderate problems with washing or dressing myself
	4	I have severe problems with washing or dressing myself
	5	I am unable to wash or dress myself
Usual activities	1	I have no problems with doing my usual activities (e.g. work, study, housework, family, or leisure activities)
	2	I have slight problems with doing my usual activities
	3	I have moderate problems with doing by usual activities
	4	I have severe problems with my usual activities
	5	I am unable to do my usual activities
Pain/discomfort	1	I have no pain or discomfort
	2	I have slight pain or discomfort
	3	I have moderate pain or discomfort
	4	I have severe pain or discomfort
	5	I have extreme pain or discomfort
Anxiety/depression	1	I am not anxious or depressed
	2	I am slightly anxious or depressed
	3	I am moderately anxious or depressed
	4	I am severely anxious or depressed
	5	I am extremely anxious or depressed

Contact developers for application details and use registration.

An English valuation survey of the EQ-5D-5L recruited 1,000 members of the general public (selected at random from residential codes); they valued 10 states by TTO and seven DCE pairs which were administered by interviewers in the respondent's own home, using the EQ-VT computer-assisted programme (Devlin *et al.* 2016). The TTO task for states better than dead specified 10 years in the ill health state (i.e. same as the MVH protocol). For states worse than dead, another 10 years of full health was added to the start (i.e. lead time) for participants to trade (see Chapter 4 for details). The final data set used in the modelling excluded 23 respondents who gave all 10 health states the same TTO value, and 61 respondents who valued the worse state, 55555, at no lower than the TTO value they gave to the mildest health state included in their block.

The remaining 912 participants provided the data form analysis. The TTO values exhibited substantial spikes at 1, 0.5, 0, and −1 at the individual level, but the mean health state values correlated highly with the severity of the state. The TTO data were subjected to various manipulations to deal with these spikes and other concerns with the data:

◆ It was accepted that those who used up their lead time (i.e. −1.0) may have given lower values (e.g. with more lead time to use), therefore it was assumed that the values had been censored at −1.0, and so could go below −1.0.

◆ The data were also assumed to be censored at 1.0. This is not common practice in the analyses of preference data, but the authors argued that current assumptions of normality are violated at the upper end as participants can mistakenly give values below 1.0, but not above 1.0. Allowing for censoring is one method for addressing this problem.

◆ Those individuals with more than two values at zero and no negative values were assumed to have been reluctant to use the task for states worse than dead (perhaps due the complexity of the task) and their true values could be negative. This was addressed by assuming the values are censored at zero (150 individuals).

◆ For those individuals with more than one negative value, but who valued state 55555 at zero or more, the value was assumed to be censored (n = 27), which increased the average values for the negative states to zero or more.

◆ Lastly, to improve the precision and consistency of the coefficients, the TTO data were then combined with the DCE data using a common maximum likelihood estimator (see Chapter 5 for a description of the method).

The least restrictive model was fitted, but with separate parameters for each level below the baseline. No interaction terms were found to signficiantly improve the model. However, heterogeneity was found in the relationship between state severity and utility, and the researchers fitted three latent groups. The final English value set (at the time of going to press) is presented in Table 7.10 (from Devlin *et al.* 2016). The complexity and subjectivity of some of these manipulations need to be subject to full and independent review. At the time of going to press, this survey has been replicated in a number of other countries, though the results were not available.

7.3.7 **SF-6D**

The SF-6D was developed by a team at the University of Sheffield (Brazier *et al.* 1998, 2002) as a means of taking advantage of the most widely used health status measure in the world at the time, the SF-36. The SF-36 was originally developed from the tools used in the RAND Health Insurance Experiment and has been refined in a series of medical outcomes studies (Ware 2000). The original SF-36 yields scores across eight dimensions and two summary scores. The British team developed the SF-6D

Table 7.10 EQ-5D-5L scoring algorithm

		Central estimate	Standard Deviation	Value for health state 23245
Constant		1.000		1.000
Mobility	slight	0.051	0.004	0.051
	moderate	0.063	0.004	
	severe	0.212	0.006	
	unable	0.275	0.006	
Self-care	slight	0.057	0.004	0.076
	moderate	0.076	0.004	
	severe	0.181	0.005	
	unable	0.217	0.005	
Usual activities	slight	0.051	0.004	0.051
	moderate	0.067	0.004	
	severe	0.174	0.005	
	unable	0.190	0.005	
Pain/discomfort	slight	0.060	0.004	0.276
	moderate	0.075	0.005	
	severe	0.276	0.007	
	extreme	0.341	0.008	
Anxiety/depression	slight	0.079	0.004	0.301
	moderate	0.104	0.005	
	severe	0.296	0.007	
	extreme	0.301	0.007	
Probability (group 1)		0.397	0.019	$0.397 \times 0.427 + 0.270$
Probability (group 2)		0.270	0.018	$\times\ 0.939 + 0.333 \times$
Probability (group 3)		0.333	0.018	1.635
Slope (group 1)		0.427	0.031	$= 0.9675$
Slope (group 2)		0.939	0.067	
Slope (group 3)		1.635	0.017	
The value for health state 23245				$1 - 0.9675 \times (0.051 + 0.076 + 0.051 + 0.276 + 0.301)$ $= 0.270$

health state classification from the SF-36 to make it amenable to valuation. There is an SF-6D based on the 36-item version of the survey (Brazier *et al.* 2002) and another based on the 12-item version (Brazier and Roberts 2004). A new version of the SF-6 has recently been developed to overcome some of the problems identified with this first version: inconsistencies in some coefficients, and the role limitation dimension only having two levels that use the SF-36 version 2 (Brazier *et al.* 2015; Mulhern *et al.* 2015).

7.3.7.1 Descriptive system

The SF-6D has six dimensions: *physical functioning, role limitation, social functioning, pain, mental health*, and *vitality*. The number of levels per dimension is between four and six, depending on the response choice categories of the original items from the SF-36. The SF-6D obtained from the SF-36 defines 18,000 states (Table 7.11) and from the SF-12, it defines 7,500 states (see Brazier and Roberts 2004). These can be derived from 11 items of the SF-36 and seven items of the SF-12, respectively, and from either version of SF-36 or SF-12.

Table 7.11 The SF-6D classification (SF-36 version)

Level		Level	
	Physical functioning		**Pain**
1	Your health does not limit you in *vigorous activities*	1	You have *no* pain
2	Your health limits you a little in *vigorous activities*	2	You have pain but it does not interfere with your normal work (both outside the home and housework)
3	Your health limits you a little in *moderate activities*	3	You have pain that interferes with your normal work (both outside the home and housework) *a little bit*
4	Your health limits you a lot in *moderate activities*	4	You have pain that interferes with your normal work (both outside the home and housework) *moderately*
5	Your health limits you *a little in bathing and dressing*	5	You have pain that interferes with your normal work (both outside the home and housework) *quite a bit*
6	Your health limits you *a lot in bathing and dressing*	6	You have pain that interferes with your normal work (both outside the home and housework) *extremely*
	Role limitations		**Mental health**
1	You have *no* problems with your work or other regular daily activities as a result of your physical health or any emotional problems	1	You feel tense or downhearted and low *none of the time*

(continued)

Table 7.11 Continued

Level		Level	
	Role limitations		**Mental health**
2	You are limited in the kind of work or other activities as a result of your physical health	2	You feel tense or downhearted and low *a little of the time*
3	You accomplish less than you would like as a result of emotional problems	3	You feel tense or downhearted and low *some of the time*
4	You are limited in the kind of work or other activities as a result of your physical health and accomplish less than you would like as a result of emotional problems	4	You feel tense or downhearted and low *most of the time*
		5	You feel tense or downhearted and low *all of the time*
	Social functioning		**Vitality**
1	Your health limits your social activities *none of the time*	1	You have a lot of energy *all of the time*
2	Your health limits your social activities *a little of the time*	2	You have a lot of energy *most of the time*
3	Your health limits your social activities *some of the time*	3	You have a lot of energy *some of the time*
4	Your health limits your social activities *most of the time*	4	You have a lot of energy *a little of the time*
5	Your health limits your social activities *all of the time*	5	You have a lot of energy *none of the time*

The SF-36 items used to construct the SF-6D are as follows: physical functioning items 1, 2, and 10; role limitation due to physical problems item 3; role limitation due to emotional problems item 2; social functioning item 2; both pain items; mental health items 1 (alternative version) and 4; and vitality item 2.

7.3.7.2 **Valuation**

A representative sample of 836 members of the UK general population (response rate 65 per cent) was interviewed and asked to value a total of 249 states defined by the SF-6D using the SG (each respondent valued six states). There were 225 respondents excluded for either failing to value the pits state, producing fewer than two values, or producing values without any variation. An SG valuation algorithm has been estimated for the SF-6D by random effects regression methods for the 36-item and

Table 7.12 Scoring for the SF-6D

SF-36	
c	1.000
PF23	−0.035
PF4	−0.044
PF5	−0.056
PF6	−0.117
RL234	−0.053
SF2	−0.057
SF3	−0.059
SF4	−0.072
SF5	−0.087
PAIN23	−0.042
PAIN4	−0.065
PAIN5	−0.102
PAIN6	−0.171
MH23	−0.042
MH4	−0.100
MH5	−0.118
VIT234	−0.071
VIT5	−0.092
MOST	−0.061

These are the published UK scoring algorithms from Brazier and Roberts (2004). See also the Bayesian non-parametric algorithms (see Kharroubi *et al.* 2005).

12-item versions (Table 7.12) (Brazier *et al.* 2002; Brazier and Roberts 2004). The methods and results of this work have been summarized in Chapter 6.

There have been valuations undertaken in Japan (Brazier *et al.* 2009), Hong Kong (Lam *et al.* 2004), Portugal (Ferreira *et al.* 2010), and Brazil (Cruz *et al.* 2011) using the same version of SG. There were significant differences found between countries. A closely related instrument is the US VR-12, which has an algorithm estimated from the UK weights (Selim *et al.* 2011).

An alternative algorithm has been estimated from the UK SG data using a non-parametric Bayesian approach that has been shown to perform better in terms of predictive ability, and overcomes the systematic patterns of overpredicting the poor states and underpredicting the better health states found in the original model (Kharroubi *et al.* 2005). It results in a lowest score of 0.2. A model has also been estimated from the rank data that was found to generate weights similar to those from SG data (McCabe *et al.* 2006). There is an algorithm estimated for the SF-6D using DCE in Australia (Norman *et al.* 2013) and a lottery equivalent variant of SG in Spain (Abellán-Perpiñán *et al.* 2012), both of which generate larger ranges in the values than the variant of SG used in the other valuation studies.

The SF-36 and SF-12 are copyrighted and can be obtained from the Medical Outcomes Trust and Quality Metric. The SF-6D algorithms are readily available and free for non-commercial applications (see https://www.shef.ac.uk/scharr/sections/heds/mvh/sf-6d for UK algorithms).

7.3.8 SF-6D Version 2 (V2)

Version 2 was developed in response to concerns that the index score does not cover the same score range as other widely used measures such as EQ-5D and HUI3. This seems to be a result of the descriptive system (e.g. Brazier *et al.* 2004) and the use of the two-stage SG valuation methodology (Abellán-Perpiñán *et al.* 2012). It was decided to revisit the item selection from the SF-36 and also to address the ambiguity in the *physical functioning* levels (between 'moderate activities' and 'bathing and dressing'), the confusion of positive wording on one item (i.e. *vitality*), and the crudeness of using two level SF-36 V1 *role limitation* items. An international SF-6D development group reviewed the decisions made using the results of new psychometric analyses and a new version of the SF-6D was constructed (Brazier *et al.* 2015; Mulhern *et al.* 2015). The group also adopted a variant of DCE with duration to estimate a scoring algorithm.

7.3.8.1 Description

It has the same dimensions as before, except: *physical functioning* has five levels (removing 'limited a lot in bathing and dressing'); *role limitation* uses the five levels of SF-36 version 2; *pain* is the *bodily pain* item (rather than the one concerned with interference with work); and 'feeling full of energy' has been replaced with 'worn out' (Brazier *et al.* 2015) (see Table 7.13). It defines 18,750 health states in total (5*5*5*6*5*5). The SF-6D is derived from the SF-36 version 2.

7.3.8.2 Valuation

The group adopted DCE with a duration attribute (set at 1, 4, 7, and 10 years) as the method of valuation to replace SG, using methods successfully applied to value the SF-6D (Norman *et al.* 2013) and EQ-5D (Bansback *et al.* 2012; Viney *et al.* 2014; Mulhern *et al.* 2014). A preliminary UK survey used 300 health state pairs with duration selected using d-optimal methods from Ngene software that was developed for designing choice experiments (Choice Metrics 2014). The survey was completed by 3,000 members of the general population, representative in terms of age and gender. The algorithm is being finalized for the United Kingdom, but initial results suggest that the coefficients are generally larger, resulting in a larger range of values (1.0 down to −0.718). Similar valuation surveys are currently planned for the United States, Canada,

Table 7.13 The SF-6D classification V2

Level	Physical functioning	Level	Pain
1	Limited in vigorous activities (such as running, lifting heavy objects, participating in strenuous sports) not at all	1	No pain
2	Limited in vigorous activities a little	2	Very mild pain
3	Limited in moderate activities (such as moving a table, pushing a vacuum cleaner, bowling, or playing golf) a little	3	Mild pain
4	Limited in moderate activities a lot	4	Moderate pain
5	Limited in bathing a dressing a lot	5	Severe pain
		6	Very severe pain
	Role limitation		**Mental health**
1	Accomplish less than you would like (at work or during other regular daily activities as a result of your physical health or emotional problems) none of the time	1	Depressed or nervous none of the time
2	Accomplish less than you would like a little of the time	2	Depressed or nervous a little of the time
3	Accomplish less than you would like some of the time	3	Depressed or nervous some of the time
4	Accomplish less than you would like most of the time	4	Depressed or nervous most of the time
5	Accomplish less than you would like all of the time	5	Depressed or nervous all of the time
	Social functioning		**Vitality**
1	Social activities are limited none of the time	1	Tired none of the time
2	Social activities are limited a little of the time	2	Tired a little of the time
3	Social activities are limited some of the time	3	Tired some of the time
4	Social activities are limited most of the time	4	Tired most of the time
5	Social activities are limited all of the time	5	Tired all of the time

The SF-36 V2 items used to construct the SF-6D are as follows: physical functioning items 1, 2, and 10; role limitation due to physical problems item 2; role limitation due to emotional problems item 2; social functioning item 2; pain item 1; mental health items 1 and 4; and vitality item 3.

Australia, Portugal, and Brazil. For the final V2 algorithm, go to https://www.shef.ac.uk/scharr/sections/heds/mvh/sf-6d.

7.3.9 The assessment of quality of life (AQoL)-8D

The AQoL-8D is an extension of two earlier versions of the AQoL, now known as AQoL-4D and AQoL-6D (Hawthorne *et al.* 1997; Richardson *et al.* 2004). It was developed in response to the apparent gaps in existing GPBMs, particularly what the authors called the 'psychosocial' aspects such as happiness, relationships, and self-worth (Richardson *et al.* 2015a). It is able to cover a substantially larger number of dimensions than the other GPBMs by using a hierarchical structure (see Fig. 7.1), and the novel use of a multistage valuation process, which is outlined next.

7.3.9.1 Descriptive system

The AQoL-8D differs from the previous GPBMs in that it has a hierarchical causal structure (Fig. 7.1). The 35 items are combined to form eight dimensions: *independent living, pain, senses, mental health, happiness, coping, relationships,* and *self-worth.* A unique feature of this design compared to conventional health state classification systems is that each dimension has more than one item (e.g. *mental health* has eight items). At the next level in the hierarchy, three dimensions come under a *physical health 'super dimension'* and five under a *psychological 'super dimension'.* The AQoL-8D defines the largest number of states of any GPBM with $2.37*10^{23}$. This presents a major challenge for valuation.

The development of the AQoL measures started with a handicap-based concept of QoL: '. . . disutility depends upon a person's capacity to achieve a productive and fulfilling life in their social environment . . .' (Richardson *et al.* 2012). The authors briefly describe the items as coming from a review of the literature, focus groups, and researcher input. Each version has gone through complex psychometric analyses. AQoL-8D used items from existing mental health measures and focus groups consisting of mental health patients and carers to generate an item pool of 250. Further reductions using research judgement resulted in a bank of 133 items administered to patient and general population samples. The data were subjected to a combination of confirmatory and exploratory analyses to reduce the number of items down to 35. While the details of the work are not always clear, the process appears more thorough than in other GPBMs.

7.3.9.2 Valuation

The size and complexity of the classification was dealt with in four stages: (i) MAUT valuation to combine the 35 items into the eight dimensions using a multiplicative form; (ii) econometric models estimated for each dimension to correct the MAUT values; (iii) MAUT valuation to estimate a multiplicative combination of the eight dimensions; and (iv) an econometric correction for the overall MAUT estimates.

General issues regarding the application of MAUT and econometric (or statistical inference) approaches have been detailed in Chapter 6. A novel element for AQoL has been to combine these approaches (Richardson *et al.* 2014b). This was justified on the grounds that MAUT requires strict orthogonality and AQoL-8D contains items and dimensions that substantially overlap and so double count. At the same time, they argue that 35 items is too many for statistical modelling. The modelling in stages two and

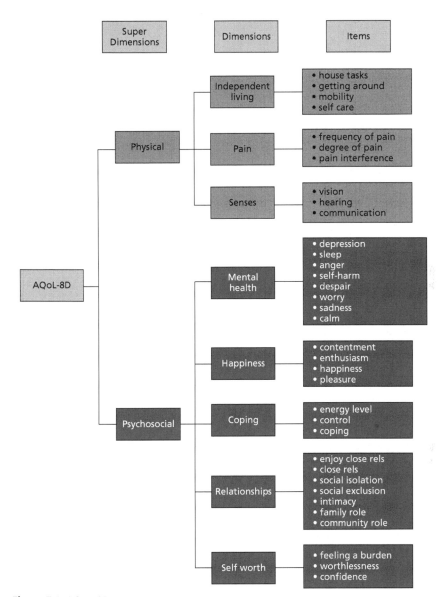

Figure 7.1 AQoL-8D structure.
Reproduced from Richardson J, Iezzi A, Khan M, and Maxwell A, 'Validity and Reliability of the Assessment of Quality of Life (AQOL)-8D multi-attribute utility instrument', *The Patient—Patient Centered Outcomes Research*, Volume 7, Issue 1, pp. 85–96, Copyright ©2013 Richardson *et al.*, with permission from Springer.

four regresses the predicted MAUT scores from stages one and three, respectively, as explanatory variables to the observed mean values to address the latter problem. They argue that the econometric correction to the MAUT estimates in stage four overcomes the double counting and preference interdependencies between items and dimensions.

VAS is used in the first three stages: the MAUT is used to estimate values for the eight dimensions (level 1); the econometric corrections to the dimension models (using 174 within dimension multi-item states) (level 2); and the AQoL multiplicative models across dimensions (level 3). The survey to value 375 multidimensional states in stage four is by TTO, and so the econometric correction process builds in a transformation of VAS into TTO. The sample used to provide the VAS and TTO values are 323 mental health patients and 347 members of the general public aged 18–65 years (no response rates reported). The 65 years or over group was underrepresented in the general public sample, as none of this age were recruited; however, the authors state that satisfactory numbers were obtained in the other age cohorts. The final predictions seem to correlate highly with average observed values.

It is usually recommended that health states contain no more than nine attributes (see Chapter 5), but in stage four respondents have states described using 35 items. The authors attempt to deal with this in the selection of states. Firstly, the levels of most health attributes did not change between states and those attributes whose levels did vary were at the same level. Secondly, the states had to be credible and not contain unlikely combinations of items. Lastly, after the first set of states were valued, respondents were asked to value states immediately above or below those states to make the task easier.

It is not possible to do this work justice in the brief description provided here, so readers are recommended to examine the references at http://www.aqol.com.au/choice-of-AQoL-instrument/58.html. The methods described here require a detailed and independent review.

7.4 Comparison of measures

7.4.1 How do the scores compare between GPBMs?

If these measures produced the same scores, much of the debate about which measure to use would be redundant. However, there is a substantial body of evidence to show that they do not produce the same values when administered to the same patients across many different conditions. Next is a summary of the main findings from a review of 24 studies that compared two or more GPBMs, covering a diverse range of populations and interventions (Brazier *et al.* 2007). This is followed by a more recent comparison across all six GPBMs using online patient panel samples from the Multi Instrument Comparison (MIC) project, covering 10 conditions (asthma, cancer, depression, diabetes, hearing loss, arthritis, heart disease, COPD, stroke) and a healthy sample (Richardson *et al.* 2014a).

The six measures have been found to have moderate-to-high product–moment correlation in the literature (see review presented in the previous edition of this book: Brazier *et al.* 2007). However, agreement is more effectively measured using the Intraclass Correlation Coefficient (ICC) which tends to be lower, with poor to moderate values at 0.3–0.5 in the 24 studies. Across 10 conditions, the MIC project produced values ranging from 0.34 to 0.82 (Richardson *et al.* 2015a), which reflected substantial variation in agreement between the measures, with EQ-5D, HUI3, and AQoL in closer agreement to each other than the others. Differences in mean scores have typically been little more than 0.05 between SF-6D, EQ-5D, HUI3, and the AQoL (Brazier *et al.* 2004; Hatoum *et al.* 2004; O'Brien *et al.* 2004; Richardson *et al.* 2015*a*), though the 15D tends to be higher and QWB lower than the other instruments by more than this amount. This suggests that the mean statistic masks considerable differences between scores and in the distribution of scores at the individual level. For example, the distribution of scores for EQ-5D, HUI3, and 15D have a strong negative skew, 19.3 per cent, 7.2 per cent, and 7 per cent on the ceiling in the MIC patient population (Gamst-Klaussen *et al.* 2016), and sharply declining proportions with decreasing scores (with a number of other modes). SF-6D and AQoL are less skewed with lower proportions at the ceiling, though the proportions do fall off with decreasing score. All five distributions differ in other ways including differences in the score range shown in Table 7.2 and different proportions with scores below 0.4 in the MIC survey.

Below, the key two-way comparisons between GPBMs from the literature are highlighted.

7.4.1.1 EQ-5D vs SF-6D

The comparison of the UK values for EQ-5D-3L and SF-6D V1 has attracted the most papers over the last decade and they have all reported similar results. A comparison across seven patient groups, for example, shows the substantial disagreement between the scores at the individual level in a plot of EQ-5D to SF-6D administered alongside each other (Brazier *et al.* 2004). This partly reflects the different ranges with an EQ-5D minimum value of −0.56 compared with the SF-6D of 0.3. Negative indices on the EQ-5D are associated with values on the SF-6D as high as 0.75. On the other hand, there is a wide range in SF-6D values for those significant numbers with EQ-5D values of 1.00 (i.e. state 11111). Some of these respondents can have SF-6D values as low as 0.56. The discrete steps in the EQ-5D distribution reflect its scoring algorithm, such as the gap between those with 1.00 and those less with than 1.00, and at around 0.45 that reflects the role of the 'N3' term. This relationship was found to vary between conditions (Brazier *et al.* 2004).

7.4.1.2 HUI3 to SF-6D

Comparisons of the HUI3 and SF-6D have also found that similarities in mean scores mask major differences in the distribution by severity, with considerable divergence at the lower end (Feeny *et al.* 2004; Hatoum *et al.* 2004; O'Brien *et al.* 2004). The differences also vary between conditions, with notable differences in vision (0.34–0.66) (Espallargues *et al.* 2005) and hearing (0.58–0.78) (Barton *et al.* 2004). The longer range in the HUI3 has been shown to result in larger mean gains from total hip arthroplasty, with HUI3 at 0.23 compared to SF-6D at 0.1 (Feeny *et al.* 2004).

7.4.1.3 EQ-5D to HUI3

Comparisons of EQ-5D and HUI3 have been more mixed, with some finding HUI3 to have higher intermittent claudication (Bosch and Hunink 2000) and spinal patients

(McDonough *et al.* 2005), one finding them to be very similar in a different study of intermittent claudication (Bosch *et al.* 2002), with another finding HUI3 scores to be lower in patients with impaired hearing (Barton *et al.* 2004) and vision (Espallargues *et al.* 2005). Such variation in findings suggests that differences depend on the condition and other characteristics of the patient group.

These differences between individual two-way studies were supported by those from the MIC project comparing the six measures. These differences have important implications for estimates of the size of impact of medical conditions, with HUI3 having the largest decrement across six of the seven conditions in the MIC project (the exception being depression where it was second after AQoL), followed by EQ-5D, AQoL, QWB, and SF-6D (Richardson *et al.* 2015a). The question to ask is: do these differences matter?

7.5 The importance of these differences

Although mean differences may seem quite small at around 0.03–0.05, differences have been shown to have potentially important implications for the incremental cost per QALY (ICERS) of health care interventions and hence the cost-effectiveness of interventions. The variations in the MIC study for the decrements from full health attributed to medical conditions were between 1.55-fold for asthma and 3.6 for hearing, and are likely to translate into large differences in ICERs. For example, the differences found between HUI3 and EQ-5D in the vision disorder macular degeneration resulted in incremental cost per QALY values of the same treatment of around £20,000 with HUI3, compared to £140,000 with EQ-5D (Bansback *et al.* 2007).

7.6 Why do these differences exist?

Given the different coverage of dimensions and methods used to value the health states (summarized in Tables 7.1 and 7.2), it is not surprising that GPBMs have been found to generate different values. The role of these two components is discussed in the next section.

7.6.1 Differences in dimensions and items

The descriptive systems are compared in Table 7.14 against a list of physical and psychosocial health (adapted from Richardson *et al.* 2015a). The measures differ in size, with EQ-5D-3L covering the least number of domains and AQoL-8D the most. There is preponderance of physical dimensions in EQ-5D, HUI3, and 15D, while SF-6D and particularly AQoL cover more psychosocial dimensions. QWB-SA is mainly concerned with symptoms or problems, and so predominantly covers physical aspects (although it covers more mental health aspects than the earlier version of QWB).

Even within the physical and psychosocial split, the instruments conceptualize health differently. There is a difference between whether the concept is described in terms of capacity (e.g. HUI) or actual behaviour and performance (e.g. QWB). The coverage of symptoms, mental health, and social health is variable. Most measures cover some of the consequences for *usual activities, work, role*, and *relationships* that are usually seen as aspects of participation. The exception is HUI3, which contains symptoms and a number of key impairments (such as *vision* and *hearing loss*) but does

Table 7.14 Content of six generic preference-based measures (number of items)

	EQ-5D	SF-6D	HUI3	15D	QWB	AQoL
Dimensions of physical health[a]						
Mobility/physical activity	1	1	1	1	7	2
Bodily function/self-care	1	1	1	3	13	1
Dexterity			1			
Coping						1
Pain/discomfort	1	1	1	1	14	2
Senses (vision/hearing)			2	2	5	2
Usual activities/work/role related to physical health	1	1		1	12	4
Communication due to speech problems			1	1	2	1
Vitality		1		1	1	1
Dimensions of psychosocial health[a]						
Sleeping				1	1	1
Well-being/depression/anxiety/happiness/calmness	1	1	1	2	4	7
Hope						
Autonomy/control/dignity					1	1
Self-esteem/identity						2
Meaning/achievement						
Safety/security						
Cognition/memory			1	1	1	
Usual activities/work/role related to psychosocial health	1	1		1	12	4
Relationships/social functioning/belonging					2	6
Family						1
Intimacy (including sexual relations)					1	1
Total number of items	5	6	8	15	68	35

[a] values in the table for dimensions are number of items (or symptoms for QWB). Some items cover two dimensions

Adapted with permission from Richardson J et al., 'Comparing and explaining differences in the content, sensitivity and magnitude of incremental utilities predicted by the EQ-5D, SF-6D, HU13, 15D, QWB & AQoL-8D multi-attribute utility instruments', *Medical Decision Making*, Volume 35, Issue 3, pp. 276–91, Copyright © 2014 Sage.

not examine participation, since this is regarded as 'out of skin' and was not deemed appropriate in a measure of individual health preferences. The SF-6D and EQ-5D have *pain* and *mood*, but no other symptoms or impairments. Of course, the fact that EQ-5D and SF-6D do not have dimensions for particular impairments should not matter, provided the impact on health-related quality of life is reflected in other dimensions such as *usual activity, role*, and *social functioning*. The extent to which this appears to be the case and the impact of other differences in coverage of the descriptive systems is examined later in this chapter.

7.6.2 Sensitivity of dimensions

The instruments differ considerably in the number of levels in each dimension and the range of severity that they cover. The AQoL, 15D, and HUI3 define many millions of states compared to the SF-6D with 18,000 and the three-level EQ-5D with just 243. However, do size and differences in range lead to different values?

There is some evidence in response to this question from comparisons of the SF-6D and EQ-5D, where many of the dimensions seem to be tapping the same underlying domains; EQ-5D *mobility* and *self-care* dimensions cover similar concepts to the *physical functioning* dimension from SF-6D, *usual activities* is related to *role* and *social activities, pain and discomfort* to *pain*, and *depression and anxiety* to *mental health*. Evidence from the SF-6D suggests that *physical functioning, role limitations*, and *social functioning* dimensions suffer from having a significant number of respondents at the lowest level for patient groups with more severe problems (Bryan and Longworth 2005; Brazier *et al.* 2004). This 'floor effect' in the SF-6D seems to be reflected in the larger differences between SF-6D and EQ-5D for conditions focused more on physical health problems, such as leg ulcers and osteoarthritis, compared with conditions such as lower back pain and irritable bowel syndrome, which are more focused on *pain*, a dimension that does not suffer from such a floor effect (Brazier *et al.* 2004).

At the other end of the scale, EQ-5D-3L was found to suffer from having a large proportion of respondents indicating no problem (i.e. state 11111), and yet many of these respondents report problems in other measures. The study of seven patient groups found that most people in state 11111 of the EQ-5D had problems according to the SF-6D (Brazier *et al.* 2004). The results indicated that milder problems are getting higher mean values (according to the EQ-5D) than the SF-6D (Petrou and Hockley 2005; Richardson *et al.* 2015a).

The limitation of having three levels per dimension has been raised in the literature (McDowell and Newell 1996). There is evidence that the EQ-5D can be insensitive in some conditions, such as chronic respiratory disease and leg reconstruction, but whether or not the low number of levels caused this problem was not examined (Harper *et al.* 1997; Burton *et al.* 2002). Indeed, there are many more cases where this apparent limitation does not seem to have impaired its sensitivity, such as in an older, chronically ill population (Gerard *et al.* 2004) and rheumatoid arthritis (Marra *et al.* 2005). Nonetheless, the EuroQol group have developed the EQ-5D-5L to address this problem and early findings suggests this does reduce the proportions in level 1 of each dimension, though a significant number remain (Herdman *et al.* 2011).

7.6.3 **Valuation methods**

The SF-6D values were obtained using SG; EQ-5D-3L AQoL used TTO; 15D and QWB used VAS; HUI3 used VAS and SG; and AQoL used VAS and TTO. These three valuation methods have been shown to generate different values for the same health states. As reported in Chapter 4, SG values consistently exceeded those of VAS in most studies, although there is a suggestion of a crossover at around 0.8, with milder health states having lower SG values than VAS rating, even after transforming onto the scale where one is full health and zero is being dead (Dolan and Sutton 1997). Studies reporting TTO and VAS results found a less consistent relationship, although in the majority of studies TTO values exceeded VAS (Green *et al.* 2000).

It has been suggested that SG would be expected to generate higher values than TTO due to risk aversion and positive time preference; this has been supported in a number of studies (Chapter 4). However, one study provides evidence for a crossover in this relationship too, with SG values exceeding TTO up to VAS values of 0.4 on the scale (where 1.0 is full health), but then TTO values exceeding SG values are above 0.4 (Dolan and Sutton 1997). They also found that the difference between TTO and SG depended on the variants of the two techniques being used.

Another source of difference is likely to be the use of 'chained' SG values (Brazier *et al.* 2002; Feeny *et al.* 2002). As described in section 5.2.2.2, the first step involves the valuation of intermediate health states with perfect health and the worst health state as anchor points. In the second step, the worst state is valued using an SG with the anchor points at 'perfect health' and 'dead'. Finally, the value for worst health in step two is used to transform the value for the intermediate states from step one onto the full health–dead scale. There is evidence that 'chained' values may be higher than values obtained directly (see review in Brazier *et al.* 1999). This would mean that the values of the SF-6D would be shifted upward compared with the unchained valuation of the EQ-5D. A final source of difference is the mapping procedures used by HUI3 and AQoL. HUI3 estimated a mapping function between VAS to SG values whereas AQoL combined VAS and TTO values in the econometric correction, which was applied to the multiplicative function for multidimensional health states. The direction of effect for these mappings is not known.

7.6.4 **Descriptive system or valuation method?**

One approach to understanding the importance of the valuation method compared to the descriptive system is to value a set of states using the same method. In one study, EQ-5D and SF-6D states were valued using both TTO and SG (Tsuchiya *et al.* 2006). It found that TTO values for milder states were higher than SG values, while there was some suggestion that TTO generated lower values for poor states. A full valuation of the two measures using a common valuation method was undertaken in a study comparing the three-level EQ-5D and SF-6D, which scored discrete choice experiments using algorithms derived from two Australian general populations (Whitehurst *et al.* 2014). It used the seven-patient data set from Brazier *et al.* (2004) (reported earlier) to compare the original scoring algorithms, but scored by applying DCE-derived algorithms. There was no improvement over the previous study, with similar ICCs (from 0.375 to 0.615). However, minimum values were more similar between the two measures and mean SF-6D scores were significantly lower than the respective mean EQ-5D score across all patient groups, which was a reversal of results using the original algorithms. This would suggest that most of the 'floor effects' in the SF-6D relative to EQ-5D were due to differences in the valuation procedures and the remaining disagreement was due to differences in their descriptive systems.

The MIC project attempted to decompose the differences between the measures into those arising from the descriptive system and those from the preference-based scoring algorithms, including the method of valuation and source of values (Richardson *et al.* 2015*b*). This was done by estimating the scaling effect caused by the valuation method by undertaking a linear transformation of five measures onto the same scale. This was found to account for nearly a third of the pairwise differences, leaving the descriptive system to explain the remaining two-thirds. While the precise estimate of the split between descriptive system and the valuation method may be disputed, this work shows that both account for the differences and that the descriptive system may in many cases be more important.

7.7 Which measure should be used?

The choice of GPBM has been a point of some contention, since the respective instrument developers have academic and, in some cases, commercial interests in promoting their own measure (including one of the authors of this book). Therefore, it is important to have a clear set of criteria for selecting the best measure for use in economic evaluation. This chapter will proceed to describe the criteria commonly used in the literature for comparing measures and their limitations with respect to comparing GPBMs, and then provide an overview of the evidence.

7.7.1 Review criteria

The criteria of practicality, reliability, and validity are important concerns for assessing the performance of any measurement instrument (Streiner *et al.* 2014). In the context of PBMs, it is more complicated because they contain a description of health that is completed by patients and a scoring algorithm based on the elicitation of preferences (usually) from the general public. The interplay of these two components is important for assessing the validity of an instrument.

7.7.1.1 Practicality

The practicality of an instrument depends on the acceptability to respondents and burden of administration from completing the health state classification (e.g. EQ-5D), or the questionnaire used to assign the patient onto the classification (e.g. 19 items for HUI3 and 35 items for AQoL). These can be assessed in terms of how long the instrument takes to complete for different modes of administration and the proportion of completed questionnaires. Response rates may vary between types of populations and there may be some for whom it is not practical or meaningful to respond (e.g. those who are extremely ill or cognitively impaired).

All the GPBMs can be administered using brief and easy-to-use self-completed questionnaires that are practical to use in most settings. They involve asking between five (EQ-5D) and 68 (QWB-SA) questions, and have been estimated to take between 1 to 10 minutes for self-completion (Richardson *et al.* 2014*a*; Seiber *et al.* 2008). As would be expected, interviewer-administered versions take longer. In many studies, completion rates were over 95 per cent for all instruments (Brazier *et al.* 2007). However, completion rates for the EQ-5D were found to be significantly better than the longer SF-6D (based on SF-36) and AQoL in two studies with older people (Gerard *et al.* 2004; Holland *et al.* 2004).

7.7.1.2 Reliability

Reliability is the ability of a measure to reproduce the same value on two separate administrations when there has been no change in health. This can be over time, between methods of administration, or between raters. Published evidence suggests an acceptable degree of test–retest reliability across the measures (Brazier *et al.* 1999; Richardson *et al.* 2014*a*). Variation by method of administration may be a threat to comparability, and existing evidence suggests that there is a difference between self-report and interviewer administration, but not between different modes of self- completion (see overview in Chapter 9). Evidence was found of differences between the assessments by patients of their own health compared with that of health professionals using HUI2 (Feeny *et al.* 1993; Barr *et al.* 1994). Where the aim is to make cross-programme comparisons, this implies that the person completing the instruments needs to be standardized (and where possible this should be self-completed).

7.7.1.3 Validity

Validity is the extent to which a measure captures what it is intended to measure (Streiner *et al.* 2014). The assessment of *validity* is rather more complex, since it involves an assessment of how well the health state classification describes health and the appropriateness of the valuation methods. Both these elements are technically complex and controversial because they involve normative judgements in addition to more technical considerations such as the methods of modelling the data. There is no agreed 'gold standard' and some health economists have been sceptical about the value of trying to demonstrate validity. Thus, Williams suggested that '. . . searching for 'validity' in this field . . . is like chasing will o' the wisp, and probably equally unproductive' (Williams 1995).

The challenge of assessing the validity of measures for many different psychological phenomena, including such diverse things as happiness, fear, experiences of heat and cold, and so forth, has been met in the psychometric literature by the development of various psychometric tests. However, it is important to take into account the valuation component of GPBMs and so these tests have been adapted by Brazier and Deverill (1999) for this purpose.

In economic theory, one source of evidence for testing the validity of preference-based measures is their ability to predict preferences *revealed* in real market transactions. For the field of health care, data on revealed preferences over health states are not available in a useable form for testing validity. As described in Chapter 3, private markets for health care are limited in many countries and where markets do exist, they are distorted in certain ways: by the nature of the agency relationship between physician and patient, and by the insurance market making health care free or low cost at the point of consumption. Furthermore, this would only tap into a welfarist concept of value, namely the extent to which individuals' stated preferences for a state are reflected in their actual decisions over health care, but these decisions may involve other attributes.

Despite these conceptual problems, it is important to examine the validity of a measure, since there is little point in having a practical and reliable measure if it cannot be shown to be measuring the right concept. A three-part approach explained below has been developed for examining the validity of preference-based measures (Brazier and Deverill 1999). The first part is to examine the validity of the health state descriptive system, the second the validity of the methods of valuation, and the third is the extent to which the overall score is shown to be an empirically valid measure of preferences over health states. The key questions for assessing the validity of GPBMs across these three areas are summarized in Table 7.15.

7.7.1.4 Description of health

The validity of the health state classification as a description of health can be assessed in terms of the standard psychometric concepts of content, face, and construct validity, along with the related concept of responsiveness to change (Bowling 2004; Streiner *et al.* 2014).

Content validity is defined as the extent to which the description comprehensively covers the different dimensions of health and is sufficiently sensitive to changes. The most fundamental question concerns the definition of health. A highly influential definition of health is provided by the World Health Organization (WHO 1948), defining it as 'a state of complete physical, mental and social well-being, and not merely the absence of disease and infirmity'. The key aspects of this definition are its inclusion of social well-being and the emphasis on more than the absence of disease. A more recent definition of health or health-related quality of life (HRQL) by researchers in the field is: 'A person's subjective perception of the impact of health status, including disease and treatment, on physical, psychological and social functioning and well-being' (Leidy *et al.* 1999). Not everyone agrees on the inclusion of social well-being in the definition of health (Torrance 1987).

Most of the dimensions of health likely to be covered by these definitions are presented in Table 7.14, though there is no universal agreement on this list. As is clear from this table, some of the GPBMs cover a comparatively narrow set of dimensions and so might miss important aspects of health, depending on the condition. There is also scope for overlap between the dimensions, particularly for the larger ones. Instrument developers typically assume independence between the dimensions, but this seems unlikely between certain dimensions such as pain or self-care and usual activities. More generally, the structural model underpinning the relationship between dimensions is rarely examined and there has been little empirical testing of dimensionality using techniques like factor analysis (see Chapter 8 for a description). For the AQoL this is explicitly recognized in a causal hierarchy, with the 35 items forming eight dimensions and then these in turn forming two super-dimensions for physical and psychological factors (see

Fig. 7.1). The econometric correction is designed to address the consequences of overlap in preferences between dimensions, but it could be argued that this overlap should be dealt with using a more parsimonious descriptive system.

The selection of content for a measure was traditionally undertaken by researchers with little input from patients or health professionals. These methods would not meet the rigorous standards for the development of patient-reported outcomes measures adopted in more recent years (e.g. Mokkink *et al.* 2010; US Food and Drug Administration 2009). This has begun to change, with the AQoL using some patient interview data, and the latest version of QWB-SA using data collected from focus groups. The ICECAP, a preference-based capability index, was based on interviews with the general population (Grewal *et al.* 2006) (which is reviewed in Chapter 8), as was a recently developed preference-based mental health measure (Brazier *et al.* 2014).

Face validity considers whether the items of each domain appear to be sensible and appropriate, mainly from the point of view of those completing the instrument (Holden 2010). It can be determined using qualitative techniques to establish whether patients, for example, understand the descriptions in the way they are intended to be understood. In health economics, these more qualitative forms of validation have not been widely adopted, but have become essential components in the literature on the development and testing measures of health outcomes (Patrick *et al.* 2010).

Construct validity is tested empirically in terms of the extent to which a measure agrees with other measures or indicators of health. A related empirical test is *responsiveness*, which is the ability of an instrument to measure changes in health. Ideally, these tests should be performed on descriptions in the health state classifications alone, not the preference-based index derived from the measure (Brazier and Deverill 1999), because a difference in health may not translate into a difference in preferences. Respondents may not value the differences sufficiently to trade-off life years. However, testing on unscored items is almost never done and these tests of construct validation are typically used on the preference-based index. The empirical testing of the validity of the index generated by GPBMs is discussed in part 3.

7.7.1.5 Validity of valuation

Assessing the validity of the valuation methods used in the development of GPBMs is highly problematic; there are substantial disagreements in the literature about the most appropriate valuation techniques, and the decision about the source of values, such as whether it should be the general public or patients, is a normative judgement. To help assess the valuation methods, a checklist has been developed by a group of researchers in the field to assess the reporting standards of valuation studies (Checklist for Reporting Valuation studies. or CREATE) (Xie *et al.* 2015). This checklist requires the developers of measures to report the following: the descriptive system used; the health states that were valued (including the method of selection); the methods for sampling the valuation sample; the technique and mode of preference data collection; the study sample; key aspects of the modelling; and the scoring algorithm. This is helpful to understanding what research has done, but cannot answer many of the questions about how it should be done.

The question of which values to use is a normative issue discussed at some length in Chapter 4. For most GPBMs, the values have been obtained from a sample of the general population and this is consistent with the requirements of a number of agencies that use the data. The measures differ in terms of valuation techniques and methods of extrapolation. The main conclusion from the review of the valuation techniques presented in Chapter 4 is that for measures purporting to be preference-based, the valuation technique should present a choice-based context; such as SG (where the choice is between a certain and risky outcome), TTO (where the choice is between some period in a chronic state and a shorter period in full health), or a Discrete Choice Experiment (where the choice is between pairs of states), rather than VAS, which asks about a person's feelings instead of their strength of preference and does not involve any choice. There is, however, considerable disagreement in the health economics literature regarding the best choice-based technique. There is also the issue of the variant of the valuation technique that has also been shown to have substantial implications for the values obtained. There is little agreement on the method of administering the techniques in terms of mode (e.g. face-to-face versus online), use of different procedures for arriving at the point of indifference in techniques such as TTO or SG, and optimal starting points in valuation tasks (see Chapters 4 and 9 for a discussion of these issues). There are also important questions regarding the quality of the data collected as part of the valuation survey, such as the representativeness of the respondents, the levels of missing data, and the extent to which respondents understand or engage with the task. The latter may be reflected in the time taken to do the task and the levels of inconsistency and evidence of spikes at certain points in the distribution (such as around zero).

The methods for modelling of health state preference data are more technical in nature and have been reviewed in Chapter 6 and earlier on in the present chapter. The predictive performance of the final model must be assessed. For two of the measures (i.e. HUI3 and AQoL) there is also a mapping from one valuation method to another that adds further potential sources of error. More evidence is needed on the relative predictive validity of alternative ways to model preference data before it is possible to use this as a means of differentiating between the instruments. However, in Chapter 5 it was argued that existing evidence suggests that statistical inference is superior to MAUT, and that some of the new methods of modelling data seem to offer worthwhile improvements.

7.7.1.6 Empirical validity

Together, the descriptive system and the methods used to value it form the basis for a measure's *empirical validity*. There are two tests for the empirical validity of preference-based measures other than examining *revealed preferences*; one is based on *stated preferences* and the other on *hypothetical preferences*.

A test of *stated preferences* is to administer a GPBM alongside another GPBM and to examine the degree of convergence, but this does become rather circular. Another is to assess convergence against values from TTO or SG directly administered in patients who have completed a GPBM (Richardson *et al.* 2015a). However, we would not expect high levels of agreement since GPBM are valued using general population respondents imagining the state, rather than patients valuing their own health. As shown in Chapter 4, there are substantial differences between them. Nonetheless, we would expect that the score from a GPBM would be correlated with the values of patients to some extent.

Hypothetical tests of validity have dominated the literature to date. Here the researcher must assume differences in preferences, such as patients or members of the general public preferring a less severe state and examine whether this is reflected in the preference-based index derived from the GPBM. The empirical tests used to do this are usually 'construct validity' and 'responsiveness' (e.g. Longworth *et al.* 2014; Brazier *et al.* 2014).

There are two commonly used approaches in the psychometric literature to examine construct validity. One approach is to examine whether it is possible to differentiate between groups thought to differ in terms of their health (known group validity), and the other is the extent to which it correlates with another measure of health (convergent validity). These tests can never prove the validity of an instrument and indeed validity is a question of degree rather than being dichotomous. All this can do is provide some evidence to support (or otherwise) the appropriateness of an instrument as a measure of health in the population of interest. For tests based on known group differences, this depends on the basis for the groupings. Where these are other self-report measures of dimensions of interest (that may not be preference-based), such as scales of mobility or self-care, they can be useful in assessing whether the EQ-5D descriptive system is sensitive to such differences. In practice, studies in the literature often use clinical measures that may have only a weak relationship to HRQL in any case, such as visual acuity, respiratory function, or symptoms of schizophrenia. Great care must be taken to scrutinize the measures being used to establish known group differences or convergence, and to establish that these are themselves appropriate indicators of preferences.

Responsiveness is the ability of a measure to reflect changes in health. This partly depends on the distribution of responses across the levels of the dimensions. A measure with a large proportion of respondents at level 1 or at the worst level of one or more dimension, means it cannot reflect improvements outside this scale. These are sometimes known as ceiling or floor effects, respectively. For example, there has been a concern that significant numbers of responders reporting level 1 across all the dimensions in the EQ-5D limits its sensitivity at the milder end for some conditions (Brazier *et al.* 1993). Responsiveness is usually tested in terms of changes in the preference-based index. There is substantial variability in GPBM scales, with some twice as large as others (e.g. UK scores of EQ-5D scale range is 1.59 compared to 0.7 for SG SF-6D), which will inevitably translate into larger differences between groups or over time, all else being equal. However, this does not necessarily result in the measure being more sensitive to differences or more responsive to change. An approach borrowed in psychometrics has been to standardize the differences for these scale effects using standardized effects sizes to test the ability of a measure, in order to distinguish the signal from the noise (Streiner *et al.* 2014). A standardized effect size equals the difference between groups divided by the standard deviation across the groups (or in some cases a normal population). Responsiveness is usually assessed using the mean change in the score divided by either the standard deviation at

Table 7.15 Checklist for judging the merits of preference-based measures of health

		Components
Practicality		How long does the instrument take to complete?
		What is the rate of completion?
Reliability		What is the test–retest reliability?
		What is the reliability between modes of administration?
		What is the reliability between different raters?
		What is the reliability between places of administration?
Validity	Description	Content validity:
		Does the instrument cover all dimensions of interest?
		Do the items appear sensitive enough?
		Face validity
		Are the items relevant and appropriate for the population?
	Valuation	Whose values have been used?
		Technique of valuation
		Is it choice-based?
		Which choice-based method has been used?
		Which variant, which mode of administration, etc.?
		Quality of data
		Is the sample representative?
		What is the rate of response and level of missing data?
		Is there evidence of the respondents' understanding of the task (e.g. level of logical inconsistency in responses, spikes in the distribution)?
		Are the coefficients for the levels within a dimension logically ordered?
		What was the predictive performance of the estimated model?
	Empirical	Is there any evidence for the empirical validity of the instrument against:
		Stated preferences?
		Hypothesized preferences?

baseline or the standard deviation of the change (Guyatt *et al.* 1987), with the latter known as the standardized response mean. Effect sizes are often assessed against cut-offs for small, moderate, and large effects, such as those published by Cohen (1978) at 0.2, 0.5, and 0.8.

A common assumption in the psychometric literature is that for a given health change or difference, the measure with the larger effect size is better (Fitzpatrick *et al.* 1993; Katz *et al.* 1994). This makes sense when the objective is to minimize the sample size for a clinical trial (e.g. Walters and Brazier 2005). However, when the purpose is to measure the size of benefit between treatments as part of an economic evaluation, it is the absolute value of the change which matters. Where two GPBMs differ, there is no objective means of determining which is right and the use of effect sizes does not help. A GPBM such as EQ-5D would be less responsive than a more narrowly focused condition-specific measure, but this is not surprising as it will be associated with more variability arising from the fact that it is picking up the impact of other conditions. This greater variability does not mean it is a less valid indicator of the value of the difference or change in health. The literature often also reports the statistical significance of any difference between groups or change over time. This is another way of establishing signal to noise, but is largely dependent on sample size.

As shown, this area is fraught with conceptual and measurement problems, but a combination of assessing the relevance of the content and simple tests of construct validity and responsiveness provide some basis for supporting (or otherwise) the validity of a measure in the population of interest. Ultimately, researchers and policy makers want to be confident that the benefits to patients from a treatment that matters to society are being reflected in the measure. These criteria have been summarized in a checklist of questions shown in Table 7.15, and are designed to guide a researcher in the selection of a preference-based instrument for use in an economic evaluation.

7.7.2 An overview of the evidence on empirical validity

The literature on the empirical validity of these GPBMs is already too large to provide a systematic review for this book. Instead, we draw heavily on a recent study of reviews by Finch and colleagues (2015) conducted across the six measures. The majority of published studies reviewed just one or two measures, with very few examples of three or more instruments being compared. For this reason, this review of reviews is complemented by the MIC project comparing the performance of all six measures using an online panel of over 8,000 patients (Richardson *et al.* 2015a).

The systematic search of the literature conducted for the review of reviews identified 30 reviews of measures across more than 30 conditions, covering several hundred studies (Finch *et al.* 2015). However, the vast majority of the evidence was for the EQ-5D (n = 29 studies), followed by SF-6D (n = 12), and then HUI3 (n = 8), with very little on the AQoL (n=3) or 15D (n = 2). The number of studies in each review varied from 5 to 22. This evidence base in part reflects the tendency for more research into the EQ-5D, following the publication of the National Institute for Health and Clinical (now Care) Excellence (NICE)'s preference for EQ-5D in 2008 (NICE 2008). This makes it very difficult to make statements about the comparative performance across the measures. Furthermore, few reviews cover three or more measures.

There is considerable variation in the way reviews report evidence. For example, many reviews did not report whether or not the statistical significance of differences was reported in the original study. Few reviews report standardized effect size (whether or not the original studies reported them). There is limited critical review of the basis for defining groups or changes over time, which are often based on clinical assessment and so cannot be guaranteed to provide a sound basis for the hypothetical differences being assumed in the original studies. More generally, for the reasons given here, any conclusions made by the reviewers regarding relative performance are subjective and may be prone to bias. Only a broad summary of findings is given here (for more details see Finch *et al.* 2015).

Whenever evidence is available, it often supports the performance of GPBMs in many conditions, with differences and changes usually in the right direction and often significant. This includes known group differences between patient populations and healthy populations and between severity groups of patients. The GPBMs have been shown to correlate with one another moderately and more highly in some cases. They have also been shown to respond to hypothesized changes in health for many conditions.

It is difficult to make many comparative statements between the measures, but there are a few findings of note. The first concerns situations where the evidence on EQ-5D suggests mixed or poor levels of performance. Three areas stand out from the literature: the senses of vision and hearing (Tosh *et al.* 2012; Yang *et al.* 2013; Longworth *et al.* 2014); elderly populations with dementia (Hounsome *et al.* 2011); and more severe and complex mental health conditions like schizophrenia and bipolar disorder (Papaioannou *et al.* 2011; Brazier *et al.* 2014). There are other areas where EQ-5D has been shown to be problematic: it was found to be less responsive in rehabilitation patients than SF-6D (Moock and Kohlman 2008), COPD (Harper *et al.* 1997), and in orthopaedic leg reconstruction (Burton *et al.* 2012). The EQ-5D has been shown to perform satisfactorily in many conditions including rheumatoid arthritis, many cancers, depression (Longworth *et al.* 2014; Brazier *et al.* 2014), and was found to be more responsive than HUI3 (Spady and Suarez-Almazo 2001) in musculoskeletal disease and more responsive than SF-6D in liver disease (Longworth and Bryan 2003). However, there is insufficient comparative evidence to draw definitive conclusions between the measures. There are huge gaps in the coverage of evidence across conditions, the quality of evidence is often poor, and there are few head-to-head comparisons.

The MIC project has comparative evidence across six GPBMs and reported substantial convergence between them, with the highest (product–moment) correlations at 0.84 for 15D to AQoL, and the lowest at 0.65 for EQ-5D and QWB-SA (Richardson *et al.* 2015a). The size of differences between the seven patient panel populations and a healthy population was largest for HUI3 for all patient groups except depression, followed by EQ-5D and AQoL, then QWB with 15D and SF-6D last or second to last in all groups (Richardson *et al.* 2015a). Ranking by effect sizes (i.e. dividing through by their standard deviations) resulted in QWB having the largest in six out of seven conditions, followed by 15D, SF-6D, and then a mix between the others with HUI3 and EQ-5D at the lower end. This has implications for sample sizes, but for the aforementioned reasons, it has limited implications for the relative validity of the measures. Finally, the authors adjusted for the differences in the scales by undertaking linear transformations onto a common scale, which resulted in SF-6D and 15D being near the top and QWB and HUI3 near the bottom across the conditions. The range of differences is substantially smaller than for the original values, but for effect sizes this does not provide an unambiguous means of ranking the performance of the GPBMs.

7.7.3 Implications for decision making

The ideal approach to selecting measures for use in clinical trials is to choose the one that appears best for the population of interest in terms of practicality, reliability, and validity. There are other considerations when selecting a measure for use in economic evaluation, whether alongside a clinical trial or in a decision analytic model (see Box 7.1). These include the appropriateness of the techniques of valuation (e.g. TTO versus SG) and its source of values (e.g. general public versus patient). Some policy makers specify a reference case set of methods for economic evaluation that includes the valuation technique, source of values, and types of measure (e.g. generic or condition specific—see Chapter 8 for a discussion of condition preference-based measures). These requirements are reviewed in Chapter 12. Only in the case of NICE is there a strong preference for one particular measure, the EQ-5D.

The rationale for selecting one measure is that the different GPBMs generate different values for the same population. This creates problems for policy makers wishing to make cross-programme comparisons, since it makes it difficult to compare scores generated by different measures. It also creates a practical problem for researchers wishing to synthesize evidence from studies that used different instruments. The NICE solution is to prescribe the use of one measure (in most cases), but there is little agreement around the world on which measure this should be. The problem with this approach is that no one measure covers all areas relevant for health policy. There are special populations where these GPBMs could be argued to be unsuitable, including children (e.g. pre-school, school, and adolescents) and those populations in receipt of social care (Netten *et al.* 2012). Indeed, NICE does not recommend a single measure in paediatrics (NICE 2013) or populations receiving social care (NICE 2014), and has been less prescriptive in public health (NICE 2012). Furthermore, evidence reviewed in the last section showed that GPBMs of health have been found to be inappropriate or insensitive in some medical conditions.

One approach for policy makers might be to select one measure that covers the most domains of health-related quality of life, such as AQoL or 15D (Table 7.14). At present, these are used infrequently outside their countries of origin (Australia and Finland, respectively). Furthermore, these two scales present substantial challenges in the valuation from overlapping domains and size of health states to value (containing well above the five to nine pieces of information recommended in stated preference research). The authors have presented solutions to these challenges that need to be independently validated (section 7.2).

Whichever measure is best, the fact remains that different measures are being used around the world (where there is no international agreement on what measure to use). The most widely used by far is the EQ-5D, with 63.2 per cent of studies employing a

Box 7.1 Selecting preference-based measures

The usual psychometric selection criteria are practicality, reliability, and validity, but these need to be considered alongside the valuation methods and requirements of different jurisdictions.

Practical: All six measures have been found to be practical for self-administration, though shorter measures may be easier to include in trials.

Reliability: All measures achieve similar levels of retest reliability.

Content validity: The aim is to select a measure that covers the dimensions of relevance to the patient population. The shorter measures are more likely to miss dimensions, but the longer measures may suffer from overlap.

Construct validity: There are too few head-to-head comparisons to select one measure over another in many cases. Evidence suggests that EQ-5D (the three-level version) is able to detect differences in many populations (despite the shorter size), but there are some important exceptions (see section 7.7.1.3 for details).

Valuation: Do the valuation methods and source of values meet the requirements of the relevant policy maker (where relevant)? For those requiring choice-based methods this would rule out 15D, HUI3, and QWB, and some jurisdictions require country-specific values. Variations in quality of valuation data have not been explored.

Requirements of jurisdictions: Some policy makers insist on one measure to achieve comparability (more on this in the discussion), but may permit submissions using other measures where this can be justified.

GPBM using it between 2005–10, followed by HUI3 (9.8 per cent), and then SF-6D (8.8 per cent) (Richardson *et al.* 2015*a*). This has been partly led by NICE's preference for EQ-5D. So, should analysts simply adopt EQ-5D to maximize comparability with previous studies? For some conditions this would be suboptimal in terms of validity, so what happens if a researcher decides to use another, more relevant generic (or condition-specific) preference-based measure?

When a different measure is selected, an answer to comparability could be to undertake an empirical mapping or cross-walking exercise between the measures. The details of this method are described in Chapter 8, but essentially it uses a statistical model to predict the preference-based single index score in the desired measure (e.g. EQ-5D) where the measure was not used in a given study. However, where one or other of the measures are not valid for the condition, this would not overcome such limitations. Another approach to mapping has been to estimate an exchange rate between measures using a common valuation method such as TTO with a generic full health upper (Rowen *et al.* 2012). This technique would preserve the benefits of the descriptive systems of the different measures. This alternative approach is also examined in the next chapter.

7.8 Generic preference-based measures of health for children

There are a growing number of economic evaluations of health care interventions in children using QALYs (Kromm *et al.* 2012; Chen and Ratcliffe 2015). The GPBMs reviewed in the previous section were all developed primarily for use in adults, but it has been argued that they are not relevant in their dimensions (content validity) or wording (face validity), particularly for young children (Stevens 2009). Consequently, measures have been developed or adapted for children and here six GPBMs are briefly described: HUI2, 16D and 17D, AQoL-6D, EQ-5D-Y, and CHU-9D (summarized in Table 7.16).

7.8.1 HUI2

The original HUI2 had seven dimensions: *sensation, mobility, emotion, cognition, self-care, pain*, and *fertility*, with three to five levels to each dimension. The first six dimensions were developed from the literature and a survey of parents (Cadman and Goldsmith 1986). The first application of the HUI2 was to childhood cancer, and so *fertility* was added in order to capture the side effects of cancer. The seven dimensions of the HUI2 define 24,000 states in all. Most applications use a six-dimensional version of the HUI2 by assuming *fertility* is normal, and this reduces the number of states to 8,000.

The original Canadian HUI2 weights were estimated from the responses of a sample of 293 parents of school-age children in Hamilton, Ontario, Canada (Torrance *et al.* 1996). The response rate in the valuation survey was 72 per cent, although 29 per cent of those interviewed were excluded because of missing data, poor quality interview, or evidence of confusion with the valuation tasks. The HUI2 has also been valued in the United Kingdom by McCabe *et al.* (2005). They used the descriptive system without *fertility*, and values were obtained from a sample of 450 adults from the general population (rather than just parents). They used the same valuation methods as the McMaster team (see section 7.3.2 on the HUI3) but with different VAS to SG mapping functions (Stevens *et al.* 2005), and estimated an additional function using statistical inference methods, which was found to perform better than the MAUT functions in terms of mean absolute error and root mean error (Stevens *et al.* 2007) (for more details see Chapter 5).

The health state classification system for pre-schoolers (HSCS-PS) was developed by adapting the HUI2 and HUI3 for application to the pre-school children (aged 2.5–5 years old) (Saigal *et al.* 2005). The classification system uses 10 HUI2/HUI3 dimensions (*vision, hearing, speech, mobility, dexterity, self-care, emotion, learning and remembering, thinking and problem solving, pain and discomfort*) and two additional dimensions (*behaviour* and *general health*). Twelve dimensions with three to five levels for each dimension will define 19,660,800 unique health states. There is no published scoring algorithm for this instrument.

7.8.2 16D and 17D

The 16D (for adolescents aged 12–15 years) and the 17D (for children aged 8–11 years) were developed in Finland and based upon the 15D (Apajasalo *et al.* 1996*a* and *b*). They have 14 common dimensions: *mobility, vision, hearing, breathing, sleeping, eating,*

Table 7.16 15D classification

Attribute	Level	Description
Mobility	1	I am able to walk normally (without difficulty) indoors, outdoors, and on stairs
	2	I am able to walk without difficulty indoors, but outdoors and/or on stairs I have slight difficulties
	3	I am able to walk without help indoors (with or without an appliance), but outdoors and/or on stairs only with considerable difficulty or with help from others
	4	I am able to walk indoors only with help from others
	5	I am completely bed-ridden and unable to move about
Vision	1	I see normally, i.e. I can read newspapers and TV text without difficulty (with or without glasses)
	2	I can read papers and/or TV text with slight difficulty (with or without glasses)
	3	I can read papers and/or TV text with considerable difficulty (with or without glasses)
	4	I cannot read papers or TV text either with glasses or without, but I can see enough to walk about without guidance
	5	I cannot see enough to walk about without a guide, i.e. I am almost or completely blind
Hearing	1	I can hear normally, i.e. normal speech (with or without a hearing aid)
	2	I hear normal speech with a little difficulty
	3	I hear normal speech with considerable difficulty; in conversation I need voices to be louder than normal
	4	I hear even loud voices poorly; I am almost deaf
	5	I am completely deaf
Breathing	1	I am able to breathe normally, i.e. with no shortness of breath or other breathing difficulty
	2	I have shortness of breath during heavy work or sports, or when walking briskly on flat ground or slightly uphill
	3	I have shortness of breath when walking on flat ground at the same speed as others my age
	4	I get shortness of breath even after light activity, e.g. washing or dressing myself
	5	I have breathing difficulties almost all the time, even when resting
Sleeping	1	I am able to sleep normally, i.e. I have no problems with sleeping

Attribute	Level	Description
	2	I have slight problems with sleeping, e.g. difficulty in falling asleep, or sometimes waking at night
	3	I have moderate problems with sleeping, e.g. disturbed sleep, or feeling I have not slept enough
	4	I have great problems with sleeping, e.g. having to use sleeping pills often or routinely, or usually waking at night and/or too early in the morning
	5	I suffer severe sleeplessness, e.g. sleep is almost impossible even with full use of sleeping pills, or staying awake most of the night
Eating	1	I am able to eat normally, i.e. with no help from others
	2	I am able to eat by myself with minor difficulty (e.g. slowly, clumsily, shakily, or with special appliances)
	3	I need some help from another person in eating
	4	I am unable to eat by myself at all, so I must be fed by another person
	5	I am unable to eat at all, so I am fed either by tube or intravenously
Speech	1	I am able to speak normally, i.e. clearly, audibly, and fluently
	2	I have slight speech difficulties, e.g. occasional fumbling for words, mumbling, or changes of pitch
	3	I can make myself understood, but my speech is, e.g. disjointed, faltering, stuttering, or stammering
	4	Most people have great difficulty understanding my speech
	5	I can only make myself understood by gestures
Elimination	1	My bladder and bowel work normally and without problems
	2	I have slight problems with my bladder and/or bowel function, e.g. difficulties with urination, or loose or hard bowels
	3	I have marked problems with my bladder and/or bowel function, e.g. occasional 'accidents', or severe constipation or diarrhoea
	4	I have serious problems with my bladder and/or bowel function, e.g. routine 'accidents', or need of catheterization or enemas
	5	I have no control over my bladder and/or bowel function
Usual activities	1	I am able to perform my usual activities (e.g. employment, studying, housework, free-time activities) without difficulty
	2	I am able to perform my usual activities slightly less effectively or with minor difficulty

(continued)

Table 7.16 Continued

Attribute	Level	Description
	3	I am able to perform my usual activities much less effectively, with considerable difficulty, or not completely
	4	I can only manage a small proportion of my previously usual activities
	5	I am unable to manage any of my previously usual activities
Mental function	1	I am able to think clearly and logically, and my memory functions well
	2	I have slight difficulties in thinking clearly and logically, or my memory sometimes fails me
	3	I have marked difficulties in thinking clearly and logically, or my memory is somewhat impaired
	4	I have great difficulties in thinking clearly and logically, or my memory is seriously impaired
	5	I am permanently confused and disoriented in place and time
Discomfort and symptoms	1	I have no physical discomfort or symptoms, e.g. pain, ache, nausea, itching, etc.
	2	I have mild physical discomfort or symptoms, e.g. pain, ache, nausea, itching, etc.
	3	I have marked physical discomfort or symptoms, e.g. pain, ache, nausea, itching, etc.
	4	I have unbearable physical discomfort or symptoms e.g. pain, ache, nausea, itching etc.
Depression	1	I do not feel at all sad, melancholic, or depressed
	2	I feel slightly sad, melancholic, or depressed
	3	I feel moderately sad, melancholic, or depressed
	4	I feel very sad, melancholic, or depressed
	5	I feel extremely sad, melancholic, or depressed
Distress	1	I do not feel at all anxious, stressed, or nervous
	2	I feel slightly anxious, stressed, or nervous
	3	I feel moderately anxious, stressed, or nervous
	4	I feel very anxious, stressed, or nervous
	5	I feel extremely anxious, stressed, or nervous
Vitality	1	I feel healthy and energetic
	2	I feel slightly weary, tired, or feeble
	3	I feel moderately weary, tired, or feeble
	4	I feel very weary, tired, or feeble, almost exhausted
	5	I feel extremely weary, tired, or feeble, totally exhausted

Attribute	Level	Description
Sexual activity	1	My state of health has no adverse effect on my sexual activity
	2	My state of health has a slight effect on my sexual activity
	3	My state of health has a considerable effect on my sexual activity
	4	My state of health makes sexual activity almost impossible
	5	My state of health makes sexual activity impossible

excretion, speech, discomfort and symptoms, school and hobbies, friends, physical appearance, depression, and *vitality*. 16D contains two additional dimensions: *mental function* and *distress*, and 17D contains three additional dimensions: *anxiety, concentration*, and *learning and memory*. The values for 16D and 17D were elicited using a combination of VAS and magnitude estimation methods. The 16D is the first measure that elicits the health states preference weights directly from a school-based adolescent sample (N = 213, aged 12–15 years old). For the 17D, which targets younger children, parents' (N = 115) preferences were used. More details can be obtained at: http://www.15d-instrument.net.

7.8.3 **AQoL-6D Adolescent**

The AQoL-6D Adolescent measure was based on the AQoL-6D that had been originally developed for use in adults (Moodie *et al.* 2010). The AQoL-6D Adolescent instrument consists of six dimensions and 20 items: *independent living* (four items), *pain* (three items), *senses* (three items), *mental health* (four items), *relationships* (three items) and *coping* (three items). The scoring is a power function of the algorithm for the adult AQoL-6D estimated from TTO values for 30 states obtained from a student adolescent sample (N = 279) from the same four countries. For more information go to: http://www.AQoL.com.au.

7.8.4 **EQ-5D-Y**

The EQ-5D-Y is based on the health state classification of the three-level EQ-5D. The EQ-5D-Y contains five dimensions: *mobility, looking after myself, doing usual activities, having pain or discomfort*, and *feeling worried, sad or unhappy* (Wille *et al.* 2010; Ravens-Sieberer *et al.* 2010). An EQ-5D-Y user guide version 1.0 (van Reenen *et al.* 2014) recommends the selection of the EQ-5D version should be based on the age classification of the respondent: for ages 4–7 they suggest a proxy-assessed version; for ages 8–11, an EQ-5D-Y self-completed version; for ages 12–15, the EQ-5D-Y or the (adult) EQ-5D for self-completion; and for ages 16 or older they suggest the (adult) EQ-5D for self-completion. A scoring algorithm for the EQ-5D-Y is currently under development but is not yet publically available. For more information go to the main EuroQol group site: http://www.euroqol.org.

7.8.5 **CHU9D**

The CHU9D was developed in the United Kingdom and, in contrast to the other measures, is not an adaptation of an existing adult measure. It was designed from its inception for use with young people (Stevens 2009). The CHU9D consists of nine dimensions: *worried, sad, pain, tired, annoyed, schoolwork/homework, sleep, daily routine,* and *ability to join in activities.* Although originally developed from qualitative analyses of interviews with school children in Sheffield (England) aged 7 to 11 years, recent studies have also validated the CHU9D for use in older adolescent populations aged 11–17 years (Ratcliffe *et al.* 2012*a*). The original CHU9D scoring algorithm was generated using an SG method in a UK adult general population (N = 300) (Stevens 2012). More recently, an Australian adolescent-specific scoring algorithm (N = 590) has been developed, based upon best–worst scaling (BWS) methods (Ratcliffe *et al.* 2012*b*). More information on the CHU-9D can be obtained from http://www.chu9d.org.

7.8.6 **Comparison of child measures**

These child measures differ from adult measures in terms of the domains they cover, how the questions are worded (even for the same dimension), the number of levels and total number of states they generate, ranging from 243 (EQ-5D) to $7.8*10^{11}$, and the valuation methods (see Table 7.3) (Chen and Ratcliffe 2015). Existing comparisons of CHU-9D, AQoL-6D, and EQ-5D-Y found moderate ICCs of 0.717 to 0.801 (Personal communication; Ratcliffe), but mean utility differences varied, ranging from between – 0.08 to 0.14 compared to CHU-9D (Ratcliffe *et al.* 2012*c*; Chen *et al.* 2015; Canaway and Frew 2013). Little is known about relative performance across conditions.

7.8.7 **Methodological issues**

There are methodological issues around valuation in children and adolescents: the importance (or not) of having child- and adolescent-specific measures, and whose values and methods for eliciting health state values in younger people should be used. The literature in these issues lags behind that in adults, but some interesting research has begun to emerge.

Adult measures can be used in children and adolescents, but a number of the measures have been modified for use in younger populations (e.g. EQ-5D-Y). The modifications have tended to be concerned with activities (like schooling) and minor wording differences, rather than a fundamental change in the dimensions covered. The CHU-9D was the first to be based exclusively on interviews with children (aged 7–12). The argument for this is that it makes the measures more relevant to what matters to children and the wording will make more sense to them. However, no one measure is likely to be suitable across all age groups, which raises problems in patients transitioning between age groups, and those who grow up with a condition into adulthood. Currently there is no consensus in the literature and policy makers have not specified requirements for one or the other, though NICE indicated a preference for standardized measures validated in children (NICE 2013).

There is an important issue of whether to elicit preferences for these child measures from adults, or from children and adolescents. A fundamental question to address is whether or not preferences of special population groups should be used in a health care priority setting. For example, different occupation groups may have different preferences across the dimensions of health, but the allocation of adult health care resources is based on one set of general public preferences. Assuming this question is answered in the affirmative, there may be further ethical barriers in regard to asking children to consider life and death scenarios, as well as a practical concern that children may not understand elicitation tasks like SG and TTO. For these reasons, researchers have tended to revert to adults to provide the values, where there are alternative perspectives that could be taken. These include adults valuing the health states as if they were experiencing them from now onward, or imaging themselves as being in the states from childhood (e.g. 10 years of age until death for the HUI2). There remains a further normative debate to be had about the appropriateness of using adults' values when they have been shown to differ significantly from those of adolescents (though there is no evidence on children) (Apajasalo *et al.* 1996*a*, 1996*b*; Ratcliffe *et al.* 2012*c*; Ratcliffe *et al.* 2016). This is no different from using general population values rather than those elicited from patients or other specially defined adult groups. Children and adolescent's views are increasingly important in clinical decision making, but even here the views of parents continue to be important until adulthood. Further research into the normative issues, the causes for the differences, and the practical implications for decision making of the differences would seem to be warranted whatever perspective is used by decision makers.

There has been some empirical research into the use of preference elicitation techniques in children. The literature is inconclusive about their practicality, with some support for the use of TTO and SG down to age 12, whereas other research found children of that age had difficulty understanding the questions (for a review see Chen and Ratcliffe 2015). An important ethical problem is the anchoring of health state values on the zero to one scale, since this requires the valuation of states equivalent to and/or worse than being dead. Research into the use of DCE (with no duration) in young adolescents found it is more easily understood than TTO or SG, but the values still require anchoring. One approach has been to use DCE or BWS to obtain health state values on a latent scale, and then to anchor them using an external value from adults or adolescents who are able to deal with length of life trade-offs and states worse than being dead (Ratcliffe *et al.* 2012*b*).

7.9 **Conclusion**

This chapter has presented a detailed description of six GPBMs for obtaining health state values off-the-shelf. They have been shown to differ in important ways, in terms of the dimensions of health they describe and the methods used to value them. The selection of a measure should be based on the criteria of practicality, reliability, and validity in the population. The concept of validity has been adapted for preference-based measures, but it continues to be ultimately a judgement in the absence of a gold standard. Furthermore, the need to be consistent in resource allocation decision has led some policy makers to require submissions to use one specific measure, or to choose from a limited selection of measures in a reference case analysis (though these requirements are not always enforced).

Those GPBMs available for children and adolescents have also been briefly described in this chapter. This literature lags behind that for adults and there are additional problems around transition between age groups and eliciting preferences from young people. This chapter has focused on GPBMs, but there are a number of important alternative methods of obtaining utility values reviewed in the next chapter.

References

Abellán-Perpiñán JM, Sánchez Martínez FI, Martínez Pérez JE, Méndez I (2012). Lowering the 'floor' of the SF-6D scoring algorithm using a lottery equivalent method. *Health Economics* **21**:1271–85.

Apajasalo M, Rautonen J, Holmberg C, Sinkkonen J, Aalberg V, Pihko H, *et al. (1996a)*. Quality of life in pre-adolescence: a 17-dimensional health-related measure (17D). *Quality of Life Research* **5**:532–8.

Apajasalo M, Sintonen H, Holmberg C, Sinkkonen J, Aalberg V, Pihko H, *et al. (1996b)*. Quality of life in early adolescence: a sixteen-dimensional health-related measure (16D). *Quality of Life Research* **5**:205–11.

Badia X, Fernandez E, Segura A (1995). Influence of socio-demographic and health status variables on evaluation of health states in a Spanish population. *European Journal of Public Health* **5**:87–93.

Badia X, Roset M, Herdman M, Kind P (2001). A comparison of United Kingdom and Spanish general population time trade-off values for EQ-5D health states. *Medical Decision Making* **21**:7–16.

Bansback N, Brazier J, Davies S (2007). Using contrast sensitivity to estimate the cost effectiveness of verteporfin in patients with predominantly classic age related macular degeneration. *Eye* **21**(12):1455–63.

Bansback N, Brazier JE, Tsuchiya A, Anis A (2012). Using a discrete choice experiment to estimate health state utility values. *Journal of Health Economics* **31**:306–18.

Barr RD, Pai MKR, Weitzman S, Feeny D, Furlong W, Rosenbaum P, Torrance GW (1994). A multi-attribute approach to health status measurement and clinical management illustrated by an application to brain tumors in childhood. *International Journal of Oncology* **4**:639–48.

Barton GR, Bankart J, Davis AC, Summerfield QA (2004). Comparing utility scores before and after hearing-aid provision. *Applied Health Economics and Health Policy* **3**:103–5.

Bombardier C, Raboud J (1991). A comparison of health-related quality-of-life measures for rheumatoid-arthritis research. *Controlled Clinical Trials* **12**:S243–56.

Bowling A (2004). *Measuring health: a review of quality of life measurement scales*. Oxford University Press, Berkshire, UK.

Bosch J, Hunink M (2000). Comparison of the Health Utilities Index mark 3 (HUI3) and the EuroQol EQ-5D in patients treated for intermittent claudication. *Quality of Life Research* **9**:591–601.

Bosch JL, Halpern EF, Gazelle GS (2002). Comparison of preference-based utilities of the short-form 36 health survey and health utilities index before and after treatment of patients with intermittent claudication. *Medical Decision Making* **22**:403–9.

Brazier JE, Jones N, Kind P (1993). Testing the validity of the Euroqol and comparing it with the SF-36 Health Questionnaire. *Quality of Life Research* **2**:169–80.

Brazier JE, Usherwood TP, Harper R, Jones NMB, Thomas K (1998). Deriving a preference based single index measure for health from the SF-36. *Journal of Clinical Epidemiology* **51**:1115–29.

Brazier JE, Deverill M, Green C, Harper R, Booth A (1999). A review of the use of health status measures in economic evaluation. *Health Technology Assessment* **3**:1–164.

Brazier JE, Deverill M (1999). A checklist for judging preference-based measures of health related quality of life: learning from psychometrics. *Health Economics* **8**:41–52.

Brazier J, Roberts J, Deverill M (2002). The estimation of a preference-based single index measure for health from the SF-36. *Journal of Health Economics* **21**:271–92.

Brazier JE, Roberts J (2004). Estimating a preference-based index from the SF-12. *Medical Care* **42**:851–9.

Brazier JE, Tsuchiya A, Roberts J, Busschbach J (2004). A comparison of the EQ-5D and the SF-6D across seven patient groups. *Health Economics* **13**:873–84.

Brazier J, Ratcliffe J, Salomon JA, Tsuchiya A (2007). *Measuring and valuing health benefits for economic evaluations*. Oxford University Press, Oxford, UK.

Brazier JE, Fukuhara S, Roberts J, Kharoubi S, Yamamoto Y, Ikeda S, *et al.* (2009). Estimating a preference-based index from the Japanese SF-36. *Journal of Clinical Epidemiology* **62**:1323–31.

Brazier JE, Connell J, Papaioannou D, Mukuria C, Mulhern B, O'Cathain A, *et al.* (2014). A systematic review, psychometric analysis and qualitative assessment of generic preference-based measures of health in mental health populations and estimating mapping functions for widely used specific measures. *Health Technology Assessment* **18**(34).

Brazier JE, Mulhern B, Rowen D (2015). Development of the SF-6D version 2. HEDS Discussion Paper (forthcoming).

Brooks R, and the EuroQol Group (1996). EuroQol: The current state of play. *Health Policy* **37**:53–72.

Bryan S, Longworth L (2005). Measuring health related quality utility: why the disparity between EQ-5D and SF-6D? *European Journal of Health Economics* **6**:253–60.

Burton M, Walters SJ, Brazier J, Saleh M (2012). Measuring outcome in leg reconstruction and complex trauma—what to use. *Quality of Life Research* **11**:660.

Cadman D, Goldsmith C (1986). Construction of social value or utility-based health indices: the usefulness of factorial experimental design plans. *Journal of Chronic Disease* **39**:643–51.

Canaway AG, Frew EJ (2013. Measuring preference-based quality of life in children aged 6-7 years: a comparison of the performance of the CHU-9D and EQ-5D-Y—the WAVES study. *Quality of Life Research* **22**(1):173–83.

Choice Metrics (2014). Ngene 1.1.2 user manual and reference guide. Available at: http://www. choice-metrics.com.

Chen G, Ratcliffe J (2015). A review of the development and application of generic multi-attribute utility instruments for paediatric populations. *Pharmacoeconomics* **33**:1013–28.

Chen G, Flynn T, Stevens K, Brazier J, Huynh E, Sawyer M, *et al.* (2015). Assessing the health related quality of life of Australian adolescents: an empirical comparison of the EQ-5D-Y and CHU9D instruments. *Value in Health* **18**:432–8.

Cohen J (1978). *Statistical power analysis for the behavioural sciences*. Academic Press, New York, NY.

Craig BM, Busschbach JJ, Salomon JA (2009). Modeling ranking, time trade-off, and visual analog scale values for EQ-5D health states: a review and comparison of methods. *Medical Care* **47**:634–41.

Cruz LC, Camey SA, Hoffman JF, Rowen D, Brazier JE, Fleck MP, Polanczyk CA (2011). Estimating the SF-6D value set for a southern Brazilian population. *Value in Health* **14**:S108–14.

Devlin N, Shah K, Feng Y, Mulhern B, van Hout B (2016). An EQ-5D-5L value set for England. HEDS Discussion Paper Series 16/02. University of Sheffield, UK. Available at: https://www.shef.ac.uk/polopoly_fs/1.546914!/file/An_EQ-5D-5L_Value_Set_for_England_DP_Final.pdf

Dolan P (1997). Modeling valuations for EuroQol health states. *Medical Care* **35**:1095–108.

Dolan P, Sutton M (1997). Mapping VAS scores onto TTO and SG utilities. *Social Science and Medicine* **44**:1289–97.

Espallargues M, Czoski-Murray C, Bansback N, Carlton J, Lewis G, Hughes L (2005). The impact of age related macular degeneration on health state utility values. *Investigative Ophthalmology and Visual Science* **46**:4016–23.

EuroQol group (1990). EuroQol—a new facility for the measurement of health-related quality-of-life. *Health Policy* **16**:199–208.

Fanshel S, Bush J (1970). A health status index and its application to health service outcomes. *Operations Research* **18**:1021–66.

Ferreira LN, Ferreira PL, Brazier J, Rowen D (2010). A Portugese value set for the SF-6D. *Value in Health* **13**:624–30.

Feeny D, Leiper A, Barr RD, Furlong W, Torrance GW, Rosenbaum P, Weitzman S (1993). The comprehensive assessment of health status in survivors of childhood cancer: application to high-risk acute lymphoblastic leukaemia. *British Journal of Cancer* **67**:1047–52.

Feeny DH, Furlong WJ, Torrance GW, Goldsmith CH, Zenglong Z, Depauw S, et al. (2002). Multiattribute and single-attribute utility function: the Health Utility Index Mark 3 system. *Medical Care* **40**:113–28.

Feeny D, Wu L, Eng K (2004). Comparing short form 6D, standard gamble, and health utilities index Mark 2 and Mark 3 utility scores: results from total hip arthroplasty patients. *Quality of Life Research* **13**:1659–70.

Finch A, Brazier J, Mukuria C (2015). A review of reviews of the performance of six generic preference-based measures of health. HEDS DP, University of Sheffield, UK.

Fitzpatrick R, Zeibland S, Jenkinson C, Mowat A (1993). A comparison of the sensitivity to change of several health status measures in rheumatoid arthritis. *Journal of Rheumatology* **20**:429–36.

Gamst-Klaussen T, Chen G, Lamu AN, Olsen JA (2016). Health state utility instruments compared: inquiring into nonlinearity across EQ-5D-5L, SF-6D, HUI-3 and 15D. *Quality of Life Research* **25**:1667–78.

Gerard K, Nicholson T, Mullee M, Mehta R, Roderick P (2004). EQ-5D versus SF-6D in an older, chronically ill patient group. *Applied Health Economics and Health Policy* **3**:91–102.

Green C, Brazier J, Deverill M (2000). A review of health state valuation techniques. *Pharmacoeconomics* **17**:151–65.

Grewal I, Lewis J, Flynn T, Brown J, Bond J, Coast J (2006). Developing attributes for a generic quality of life measure for older people: preferences or capabilities? *Social Science and Medicine* **62**:1891–901.

Guyatt GH, Walter S, Norman G (1987). Measuring change overtime: assessing the usefulness of evaluative instruments. *Journal of Chronic Disease* **40**:171–8.

Harper R, Brazier JE, Waterhouse JC, Walters SJ, Jones NMB, Howard P (1997). A comparison of outcome measures for patients with chronic obstructive pulmonary disease (COPD) in an outpatient setting. *Thorax* **52**:879–87.

Hatoum H, Brazier JE, Ahkras K (2004). Comparison of the HUI3 with the SF-36 preference based single index in a clinical setting. *Value in Health* **7**:602–9.

Hawthorne G, Richardson J, Osborne R, McNeil H (1997). *The Australian Quality of Life (AQoL) instrument.* Monash University Working Paper 66.

Herdman M, Gudex C, Lloyd A, Janssen B, Kind P, Parkin D, et al. (2011). Development and preliminary testing of a new five level version of the EQ-5D—the EQ-5D-5L. *Quality of Life Research* **20**:1727–36.

Holden, RB (2010). Face validity. In: Weiner IB, Craighead WE (eds). *The Corsini encyclopedia of psychology* (4th edn.). Wiley, Hoboken, New Jersey, NY, pp. 637–38.

Holland R, Smith RD, Harvey I, Swift L, Lenaghan E (2004). Assessing quality of life in the elderly: a direct comparison of the EQ-5D and AQoL. *Health Economics* **13**:793–805.

Hounsome N, Orrell M, Tudor Edwards R (2011). EQ-5D as a quality of life measure in people with dementia and their carers: evidence and key issues. *Value in Health* **14**:390–9.

Kaplan RM, Sieber WJ, Ganiats TG (1997). The quality of well-being scale: comparison of the interviewer-administered version with a self-administered questionnaire. *Psychological Health* **12**:783–91.

Kaplan RM (1994). Using quality-of-life information to set priorities in health policy. *Social Indicators Research* **33**:121–63.

Kaplan RM, Anderson JP (1988). A general health policy model: update and application. *Health Services Research* **23**:203–35.

Katz JN, Phillips CB, Fossel AH, Liang MH (1994). Stability and responsiveness of utility measures. *Medical Care* **32**:183–8.

Kharroubi SA, O'Hagan A, Brazier JE (2005). Estimating utilities from individual health preference data: a nonparametric Bayesian method. *Applied Statistics* **54**:879–95.

Kind P (1996). The Euroqol instrument: an index of health-related quality of life. In: Spilker B (ed.). *Quality of life and pharmacoeconomics in clinical trials*, 2nd edn. Lippincott-Rivera, Philadelphia, PA, pp. 191–201.

Kromm SK, Bethell J, Kraglund F, Edwards SA, Laporte A, Coyte PC, Ungar WJ (2012). Characteristics and quality of pediatric cost-utility analyses. *Quality of Life Research* **21**:1315–25.

Lam C, Brazier J, McGhee S (2004). Feasibility, reliability and validity of valuation of the SF-6D health states in a Chinese. *Quality of Life Research* **13**(9):1509.

Le Gales C, Buron C, Costet N, Rosman S (2002). Development of preference-wieghted health status clasifiction system in France: the Health Utilities Index 3. *Health Care Management Science* **5**:41–51.

Leidy NK, Revicki DA, Geneste B (1999). Recommendations for evaluating the validity of quality of life claims for labeling and promotion. *Value in Health* **2**:113–27.

Longworth L, Bryan S (2003). An empirical comparison of EQ-5D and SF-6D in liver transplantation patients. *Health Economics* **12**:1061–7.

Longworth L, Yang Y, Young T, Mulhern B, Hernández Alava M, Mukuria C, et al. (2014). Use of generic and condition specific measures of Health Related Quality of Life in NICE decision making. *Health Technology Assessment* **18**:1–224.

Marra CA, Woolcott JC, Kopec JA, Shojania KI, Offer R, Brazier JE, et al. (2005). A comparison of generic, indirect utility measures (the HU12, HU13, SF-6D, and the EQ-5D) and disease-specific instruments (the RAQoL and the HAQ) in rheumatoid arthritis. *Social Science and Medicine* **60**:1571–82.

McCabe C, Stevens K, Roberts J, Brazier JE (2005). Health state values from the HUI-2 descriptive system: results from a UK survey. *Health Economics* **14**:231–44.

McCabe C, Brazier J, Gilks P, Tsuchiya A, Roberts J, O'Hagan A, Stevens K (2006). Estimating population cardinal health state valuation models from individual ordinal (rank) health state preference data. *Journal of Health Economics* **25**:418–31.

McDonough CM, Grove MR, Tosteson TD, Lurie JD, Hilibrand AS, Tosteson ANA (2005). Comparison of EQ-5D, HUI, and SF-36-derived societal health state values among spine patient outcomes research trial (SPORT) participants. *Quality of Life Research* **14**:1321–32.

McDowell I, Newell C (1996). *Measuring health: a guide to rating scales and questionnaires.* Oxford University Press, Oxford, UK.

Moock J, Kohlman T (2008). Comparing preference-based quality-of-life measures: results from rehabilitation patients with musculoskeletal, cardiovascular or psychosomatic disorders. *Quality of Life Research* **17**:485–95.

Mokkink LB, Terwee CB, Patrick DL, Alonso J, Stratford PW, Bouter LM, de Vet HCW (2010). The COSMIN checklist for assessing the methodological quality of studies on measurement properties of health status measurement instruments: an international Delphi study. *Quality of Life Research* **19**:539–49.

Moodie M, Richardson J, Rankin B, Iezzi A, Sinha K (2010). Predicting time trade-off health state valuations of adolescents in four Pacific countries using the Assessment of Quality-of-Life(AQoL-6D) instrument. *Value in Health* **13**:1014–27.

Mulhern B, Brazier JE, Bansback N, Norman R (2015). UK Valuation of the SF-6D V2. HEDS Discussion Paper.

Mulhern B, Bansback N, Brazier J, Buckingham K, Cairns J, Devlin N, *et al.* (2014). Preparatory study for the revaluation of the EQ-5D tariff: methodology report. *Health Technology Assessment* **18**:1–191.

National Institute for Health and Care Excellence (NICE) (2008,13). *Guide to the methods of technology appraisal.* National Health Service, London, UK.

National Institute of Health and Care Excellence (NICE) (2012). *Methods for the development of NICE public health guidance.* NICE, London, UK.

National Institute of Health and Care Excellence (NICE) (2014). *Developing NICE (social care) guidelines.* NICE, London, UK.

Netten A, Burge P, Malley J, Potoglou D, Towers A, Brazier J, *et al.* (2012). Outcomes of social care for adults: developing a preference weighted measure. *Health Technology Assessment* **16**:1–166.

Norman R, Viney R, Brazier J, Cronin P, King MT, Ratcliffe J, Street D (2013). Valuing SF-6D health states using a discrete choice experiment. *Medical Decision Making* **34**;773–86.

O'Brien BJ, Spath M, Blackhouse G, Severens JL, Brazier JE (2004). A view from the bridge: agreement between the SF-6D utility algorithm and the health utilities index. *Health Economics* **12**:975–82.

Oppe M, Devlin NJ, Hout van B, Krabbe PFM, de Charro F (2013). A programme of methodological research to arrive at the new international EQ-5D-5L valuation protocol. *Value in Health* **17**:445–53.

Papaioannou D, Brazier J, Parry G (2011). How valid and responsive are generic health status measures, such as the EQ-5D and SF-36, in schizophrenia? A systematic review. *Value in Health* **14**:907–20.

Patrick DL, Bush JW, Chen MM (1973). Methods for measuring levels of well-being for a health status index. *Health Services Research* **8**:228–45.

Patrick DL, Burke LB, Gwaltney CJ, Leidy NK, Martin ML, Molsen, Ring L (2010). Content validity—establishing and reporting the evidence in newly developed patient-reported outcomes (PRO) instruments for medical product evaluation: ISPOR PRO good research practices task force report: part 1—eliciting concepts for a new PRO instrument. *Value in Health* **14**:967–77.

Petrou S, Hockley C (2005). An investigation into the empirical validity of the EQ-5D and SF-6D based on hypothetical preferences in a general population. *Health Economics* **14**:1169–89.

Ratcliffe J, Stevens K, Flynn T, Brazier J, Sawyer M (2012*a*). An assessment of the construct validity of the CHU9D in the Australian adolescent general population. *Quality of Life Research* **21**:717–25.

Ratcliffe J, Flynn T, Terlich F, Brazier J, Stevens K, Sawyer M (2012*b*). Developing adolescent specific health state values for economic evaluation: an application of profile case best worst scaling to the Child Health Utility-9D. *Pharmacoeconomics* **30**:713–27.

Ratcliffe J, Stevens K, Flynn T, Brazier J, Sawyer M (2012*c*). Whose values in health? An empirical comparison of the application of adolescent and adult values for the CHU9D and AQOL-6D in the Australian adolescent general population. *Value in Health* **15**:730–6.

Ratcliffe J, Flynn T, Huynh E, Stevens K, Brazier J, Sawyer M (2016). Nothing about us without us? A comparison of adolescent and adult health state values for the Child Health Utility-9D using profile case best worst scaling. *Health Economics* **25**:486–96.

Ravens-Sieberer U, Wille N, Badia X, Bonsel G, Burström K, Cavrini G, *et al.* (2010). Feasibility, reliability, and validity of the EQ-5D-Y: results from a multinational study. *Quality of Life Research* **19**:887–97.

van Reenen M, Janssen B, Oppe M, *et al.* (2014) EQ-5D-Y user guide (Version 1.0). Avaialble at: http://www.euroqol.org/about-eq-5d/publications/user-guide.html. Accessed 12 May 2015.

Read JL, Quinn RJ, Hoefer MA (1987). Measuring overall health: an evaluation of three important approaches. *Journal of Chronic Disease* **40** Supplement 1:7S–26S.

Richardson J, Atherton Day N, Peacock S, Iezzi A (2004). Measurement of the quality of life for economics evaluation and the Assessment of Quality of Life (AQoL) Mark 2 instrument. *The Australian Economic Review* **37**:62–88.

Richardson J, Peacock S, Hawthorne G, Iezzi A, Elsworth G, Day N (2012). Construction of the descriptive system for the assessment of quality of life AQoL-6D utility instrument. *Health and Quality of Life Outcomes* **10**:38.

Richardson J, Iezzi A, Khan MA, Maxwell A (2014*a*). Validity and reliability of the Assessment of Quality of Life (AQoL-8D) multi attribute utility instrument, *The Patient: Patient-Centered Outcomes Research* **7**:85–96.

Richardson J, Khan MA, Iezzi A, Maxwell A (2015*a*). Comparing and explaining differences in the content, sensitivity and magnitude of incremental utilities predicted by the EQ-5D, SF-6D, HUI 3, 15D, QWB and AQoL-8D multi attribute utility instruments. *Medical Decision Making* **35**(3):276–91.

Richardson J, Sinha K, Iezzi A, Khan MA (2014*b*). Modelling utility weights for the Assessment of Quality of Life (AQoL)-8D. *Quality of Life Research* **23**: 2395–404.

Richardson J, Iezzi A, Khan MA (2015*b*). Why do multi-attribute utility instruments produce different utilities: the relative importance of the descriptive systems, scale and 'micro utility' effects. *Quality of Life Research* **24**:2045–53.

Rosser RM, Kind P (1978). A scale of valuations of states of illness: is there a social consensus? *International Journal of Epidemiology* 7:347–58.

Rowen D, Brazier JE, Tsuchiya A, Hernández M (2012). Valuing states from multiple measures on the same VAS: A feasibility study. *Health Economics* 21:715–29

Saigal S, Rosenbaum P, Stoskopf B, Hoult L, Furlong W, Feeny D, Hagan R (2005). Development, reliability and validity of a new measure of overall health for pre-school children. *Quality of Life Research* 14:243–57.

Salomon JA (2003). Reconsidering the use of rankings in the valuation of health states: a model for estimating cardinal values from ordinal data. *Population Health Metrics* 1:12.

Seiber WJ, Groessl EJ, Kristen MD, Ganiats TG, Kaplan RM (2008). Quality of wellbeing—self-administered (QWB-SA) scale: user's mannual. Health services research center, University of California, San Diego. Available at: https://hoap.ucsd.edu/qwb-info/QWB-Manual.pdf

Selai C, Rosser R (1995). Eliciting EuroQol descriptive data and utility scale values from inpatients—a feasibility study. *Pharmacoeconomics* 8:147–58.

Selim AJ, Rogers R, Qian SX, Brazier J, Kazis L (2011). The VR-6D derived from the veterans rand 12 item health survey. *Quality of Life Research* 20:1337–47.

Shaw JK, Johnson JA, Coons SJ (2005). US valuation of the EQ-5D health states: development and testing of the D1 model. *Medical Care* 43:203–20.

Sintonen H (1994). *The 15D measure of HRQoL: reliability, validity, and the sensitivity of its health state descriptive system.* NCFPE Working paper 41, Monash University/The University of Melbourne.

Sintonen H, Pekurinen M (1993). A fifteen-dimensional measure of health-related quality of life (15D) and its applications. In: Anonymous, *Quality of life assessment: key issues in the 1990s*, pp. 185–95. Kluwer Academic Publishers, Dordrecht, the Netherlands.

Spady B, Suarez-Almazor M (2001). *A comparison of preference-based health status tools in patients with msculosketal disease.* Proceedings of the 18th Plenary Meeting of the Euroqol Group.

Stevens KJ, McCabe CJ, Brazier JE (2005). Mapping between visual analogue and standard gamble data; results from the UK Health Utilities Index 2 valuation. *Health Economics* 15:527–34.

Stevens KJ, McCabe CJ, Brazier JE. Roberts J (2007) Multi-attribute utility function or statistical inference models: a comparison of health state valuation models using the HUI2 health state classification system. *Journal of Health Economics* 26:992–1002.

Stevens KJ (2009). Developing a descriptive system for a new preference-based measure of health-related quality of life for children. *Quality of Life Research* 18:1105–13.

Stevens K (2012). Valuation of the child health utility 9D index. *Pharmacoeconomics* 30:729–47.

Streiner DL, Norman GR, Cairney J (2014). *Health Measurement Scales: a practical guide to their development and use*, 5th edn. Oxford University Press, Oxford, UK.

Torrance GW (1982). Multi-attribute utility theory as a method of measuring social preferences for health states in long-term care. In: Kane RL, Kane RA (eds). *Values in long-term care.* Lovington Books, DC Heath & Co., pp. 127–56.

Torrance GW (1987). Utility approach to measuring health-related quality of life. *Journal of Chronic Diseases* 40:593–600.

Torrance GW, Feeny DH, Furlong WJ, Barr RD, Zhang Y, Wang Q (1996). A multi-attribute utility function for a comprehensive health status classification system: health utilities mark 2. *Medical Care* **34**:702–22.

Tosh J, Brazier J, Evans P, Longworth L (2012). A review of generic preference-based measures of health-related quality of life in visual disorders. *Value in Health* **15**:118–27.

Tsuchiya A, Ikeda S, Ikegami N, Nishimura S, Sakai I, Fukuda T, *et al.* (2002). Estimating an EQ5D population value set: The case of Japan. *Health Economics* **11**:341–53.

Tsuchiya A, Brazier JE, Roberts J (2006). Comparison of valuation methods used to generate the EQ5D and the SF6D value sets in the UK. *Journal of Health Economics* **25**:334–46.

US Food and Drug Administration (2009). Patient reported outcome measures: use in medical product development to support labeling claims. Available at: http://www.fda.gov/downloads/drugs/guidancecomplianceregulatoryinformation/guidances/ucm193282.pdf

van Agt HM, Essink-Bot ML, Krabbe PF, Bonsel GJ (1994). Test–retest reliability of health state valuations collected with the EuroQol questionnaire. *Social Science and Medicine* **39**:1537–44.

van Hout B, Janssen MF, Feng YS, Kohlmann T, Busschbach J, Golicki D, *et al.* (2012). Interim scoring for the EQ-5D-5L: mapping the EQ-5D-5Lto EQ-5D-3L value sets. *Value in Health* **15**:708–15.

Viney R, Norman R, Brazier J, Cronin P, King MT, Ratcliffe J, Street D (2014). An Australian discrete choice experiment to value EQ-5D health states. *Health Economics* **23**:729–42.

Ware JE (2000). SF-36 health survey update. *Spine* **25**:3130–9.

Walters S, Brazier JE (2005). Comparison of the minimally important difference for two health state measures: EQ-5D and SF-6D. *Quality of Life Research* **14**:1523–32.

Whitehurst DGT, Norman R, Viney R, Brazier JE (2014). Comparison of contemporaneous EQ-5D and SF-6D responses using scoring algorithms derived from similar valuation exercises. *Value in Health* **17**:570–7.

Wille N, Badia X, Bonsel G, Burström K, Cavrini G, Devlin N, *et al.* (2010) Development of the EQ-5DY:a child friendly version of the EQ-5D. *Quality of Life Research* **19**:875–86.

Williams A (1995). The measurement and valuation of health: a chronicle. Centre for Health Economics, Discussion Paper 136, University of York. Available at: http://www.york.ac.uk/che/pdf/DP136.pdf

World Health Organization (1948). Constitution of the World Health Organization. Basic documents. World Health Organization, Geneva, Switzerland.

Xie F, Pickard AS, Krabbe PF, Revicki D, Viney R, Devlin N, Feeny DA (2015). Checklist for reporting valuation studies of multi-attribute utility-based instruments (CREATE). *Pharmacoeconomics* **33**:867–77.

Yang Y, Longworth L, Brazier J (2013). An assessment of the validity and responsiveness of generic measures of health related quality of life in hearing impairment. *Quality of Life Research* **22**:2813–28.

Chapter 8

Alternatives to generic preference-based measures: mapping, condition-specific measures, bolt-ons, vignettes, direct utility assessment, and well-being

8.1 Introduction to alternatives to generic preference-based measures

The argument for using *generic* preference-based measures of health in economic evaluation is that they enable comparisons between health care programmes, even when they involve different medical conditions and treatments (Gold *et al.* 1996). This is achieved by using a standardized generic health state classification system and a preference-based scoring algorithm for estimating a health state utility value. Generic preference-based measures (GPBMs) are widely accepted around the world for use in economic evaluation to inform health care decision making, including pharmaceutical reimbursement decisions (see Chapter 12).

There is considerable evidence for the validity and responsiveness of GPBMs of health for many common medical conditions (see Chapter 7). Despite this, generic measures are not often used in key clinical trials because they are usually designed to inform licensing decisions taken by agencies, which typically do so on the basis of clinical measures (though there is a strong argument for using GPBMs to inform licensing decisions in order to determine overall effectiveness across the different clinical outcomes and side effects). One solution to this is to undertake mapping (or cross-walk) studies between patient-reported measures, or other measures, of health and generic preference-based measures in order to predict the latter even when they have not been used. Methods for undertaking mapping are described in this chapter.

Problems arise in conditions where a particular GPBM has been shown to be inappropriate or insensitive, such as in visual impairment in macular degeneration, hearing loss, leg ulcers, dementia, and schizophrenia (e.g. Tosh *et al.* 2012; Barton *et al.* 2004; Espallargues *et al.* 2006; Papaioannou *et al.* 2011). This problem can be approached by using another generic measure, for example to use the HUI3 instead of EQ-5D in vision. Another approach would be to devise condition-specific preference weights, using either an existing condition-specific health state classification, where health is described across a set of multilevel dimensions relevant to the condition (and treatment), or by using a bespoke vignette or scenario describing the impact of the condition in more narrative form, where either of these can be valued using health state valuation techniques such as standard gamble (SG) or time trade-off (TTO). There has been a growing cottage industry in developing condition-specific preference-based measures of health (CSPBMs) with a recent review finding 28 such measures (Rowen and Brazier 2014).

The vignette approach uses narrative descriptions of the impact of a condition and its treatment, rather than a standardized questionnaire. It was more prevalent before the emergence of the GPBMs in the 1970s and 80s (e.g. Sackett and Torrance 1978), but continues to be used in economic evaluations and submissions to agencies like the National Institute for Health and Clinical Excellence (NICE), where generic or condition-specific questionnaire data are not available or simply not used (e.g. rare conditions, children) (Tosh *et al.* 2011).

Finally, there has been a growing interest in the measurement of well-being, in particular subjective well-being, to help extend the metrics used to inform government policies beyond economic growth to the less tangible human concerns of quality of life (e.g. Stiglitz *et al.* 2009; O'Donnell *et al.* 2014; OECD 2013). Subjective well-being is now being considered as an alternative measure of benefit in health care (Dolan and Kahneman 2008; All-Party Parliamentary Group on Well-being Economics 2014). This has partly come from a belief that many health care interventions have an impact on things beyond what is traditionally regarded as health such a dignity, autonomy, and meaning. These broader and less tangible impacts of health care may be missed by existing generic measures of health states like EQ-5D or HUI3, and therefore result in an undervaluation of the benefits of health care. At the same time, public sector spending on health care has to compete with other sectors such as social care, education, transport, and environment, which can all claim to influence population well-being. Judgements about the allocation of resources across sectors could be better informed with the development of generic well-being measures, rather than sector specific measures such as EQ-5D.

This chapter reviews these alternatives and their advantages and disadvantages compared to using GPBMs of health.

8.2 Mapping onto generic preference-based measures (aka cross-walking)

Key clinical trials are often designed for purposes other than undertaking economic evaluation or populating cost-effectiveness models, such as supporting the licensing of a drug or a labelling claim. The primary outcome for these studies tends to be a clinical measure of outcome, and while this may be a patient-reported outcome measure, it is rarely a GPBM. Despite their modest size and intrusiveness, some designers of clinical trials argue that there is insufficient space for GPBMs like EQ-5D, or that such measures are simply not relevant from a clinical perspective.

One practical solution to this problem is to use mapping (also known as cross-walking). This has been defined as 'the development and use of an algorithm (or algorithms) to predict health state utility values using data on other indicators or measures of health. The algorithm can be applied to data from clinical trials, other studies or economic models containing the source predictive measure(s) to predict utility values even though the target measure was not included in the original source study of effectiveness' (Longworth and Rowen 2013). Typically this means estimating a relationship between a source measure, such as a condition-specific measure of health and a target measure like EQ-5D; this is done by regression, using an estimation data set that contains both measures administered alongside each other to one patient sample. The regression equation is then used to predict the target measure (e.g. EQ-5D) in another data set, such as a key clinical trial. The objective is to help inform an economic evaluation, and the resulting predictions may be used in an economic evaluation alongside a clinical trial, or more commonly, to estimate utility values for health states being used in cost-effectiveness models. There are numerous examples of mapping studies, including submissions to agencies like NICE (Tosh and Longworth 2011).

In the past, mapping has been undertaken by judgement rather than empirically, by assigning components of a health measure to specific domains and levels of a generic preference-based measure (such as the EQ-5D) (e.g. Coast 1992). For a valid translation process to be possible, the starting measure must include the dimensions of the preference-based measure and have items that readily correspond to the dimension levels of the preference-based measure. This mapping can be undertaken by dimension or by item. Another method is to take some specific health states described in terms of the starting measure and to assign them onto a generic health state descriptive system. Gerard *et al.* (1999), for example, identified four states associated with breast cancer screening and asked patients to indicate the levels on the EQ-5D dimensions that correspond to each of the four states. The main criticism of this approach is the arbitrariness of the judgements being made, which are based on guesswork rather than empirical evidence. Furthermore, these judgements account for neither the variability nor the uncertainty in any estimates. This could be addressed by testing the judgements against real data (if there were any); for example, to see whether or not patients who score between 30 to 50 on the pain dimension of the SF-36 report themselves as being on level 2 for pain in EQ-5D. However, it would be better to estimate a relationship between the measures empirically (say by regression) in the first place, and this method takes up the remainder of this section.

The process of mapping requires a number of questions to be answered: what measures are we mapping from and to; what is the estimation data set; how is the model to be specified; what model type is to be used in the estimation; how is model performance to be assessed; and how is uncertainty to be reported? An overview of the mapping process and some recommendations are given on Table 8.1.

1. The starting and the target measure(s)

The starting measure(s) is determined by what was being used in the economic evaluation. In the case of cost-effectiveness models, this is often a simple severity grouping like mild, moderate, and severe and the aim is to obtain a mean health state utility

Table 8.1 Overview of mapping process and recommendations

Target needs to be moved up a line	GBPM index (e.g. EQ-5D)
Target (or dependent variable)	GBPM dimension levels
Starting measure (or independent variables)	Generic or condition-specific measure of health: overall score, summary scores, item level scores, item level dummies, interaction terms, squared terms, cubic terms
	Clinical measures: overall score, summary score, categorical dummies
	Socio-demographic variables and other relevant health data
Estimation sample	Clinical and demographic characteristics in the estimation sample should be similar to the characteristics of the 'target' sample to which the mapping algorithm will be applied
	Covariates used in the mapping function should be overlapping in distribution for the estimation and target samples
	Variables included within the target sample thought likely to impact on health state values should be included in the estimation sample
	If no existing data set is available that includes both the independent variables and target measure data needs to be collected to estimate the mapping regression
Model selection and specification	Use prior knowledge of clinical relationships
	Use standard statistical techniques to examine the data prior to mapping estimation (e.g. frequency tables and correlations)
	Fully describe the data set used to estimate the regression model including both range of values and plots showing the distribution
	Fully describe the range of predicted values used in the cost-effectiveness model
Method of estimation	Linear ordinary least squares (OLS)
	Tobit
	Censored least absolute deviation (CLAD)
	Two-part model (TPM)
	Generalized linear model (GLM)
	Latent class mixture model
	Censored mixture model
	Multinomial logit model
Performance	*Goodness of fit:* Statistical significance, sign, and relative size of coefficients
	R-squared and adjusted R-squared
	Information criterion of AIC and BIC
	Further tests of model fit such as Ramsey RESET test, Park test, Jarque–Bera test
	Plots to examine whether model assumptions are valid

Table 8.1 Continued

	Predictive ability: Root mean squared error (RMSE) and mean squared error (MSE)
	RMSE, MSE, mean error, mean absolute error by subset of severity range of EQ-5D and/or predictive measure(s)
	Plots of observed and predicted EQ-5D scores
	Performance should be assessed using a validation sample that can be a separate patient sample to the estimation data set or the data set used to estimate the mapping function can be randomly separated into estimation and validation samples or by bootstrapping
Uncertainty	Uncertainty in health-related utility values should be incorporated into economic analyses. Multiple possible mapping functions can be used to produce utility values for sensitivity analyses

Adapted with permission from *Value in Health*, Volume 16, Issue 1, Longworth L and Rowen D, 'Mapping to obtain EQ-5D health utility values for use in NICE HTAs', pp. 202–10, Copyright © 2013 Elsevier, http://www.journals.elsevier.com/value-in-health/.

Note: AIC—Akaike Information Criterion, BIC—Bayesian Information Criterion✓

value with standard errors across these groupings (Drummond *et al.* 2015). However, these crude groupings are likely to hide important variability and the overall mean values in each group may change following intervention. The starting measure(s) can be: another patient-reported outcome measure, often condition specific (e.g. Asthma Quality of Life Questionnaire), and/or other clinical indicators (none of which with preference-based weights); and potentially a variety of background characteristics, provided they are all collected in the data set to which the mapping function will be applied.

For the best results, there needs to substantial overlap between the starting and target measures in terms of the dimensions covered and the severity range within each dimension. Failure to achieve sufficient overlap will impair the performance of any mapping function and may result in systematic errors across the severity range of the target measure. However, the choice of target measure may be determined by the requirements of the reimbursement agency (e.g. NICE have a preference for EQ-5D; NICE 2013*a*). Where the target measure is not appropriate for the condition, one of the alternatives described in the next chapter (i.e. another generic, condition-specific measure or vignette) should be used, although this may be at the expense of comparability across studies and consistency across decisions.

2. Estimation data set

Ideally, the patient sample in the estimation data set should be similar to the patient population to which it is going to be applied. It should cover the mix and range of important characteristics of the patient population, such as disease severity, in order for the predicted target value to be based upon estimation rather than extrapolation. A mapping function estimated on one type of cancer, for example, may not transfer to another cancer type, even if the starting measure was validated for both. Similarly, an estimation data set that does not cover patients with comparable severity to those in the application sample will struggle to accurately predict the value of those states (e.g. the obvious case of a function estimated on patients with mild problems being applied to those with more severe problems). The estimation data is often pre-existing, but it can be collected post hoc for this purpose and provides an opportunity to collect a data set that is better suited to the task. The estimation data set needs to be fully described in terms of the distribution of the target measure's values and plots, and the severity range of the source measure(s) compared with the data set to which the algorithm will be applied, to ensure there are no major gaps at either end of the range.

3. Model specification

The econometric mapping model can take many forms. The dependent variable can be the preference-based single index value, or the dimension levels of the target measure. The independent variables can take the form of a total score, dimension scores, or dummies for each dimension of the starting measure; each are associated with different sets of assumptions about the relative importance of dimensions (and items) of the nature of the starting measure. The model can be simply additive, or it can incorporate squared or interaction terms. These can be tested in the development of a model. However, the selection should depend based on what best suits the data. Longworth and Rowen (2013) recommend a consideration of any previous clinical expectations and a careful examination of the data prior to undertaking any map in order to fully understand the data set and the relationship between the target measure, start measure, and any other potential explanatory variables. The ultimate decision about the variables and the specification should be based on pre-specified decision rules on statistical significance of coefficients and performance.

4. Method of estimation

Many mapping functions have been estimated by ordinary least squares (OLS), though researchers have explored a range of more sophisticated model types in order to improve model performance. The choice of model type should be based on a careful examination of the distribution of the target measure. Some preference-based measures have been shown to suffer from ceiling effects, such as EQ-5D, or are multimodal. OLS is unlikely to predict such distributions accurately, particularly at the upper/milder and lower/severer ends of the distribution. Indeed, published studies reporting the relationship between observed and predicted values have shown a tendency to underpredict at the upper end and overpredict at the lower end (Brazier *et al.* 2010). Furthermore, preference-based measures are bounded at the upper end at one and a minimum value, but OLS can predict outside these bounds.

There is ongoing research exploring a range of alternative methods for estimating models for mapping (mainly onto the EQ-5D). Earlier work examined Tobit (Rowen *et al.* 2009; Sullivan *et al.* 2006) and CLAD (censored least absolute deviation) (Sullivan *et al.* 2006; Payakachat *et al.* 2009). Evidence on the impact of these models is mixed (Longworth and Rowen 2013; Brazier *et al.* 2010). Furthermore, CLAD has the feature of predicting median values, and for most applications in economic models it is the mean that is required (though in principle a median value could be used). Ongoing research has been looking at the use of other model types such as a generalized linear model (Dakin *et al.* 2010), a two-part model (Versteegh *et al.* 2010), geometric mean regression (Lu *et al.* 2013), and a random effects censored mixture model (Hernández *et al.* 2012). Further details of these models are provided in Longworth and Rowen (2013) and in the references provided. Evidence of the impact of these different types of model is mixed, but the geometric mean model substantially increases the coefficient of the starting measure to reduce the overprediction at the lower end, and the random censored mixture model does seem to offer an improvement for predicting the multimodal EQ-5D distribution. For models with a discrete dependent variable (e.g. EQ-5D dimension level), researchers have used techniques such as multinomial logistic regression models to predict the probability of achieving different levels of the classification of the GPBM (Gray *et al.* 2006). Again, evidence on the benefits of using this response mapping approach is mixed, though with larger data sets there is evidence of some improvement (Rowen *et al.* 2009; Chuang *et al.* 2009; Longworth *et al.* 2014). This method requires a significant number of responses at each level of each dimension.

As for any statistical modelling problem, the appropriate method is likely to vary by the target measure, explanatory variables and data set, and therefore due care must be taken to examine the features of the variables. This is an area where there is a considerable amount of ongoing research.

5. Performance

Studies commonly report model explanatory power in terms of adjusted R-squared, but this statistic cannot be used for some methods of estimation. A more useful test of performance is to examine the difference between predicted and observed values by calculating the mean absolute error (MAE) or the root mean squared error (RMSE). These are often used to describe individual level error, but the values are going to be applied in cost-effectiveness models to groupings of patients. MAE or RMSE can be calculated for severity groups, where the size of the errors in predicting mean EQ-5D indices is substantially less (Ara and Brazier *et al.* 2008). However, it is important to understand how the errors vary in severity by reporting for ranges of the preference-based measure (e.g. EQ-5D < 0, 0 ≤ EQ-5D < 0.25, 0.25 ≤ EQ-5D<0.5, 0.5 ≤ EQ-5D < 0.75, 0.75 ≤ EQ-5D ≤ 1). The pattern of error can also be viewed using plots of predicted against observed. The existence of bias can impact upon the cost-effectiveness of interventions. For example, underpredicting for more severe states will increase the incremental cost-effectiveness ratio of interventions that move patients from the poor states to more moderate states.

6. Validation

Model performance can be tested in a separate validation data set to better understand how well the model will predict values in other data sets. Most studies report model performance in the estimation data set, but this may be misleading because models usually perform better in the sample in which they have been estimated. The validation data set may be obtained from the same pool as the estimation data set by randomly allocating the data between estimation and validation data sets, or from an entirely independent sample with similar characteristics. The latter would provide a better test of performance.

7. Uncertainty

The act of mapping introduces an additional uncertainty in the estimated health state utility value used in economic models. Surprisingly, researchers have found that the confidence intervals around mean values from predicted health state utility values tend to be narrower than observed values (Rivero-Arias *et al.* 2010). This is in part due to a failure to take sufficient account of measurement error in the two measures involved and the estimated function (Lu *et al.* 2013). This is an area of further research, but in the meantime different mapping functions should be explored in sensitivity analyses to understand the impact of uncertainty.

8.2.1 Mapping using preferences rather than statistical association between measures—a new development

Mapping by statistical association between GPBMs and other patient-reported outcome measures assumes that it is appropriate to use the different measures on the same population. For reasons discussed next, this may not always be the case in certain patient groups and conditions. 'Preference-based mapping' is another method for estimating the relationship between measures (Rowen *et al.* 2009; Hernández *et al.* 2013). Preference-based mapping uses general population values for states defined by the descriptive systems of different measures, using the same valuation method with the same anchor points. It is argued that this generates a common yardstick for conversion between measures, while also preserving the distinct advantages of the descriptive system of each measure. The relationship between the preference-based measures is determined directly by people's preferences for different states selected deliberately by an experimental design, and not by associations in scores of self-reported states observed in nature. This enables researchers and policy makers to estimate EQ-5D utility values using available data from other preference-based measures.

The feasibility of this novel approach has been examined using a simple visual analogue scale on which states defined by different measures are rated on the same scale (Rowen *et al.* 2012*a*), and are ranked (Hernández *et al.* 2013). These studies demonstrated the feasibility of the approach, but encountered some technical difficulties in the mapping process. More recently, this approach has been used to estimate the relationship between the EQ-5D and the Adult Social Care Outcomes Toolkit (ASCOT) (a measure of social care-related quality of life) using TTO to estimate a linear relationship between the preference-based index scores of the two measures which reflects their value to members of the general public (Stevens and Brazier 2016).

8.2.2 Conclusion to mapping

This section has described commonly used methods of mapping and provided recommendations on better practice where this is possible. Mapping functions are best obtained empirically rather than by judgement, using estimation data sets that cover the range of severity and patient covariates in the intended data set, between measures that have sufficiently overlapping dimensions with each other. This can be done by using an appropriate method for estimating the model and specification, which is subjected to rigorous statistical testing of performance across the relevant range of application and where the uncertainties are fully explored. This is all good statistical practice, but no model is perfect and there will be a judgement to be made as to whether the mapping is good enough. This is problematic, as the degree of uncertainty is often not adequately accounted for in the reporting of mapping functions. In a situation where the analyst does not have any other data, a poor model may be better than no values at all, but care must be taken to fully account for the uncertainty.

The use of mapping to derive preference-based generic indices raises a more fundamental concern. The strength of the mapping function depends upon the degree of overlap between the two descriptive systems. The model may be undermined when there are important dimensions of one instrument not covered by the other. There could be a weakness if the generic measure does not cover certain dimensions of the starting measures that are regarded as important. For example, EQ-5D does not contain a dimension for energy or vitality. Therefore, it is not surprising that in published mapping functions from any of the SF instruments to EQ-5D, energy has a small and non-significant coefficient (Rowen *et al.* 2009). Another source of weakness can arise from differences in the severity range covered for a given health dimension. When generic measures are not regarded as appropriate for the condition, due to a lack of relevance and/or sensitivity, then mapping from the condition-specific measure onto a generic measure does not solve this problem and the mapping function is likely to perform poorly. An alternative approach in these circumstances is to estimate a preference-based index directly from the starting measure (e.g. a condition-specific measure), as described in the next section.

8.3 Constructing (condition-specific) preference-based measures of health

A preference-based measure of health, whether it is generic or specific to a condition, can be developed from an existing measure of health such as the cancer-specific EORTC-8D from the EORTC-QLQC30 (Rowen *et al.* 2011) or the dementia-specific DEMQoL-U from the DEMQoL (Mulhern *et al.* 2012). Alternatively, a measure can be developed *de novo*, such as the CHU-9D in children (Stevens 2009) or the Cambridge Pulmonary Hypertension Outcome Review (CAMPHOR) for people with pulmonary hypertension (McKenna *et al.* 2008). This section focuses on deriving CSPBMs from existing measures, but then moves onto developing measures *de novo*.

Why would a researcher want to estimate a preference-based measure from an existing measure of health? One reason is that the measure may have been widely used in clinical trials, such as the SF-36, and so using it to derive a preference-based measure considerably extends the scope for undertaking economic evaluation in health care. In some medical areas, there is a standard measure that is widely accepted in the clinical community for use in trials. Pragmatically, whether or not it is the most sensitive or responsive measure is less important than the extent of the instrument's use in clinical studies. The downside is that it may not measure what is of most interest to policy makers.

8.3.1 **The problem**

The main problem faced when deriving preference-based indices from existing generic and condition-specific measures (CSMs) is their size and complexity. For example, the Asthma Quality of Life Questionnaire (AQLQ) is a typical CSM designed to assess health in patients with asthma (Juniper *et al.* 1993) and consists of 32 items that measure health-related quality of life (HRQL) across four dimensions: symptoms (12 items); activity limitations (11 items); emotional function (five items); and environmental stimuli (four items). For each item in the AQLQ, respondents are asked to choose from a series of seven responses, ranging from extreme problems to no problems. Scores are then summed to obtain a dimension score and an overall score across all 32 items. It defines many millions of potential health states, and each state involves too much information for valuation by respondents. It has been suggested that individuals can only process between five and nine pieces of information at a time in a valuation task (Miller 1956; Dolan *et al.* 1996). There is evidence of respondents adopting simplifying heuristics when undertaking preference elicitation tasks (Lloyd 2003). Larger and more complex descriptions are more likely to result in respondents adopting heuristics, such as focusing on one of the dimensions. This may invalidate the valuation obtained since respondents are not valuing the entire content of the states, as is usually assumed by the analysis.

Methods have been developed for dealing with this problem by deriving a health state classification consisting of a single item for each dimension with a number of severity levels. The AQL-5D, for example, which was based on the AQLQ mentioned here, has five dimensions each containing five severity levels, and is able to define 3,125 states (Yang *et al.* 2011). This approach of developing a health state classification from a larger instrument has been widely applied and resulted in the development of many preference-based measures; these include the generic SF-36 (Brazier *et al.* 2002) and many condition-specific measures, such as CORE-OM for common mental health problems (Mavranezouli *et al.* 2011, 2013), OABq in overactive bladder (Yang *et al.* 2009), NEWQoL in epilepsy (Mulhern *et al.* 2014), Glaucoma Profile Instrument (Burr *et al.* 2007), and the Audit of Diabetes-Dependent Quality of Life (Sundaram *et al.* 2009).

8.3.2 **Methods**

The application of the health state classification approach to constructing a CSPBM from an existing measure has been described in six stages (Fig. 8.1) (Brazier *et al.* 2012). These stages are a guide to the development of a preference-based measure rather than a prescriptive methodology; it is not always practical or possible to follow each stage separately or sequentially, and the precise technique used may differ depending on the size and structure of the original instrument. However, they highlight the key components of the process.

8.3.2.1 **Stage I: establishing dimensions**

Conventionally, preference-based measures of health use a health state classification where the dimensions are structurally independent. This is important for the application of the design of valuation studies using statistical inference or multiattribute

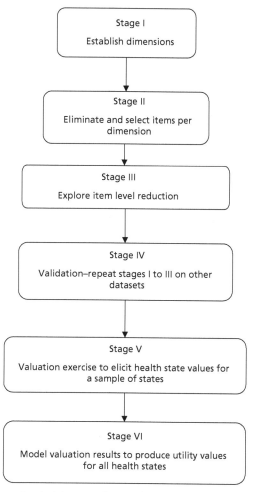

Fig. 8.1 The six stages for deriving a preference-based health-related quality of life measure.

Reproduced with permission from Brazier J *et al.*, 'Developing and testing methods for deriving preference-based measures of health from condition specific measures (and other patient based measures of outcome)', *Health Technology Assessment*, Volume 16, Issue 32, Copyright © 2012 NETSCC, DOI http://dx.doi.org/10.3310/hta16320.

utility theory (stage VI). As described in Chapter 5, the use of statistical methods requires a design such as an orthogonal array to generate health states. The resultant health states to be valued will contain mixtures of severity levels across dimensions. Multiattribute utility theory (MAUT) requires the valuation of extreme combinations or corner states, where one dimension is at the worst level and all others are at the best level (or those that are near to the corners). This requires dimensions that are sufficiently independent to allow for such combinations of states.

One method of developing independent dimensions or at least confirming their independence is factor analysis; either exploratory for the former, or confirmatory for the latter. This can be helpful to confirm the original dimension structure of a measure, or to show where dimensions are not sufficiently independent and suggest ways to reduce the number of dimensions. It can also be used to suggest a possible dimensional structure where none was proposed by the original instrument developer (Young *et al.* 2009). Alternatively, it can suggest modifications to the dimension structure proposed by the instrument developer; for example, in a study deriving the AQL-5D from the Asthma Quality of Life Questionnaire, factor analysis suggested there were five dimensions when the original instrument had four (Young *et al.* 2011). However, factor analysis needs to be used with care, as the factors it suggests may not make conceptual sense. Other techniques that have been used to inform this process have included cluster analysis and Rasch analysis to establish whether items belong to a single dimension (see next section for more details).

8.3.2.2 Stage II: selecting items

A dimension in a health state classification is usually represented by one or occasionally two items from the original instrument. The selection of items must be undertaken with great care. This process has been assisted in previous studies by a combination of conventional psychometric testing looking at the validity and responsiveness of items, Rasch analysis, and qualitative work with patients to understand their content and face validity.

Rasch is a helpful technique in the process of item selection, based on patient-reported outcome data. This is a mathematical technique that converts qualitative (categorical) responses to a continuous (unmeasured) latent scale using a logit model. The intuition underlying this approach is that the probability of an affirmative response to each item (or each response to each item) depends on the degree of severity of the item and the perceived health of the respondent. It should be applied to items thought to belong to the same underlying latent variable or dimension. In the development of a health state classification, Rasch analysis can be used to eliminate items that seem to poorly represent the dimension (see next section for details) (Young *et al.* 2009). Item response theory (IRT), based on similar principles, can also be used for this task.

In a number of studies, the process of selecting items has been broken down into two steps. The first has been the elimination of poorly performing items that do not meet key criteria. However, for the larger measures this will leave a number of items in certain dimensions and so a second step is required that involves selecting the best item for each dimension.

Step 1: eliminating items Some items may be regarded as unsuitable for the health state classification due to their poor psychometric performance, including: high levels of missing data (feasibility); poor consistency with the overall dimension (e.g. this may be revealed in the factor analysis); failing to reflect known group differences (known group validity); or being unresponsive to known changes in health. These criteria should be applied without regard to any specific intervention; otherwise, the selection may be biased in favour of the intervention. When patients are being consulted, they may identify items that they cannot understand or that do not measure what the instrument developer intended them to measure. Finally, the results of Rasch analysis (or IRT) can also help to eliminate items using specific tests. In the derivation of the five-dimensional AQL-5D from the AQLQ, for example, a Rasch model was fitted to each of the dimensions and items eliminated using three criteria:

1. Items unable to display item level ordering—these are items where the Rasch model indicates that respondents' answers were not consistent with the hierarchy of the response choices.

2. Items perform differently across populations—differential item functioning (DIF) is a technique that seeks to establish whether respondents with different characteristics respond differently to items. Items that display DIF are of limited value across subgroups of patients defined by the characteristic (as often would be required in an economic evaluation) and are therefore usually excluded.

3. Items not consistent with the dimension—items that do not fit the underlying Rasch model should be eliminated as they do not represent the underlying dimension; these items can be identified using goodness of fit statistics.

Step 2: selecting the best item per dimension Once items have been eliminated from the selection process, the same psychometric methods can be applied to select the 'best' items for the health state classification. The performance of items in each dimension can be compared against the criteria of feasibility, consistency, validity, and responsiveness (see Chapter 7). Patient views can play an important role. Finally, Rasch or IRT can help identify items that best reflect the severity range of the dimension using various statistics, such as item range. The process of selection at this stage benefits from the full involvement of researchers, clinicians, and patients in making the final judgements. This judgement will involve weighing up the aforementioned evidence, along with considerations of how well the selected items combine to form health states for valuation in stage V.

8.3.2.3 Stage III: exploring item level reduction

In practice, patients may not be able to distinguish between item response choices. Therefore, we recommend including this as an exploratory stage to examine the possibility of reducing the number of item levels in stage II. Item threshold probability curves from Rasch and response frequencies can be examined when selecting potential item levels for collapsing. Items for the AQL-5D, for example, were collapsed from seven to five using evidence from the Rasch analysis. The results of interviews with patients may also help to inform this process.

8.3.2.4 Stage IV: validation

The application of stages I to III will generate a health state classification suitable for valuation. However, prior to proceeding with the valuation process we recommend validating the selected items by repeating the analysis on alternative samples from the same data set used in stages I to III, or at alternative time points.

Before proceeding to the valuation, it is important to examine whether respondents are able to understand the states defined by the health state classification and undertake the task. Comprehension can be tested in cognitive de-briefing studies and piloting prior to embarking on a large valuation survey (see examples reported in the context of a discrete choice experiment (DCE) in Ryan and Gerard 2003).

8.3.2.5 Stage V: valuation survey

The health state classifications derived in stages I–IV typically define thousands of health states; therefore, a sample of states must be selected for valuation using one of the cardinal choice-based techniques described in Chapter 4, or valued by ordinal choice-based methods as described in Chapter 6. These methods use designs that select states for valuation with various combinations of levels across the dimensions, many of which will involve mild levels on some dimensions and severe levels for others. As explained already, this requires the dimensions to be independent, though there are methods for dealing with situations where this is not the case, as will be explained in the next section.

8.3.2.6 Stage VI: modelling health state values

The purpose of modelling health state valuation data is to predict mean values (and distributions about the mean) for all health states defined by the health state classification. This has been fully described in Chapter 5 for cardinal preference data, and in Chapter 6 for ordinal preference data.

These six stages of developing preference-based health state classification systems have been successfully applied to many instruments, but one problem has emerged when the health state classification does not have independent dimensions. Dimensions may be highly correlated and, when examined using factor analysis, were found to load onto the same factor(s). This may be causal, such that someone who is in severe pain may not be able to undertake certain activities, or they may simply tend to appear together as part of a condition (e.g. diarrhoea and vomiting). A lack of independence between items in a health state classification system creates challenges in both the valuation (V) and modelling (VI) stages of the process. Many of the states that need to be valued to estimate models, generated using techniques such as orthogonal or balanced designs, would involve combinations of dimension levels that would not be plausible (e.g. feeling downhearted and low *and* happy most of the time). One solution to this problem is described in the next section.

8.3.2.7 An alternative to the health state classification approach where dimensions are not independent

In the development of preference-based measures in common mental health problems and in vision, the results of the Rasch analysis found that the set of items used in the health state classification system were uni-dimensional (i.e. tapping the same latent variable). However, they represented significantly different qualitative information about the impact of the condition (Mavranezouli *et al.* 2011, 2013; Rentz *et al.* 2014). A condition may influence a number of related areas of life, and using more than one item, even if they are highly correlated, provides a richer picture. The solution is to select states for the valuation survey that make sense; one method for doing this was pioneered by Sugar, Lenert, and others using *k*-means cluster analysis to break up the data into states. In one study, they identified patterns of the physical and mental health summary scores of the SF-12 in models with varying numbers of discrete states (Sugar *et al.* 1998). They selected six states from the SF-12 data in a sample of depressed patients who were defined in terms of scores; therefore, the process of turning the score distributions of each state into words taken from the original 12 items to define the states had to be developed based on expert judgement.

The use of cluster analysis in this way is an interesting approach, but it suffers from three limitations. Firstly, the derivation of the states uses essentially arbitrary cut-offs in the cluster analysis. Secondly, it uses dimensions scores that then need to be related to the item descriptions to generate the states, and this requires judgement. While some judgement is always needed in this type of work, it should be minimized where possible. Finally, this method has only been used to identify a small sample of states that may poorly describe and differentiate patients with the condition and some patients may not fit into them at all.

A method has been developed that avoids these problems and uses the results of Rasch or IRT modelling to generate states to describe typical respondents at different points along the latent variable of severity. As well as providing a method for assisting in the selection of items, Rasch helps select health states for valuation that represent different levels of severity. This 'Rasch vignette approach' generates states that are more plausible and easier to imagine, based on the natural occurrence of states in the data set, and it avoids the implausible combinations generated by statistical designs (e.g. an orthogonal array) from a health state classification system (Young *et al.* 2011; Mavranezouli *et al.* 2013; Brazier *et al.* 2012). This approach offers a better solution than cluster analysis, as it uses the health utility values for these states to estimate the relationship between the health state utility values and the latent variable produced by the Rasch model using regression techniques (Young *et al.* 2010). This permits the estimation of utility values for all points on the latent scale and hence all other states that will be observed.

The Rasch vignette approach can also be extended, by combining items from one dimension with other dimensions. For example, a preference-based measure of common mental health problems was developed with a physical health item that was combined with the Rasch score for the emotional health component, in order to estimate a preference function to cover all physical and mental health combinations (Mavranezouli *et al.* 2013).

8.3.2.8 Developing a new measure

The stages in developing a preference-based measure *de novo* are broadly the same as those outlined in Figure 8.1. The measure's dimensions, items, and levels need to be determined to form a health state classification (or vignette), and then a sample of states needs to be valued and modelled.

Historically the development of generic measures has been to use expert opinion that is based upon a review of previous measures. This 'expert' approach to generating dimensions and items could be criticized for not accurately reflecting the views of those concerned, such as the patients or their carers. An exception was the development of HUI2, where parents were asked to rank statements describing the health of children, and this information was used to inform the final choice of dimensions (Cadman *et al.* 1986). More recently, a generic preference-based measure for children has been developed from interviews with children (Stevens 2009). Another approach has been to interview members of the general population, such as in the development of capability measures for older people and adults more generally (Coast *et al.* 2006; Al-Janabi *et al.* 2012). These authors used qualitative techniques to develop the dimensions and the wording of a classification system that defined quality of life from interview data. A mixed method approach is to use qualitative techniques on the interview data to generate potential items for each dimension, and then use psychometric methods to reduce the number of items for developing a classification system.

8.3.3 Description of existing condition-specific preference-based measures

Tables 8.2 and 8.3 describe the health state classification systems and valuation methods for existing CSPBMs identified in a review of published studies (Rowen and Brazier 2014). There are 28 instruments covering 27 different conditions, ranging from specific diagnoses, such as glaucoma and lung cancer, to more general conditions, such as visual impairment and cancer. The size of a health state classification system (the number of possible health states) varies greatly by measure, ranging from 10 to 390,625. The focus of the dimensions differs across instruments: some instruments only have dimensions capturing symptoms or health-related quality of life related to symptoms, whereas other instruments include dimensions covering both symptoms and HRQL.

The valuation process used to produce utility values for all states defined by the health state classification system also varies by measure. Table 8.3 indicates that 14 instruments use the statistical inference approach to value selected states and model utilities; eight instruments use a decomposed approach, which is either a pure MAUT approach or an approach combining statistical inference and MAUT. Three instruments directly value all health states defined by the classification system, and thus require no modelling to produce utility values for all health states. TTO, visual analogue scale (VAS), SG, and combinations of these were commonly used to elicit utility values. Twelve instruments have values elicited using TTO, six used VAS with mapping onto SG, four used VAS alone, while two used SG alone. Although VAS was used in 13 instruments and is the most commonly used technique, its usage differs across studies varying from valuing health states to valuing severity levels within a dimension, or valuing different dimensions. Eight instruments, though preference-based, cannot be used to estimate quality-adjusted life years (QALYs) as they are not anchored onto the required full health–dead 1–0 scale. Only half of the measures are valued using an entirely general population sample as recommended by most jurisdictions who use QALYs, with ten measures valued by patients and one by patients and carers. The majority of instruments have been valued only in the United Kingdom (18) and valuation studies across all measures have only been conducted in United Kingdom, United States (6), the Netherlands (2), and Canada (1).

8.3.4 Performance of condition-specific preference-based measures

There are two issues addressed here: how the preference-based versions compare to the original measure (where relevant) and how they compare to generic measures.

Table 8.2 Condition-specific utility instrument descriptive systems

Condition	Non-preference-based measure (where relevant)	No. of dimensions	Severity levels	No. of states defined by system	Dimensions
Amyotrophic lateral sclerosis (ALS)	Amyotrophic Lateral Sclerosis Functioning Rating Scale—revised (ALSFRS-R)	4	5–6	750	Speech and swallowing; eating, dressing and bathing; leg function; respiratory function
Asthma	N/A	5	10	100,000	Cough; wheeze; shortness of breath; awakening at night; side effects of asthma treatment
Asthma	Asthma Quality of Life Questionnaire (AQLQ)	5	5	3,125	Concern about asthma; shortness of breath; weather and pollution stimuli; sleep problems; activity limitation
Cancer	EORTC QLQ-C30	8	4–5	81,920	Physical functioning; role functioning; pain; emotional functioning; social functioning; fatigue and sleep disturbance; nausea; constipation and diarrhoea
Common mental health problems	Clinical Outcomes in Routine Evaluation—Outcome Measure (CORE-OM)	6	3	729	Functioning—close relationships; functioning—social relationships; functioning—general; symptoms—anxiety; risk/harm to self; physical health
Dementia	DEMQoL (self-report)	5	4	1,024	Positive emotion; memory; relationships; negative emotion; loneliness
	DEMQoL-Proxy (carer proxy report)	4	4	256	Positive emotion; memory; appearance; negative emotion; loneliness
Diabetes	Audit of Diabetes-Dependent Quality of Life (ADDQoL) plus additional items	5	3–4	768	Physical ability and Energy level; relationships; mood and feelings; enjoyment of diet; satisfaction with managing diabetes

(continued)

Table 8.2 Continued

Condition	Non-preference-based measure (where relevant)	No. of dimensions	Severity levels	No. of states defined by system	Dimensions
Epilepsy	Quality of Life in Newly Diagnosed Epilepsy measure (NEWQOL)	6	4	4,096	Worry about attacks; depression; memory; cognition; stigma; control
Erectile (dys) functioning	Index of Erectile Function (IIEF)	2	5	25	Ability to attain an erection sufficient for satisfactory sexual performance; ability to maintain an erection sufficient for satisfactory sexual performance
Flushing	Flushing Symptoms Questionnaire (FSQ)	5	4–5	2,500	Redness of skin; warmth of skin; tingling of skin; itching of skin; difficulty sleeping
Glaucoma	Glaucoma Profile Instrument	6	4	4,096	Central and near vision; lighting and glare; mobility; activities of daily living; eye discomfort; other effects
Handicap	International Classification of Impairments, Disabilities, and Handicaps (ICIDH)	6	6	46,656	Handicap mobility; occupation; physical independence; social integration; orientation; economic self sufficiency
Head and neck cancer	N/A	8	5	390,625	Social function; pain; physical appearance; eating problems; speech problems; nausea; donor site problems; shoulder function
Lung cancer	FACT-L	6	2	64	Physical; social/family; emotional; functional; symptoms—general: symptoms—specific

Condition	Questionnaire				Domains
Menopause	Menopause-specific quality of life questionnaire	7	3–5	6,075	Hot flushes; aching joints/muscles; anxious/frightened feelings; breast tenderness; bleeding; vaginal dryness; undesirable androgenic signs
Menorrhagia	N/A	6	4	4,096	Practical difficulties; social life; psychological health; physical health; working life; family life
Minor oral surgery	N/A	5	4	1,024	General health and well-being; health and comfort of mouth, teeth, and gums; impact on home/social life; impact on job/studies; appearance
Overactive bladder	Overactive bladder questionnaire (OABq)	5	5	3,125	Urge to urinate; urine loss; sleep; coping; concern
Paediatric asthma	N/A	3	2-3	12–but only 10 are valid	Symptoms; emotion; activity
Paediatric atopic dermatitis	Un-named questionnaire on atopic dermatitis	4	2	16	Activities; mood; settled; sleep
Parkinson's disease	N/A	2	2-5	10	Disease severity; proportion of the day with 'off-time' (impact on QOL due to condition covering domains: social function, ability to carry out daily activities, psychological function)
Pulmonary hypertension	Cambridge Pulmonary Hypertension Outcome Review (CAMPHOR)	4	2-3	36	Social activities; travelling; dependence; communication
Rhinitis	N/A	5	10	100,000	Stuffy or blocked nose; runny nose; sneezing; itchy watery eyes; itchy nose or throat

(continued)

Table 8.2 Continued

Condition	Non-preference-based measure (where relevant)	No. of dimensions	Severity levels	No. of states defined by system	Dimensions
Sexual quality of life	Sexual quality of life questionnaire (SQOL)	3	4	64	Sexual performance, sexual relationship, sexual anxiety
Stroke	N/A	10	3	59,049	Walking; climbing stairs; physical activities/sports; recreational activities; work; driving; speech; memory; coping; self-esteem
Urinary incontinence	The King's Health Questionnaire (used for urinary incontinence and lower urinary tract symptoms)	5	4	1,024	Role limitations; physical limitations; social limitations/family life; emotions; sleep/energy
Venous ulceration	N/A	5	3-5	720	Pain; mobility; mood; smell; social activities
Vision/visual impairment	N/A	6	5-7	45,360	Physical well-being; independence; social well-being; emotional well-being; self-actualization; planning and organization

Reproduced with permission from Rowen D and Brazier J, 'Multi-attribute Utility Instruments: Condition-Specific Versions', pp. 358–65 in Anthony J. Culyer (Ed.), *Encyclopedia of Health Economics*, Volume 2, Elsevier, San Diego, USA, Copyright © Elsevier 2014.

Table 8.3 Condition-specific utility instrument valuation

Condition	Theory and model type	Preference elicitation technique	Anchored on 1–0 full health–dead scale	Population	Country
Amyotrophic lateral sclerosis (ALS)	Decomposed—multiplicative	VAS both for each level of each dimension alone and health states, and SG	Yes	General population	US
Asthma	Decomposed—multiplicative	VAS and SG both for states and for the levels per dimension	No	Patients	US
Asthma	Statistical—additive	TTO	Yes	General population	UK
Cancer	Statistical—additive	TTO	Yes	General population	UK
Common mental health problems	Statistical—additive	TTO	Yes	General population	UK
Dementia	Statistical—additive	TTO	Yes	General population	UK
Diabetes	Decomposed—multiplicative	VAS and SG	Yes	Patients	US
Epilepsy	Statistical—additive	TTO	Yes	General population	UK
Erectile (dys) functioning	All states valued	TTO	Yes	General population and students	Netherlands
Flushing	Maps Rasch logit scores onto mean utilities—additive	TTO	Yes	General population	UK
Glaucoma	Statistical—additive	DCE	No	Patients	UK
Handicap	Statistical—additive	VAS	No	Patients	UK
Head and neck cancer	Decomposed—additive	VAS both for dimensions relative to each other and for the levels per dimension	No	Surgeons	UK

(continued)

Table 8.3 Continued

Condition	Theory and model type	Preference elicitation technique	Anchored on 1–0 full health–dead scale	Population	Country
Lung cancer	Statistical—additive	VAS	Yes	General population	UK, Netherlands
Menopause	Statistical—additive	TTO	Yes	Patients	UK
Menorrhagia	Decomposed—additive	Two tasks: distribute 21 counters across the dimensions in proportion to their importance; VAS of the levels per dimension	No	Patients	UK
Minor oral surgery	Decomposed—additive	Two tasks: distribute 100 counters across the dimensions in proportion to their importance; VAS of the levels per dimension	No	Patients	UK
Overactive bladder	Statistical—additive	TTO	Yes	General population	UK
Paediatric asthma	Power function used to convert VAS to SG, all states valued using VAS	VAS and SG	Yes	General population	US
Paediatric atopic dermatitis	All states valued	SG	Yes	General population	UK
Parkinson's disease	All states valued	VAS and SG	Yes	Patients	US
Pulmonary hypertension	Statistical—additive	TTO	Yes	General population	UK
Rhinitis	Decomposed—multiplicative	VAS and SG both for states and for the levels per dimension	No	Patients	US

Sexual quality of life	Statistical—additive	TTO	General population	Yes	UK
Stroke	Unclear	VAS	Patients and caregivers	No	Canada
Urinary incontinence	Statistical—additive	SG	Patients	Yes	UK
Venous ulceration	Statistical—additive	TTO	General population	Yes	UK
Vision/visual impairment	Decomposed—multiplicative	TTO, VAS for the levels per dimension	Unclear	Yes	Unclear

Notes: Statistical = statistical inference, decomposed = MAUT or combination of MAUT and statistical inference. Preference elicitation technique is reported only if it was used to produce the recommended utility values for all health states. TTO = time trade-off, SG = standard gamble, VAS = visual analogue scale, DCE = discrete choice experiment.

8.3.4.1 Do preference-based measures lose information compared to the original instrument?

There is little published analysis examining the extent of information loss caused by moving from a larger original condition-specific measure to a much smaller CSPBM. When information loss was examined in terms of ability to discriminate across severity groups and responsiveness to change over time using patient data sets in asthma, cancer, common mental health problems, and overactive bladder, it was found that there is either no information loss, or at least a minimal degree of information loss of the preference-based index compared to the total scores based on all items (Brazier *et al.* 2012). This is reassuring, given that the rationale for deriving a preference-based measure from an existing measure is due to its relevance and sensitivity, which means that this informational advantage is retained.

8.3.4.2 How do the estimated condition-specific values compare to generic instruments?

It was discussed in Chapter 7 that GPBMs produce different scores due to differences both in the health state classification system and valuation methods used to produce preference weights for each instrument. There is a concern that CSPBMs will add to the heterogeneity of health state utility values, and that these differences may have an impact on the results of economic evaluation. Therefore, it is important to understand the extent of agreement between measures.

There is little published evidence comparing CSPBMs and generic measures. One study compares the three-level EQ-5D to CSPBMs for asthma (AQL-5D), cancer (EORTC-8D), and common mental health problems (CORE-6D) using patient self-reported data (Brazier *et al.* 2012). The three CSPBMs were valued using the same variant of TTO as the EQ-5D. Figure 8.2 plots pairwise comparisons and these demonstrate that CSPBMs have a narrower range of utility values than EQ-5D. EQ-5D suffers from a ceiling effect (where patients do not report any problems in EQ-5D), failing to discriminate across patients as a CSPBM can. This suggests that CSPBMs are more responsive for patients at the upper end of HRQL. Outside this cluster, the CSPBMs on average produce higher values at the individual level than EQ-5D (the only one for which these comparisons have been done). CSPBMs may produce higher values for a variety of reasons; for example, generic measures may also be reflecting comorbidities that are not captured by the CSPBM.

The three CSPBMs were better at discriminating between groups with different severity levels. While the absolute size of the differences between severity groups was smaller compared to the EQ-5D, the standard deviation (SD) was even smaller, which resulted in larger effect sizes. The same was true for the responsiveness to change following treatment (measured using standardized response means, that is, mean change divided by the SD of the change) of the CSPBM in common mental health conditions and asthma, though not cancer. This is important for trials and for the reduced uncertainty in utility values for different time periods or severity groups.

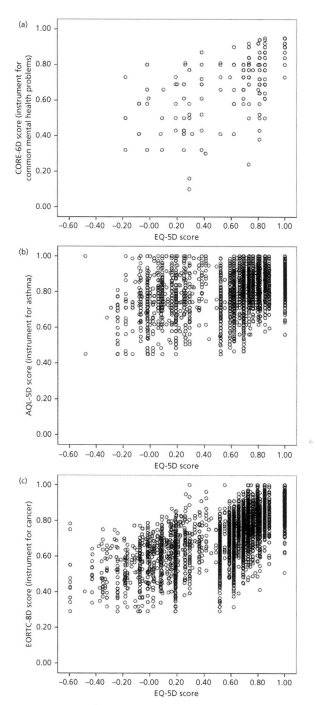

Fig. 8.2 Pairwise comparisons of the condition-specific utility instruments and generic three-level EQ-5D.

These results confirm that CSPBMs are not comparable to EQ-5D. The smaller absolute size in the differences is perhaps surprising, since condition-specific measures are designed to better reflect differences and changes over time in patients with the relevant medical condition. However, it should be noted that comparing absolute sizes between measures is problematic, since observations based on CSPBMs have a smaller range than observations from the same patients based on EQ-5D. While standardized effects sizes provide a better metric for comparison, it is absolute differences that drive cost-effectiveness models, and the results suggest that the use of CSPBMs in these conditions would increase the incremental cost per QALY (by up to twofold in these examples). The evidence is limited to three CSPBMs measures and one GPBM, so it is not possible to make any generalizations, but this evidence suggests that using CSPBMs does not necessarily lower incremental cost per QALY gained.

8.3.5 Should condition-specific preference-based measures be used at all?

The arguments for and against using CSPBMs are summarized in Box 8.1. One argument for using condition-specific descriptions is that they are expected to be more sensitive to the consequences of the condition suffered by the patient, because they focus on the most important dimensions pertinent to that condition. CSPBMs should achieve greater precision and so more effectively reflect differences in the severity of the condition and changes over time. A crude generic measure may miss more subtle changes, or require a larger sample size to be able to pick them up. This has been reflected in the aforementioned evidence, where the CSPBM had less variability and yet achieved larger effect sizes in some situations.

Another argument in favour of CSPBMs is that generic measures do not cover all dimensions of relevance to a condition. GPBMs were designed to cover the more common dimensions of health, and not all dimensions of health (Ware and Sherbourne 1992; Brooks and the EuroQol Group 1996; Richardson *et al.* 2014). On the other hand, CSPBMs may fail to capture the impact on comorbidities suffered by patients or the side effects of treatment. Patients commonly have comorbidities, particularly in older age, and these conditions can be more important to the patient's health than the condition being treated (but may be affected by the treatment). Most health care interventions have side effects which have little to do with the conditions being treated, and indeed in some cases, the main differences between pharmaceutical products is their side-effect profile rather than their consequences for the underlying condition. Therefore, a condition-specific measure could give a partial and potentially misleading view.

The final criticism for using CSPBMs is that they cannot be used to make comparisons between interventions across conditions or programmes. Is a QALY estimated from a dementia-specific measure comparable to one estimated from a cancer measure? It was an implicit assumption of the monetary willingness to pay in health care and early QALY literatures of the 1970s and 1980s that this was not a problem. Comparability was assumed to be achieved by the use of a common numeraire such as money, or a year in full health. It can be argued that a common numeraire is being

Box 8.1 Arguments for and against using condition-specific measures in economic evaluation

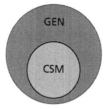

Fig. 8.3 Condition-specific measures (CSM) focuses.

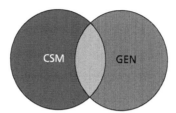

Fig. 8.4 CSM covers different dimensions.

There are two possible ways to perceive the relationship between generic and CSMs. One is characterized in Figure 8.3, where CSMs are seen to focus on a subset of generic dimensions, and the other in Figure 8.4, where CSMs are seen to cover different dimensions.

Arguments for specific measures:

- Sensitivity: by focusing on the condition, they are able to be more sensitive for a given dimension (consistent with the view in Fig. 8.3).
- Relevance: by focusing on the condition, they cover important dimensions of the condition missed by generic measures (consistent with the view in Fig. 8.4).

Arguments against condition-specific measures:

- Comorbidities: fail to reflect the impact of comorbidities (consistent with the view in Fig. 8.4).
- Side effects: fail to reflect side effects (consistent with the view in Fig. 8.4) (though some measures include side effects of common treatments).
- Focusing effects: the symptom effects are presented in isolation from other dimensions, which results in lower values.
- Labelling and naming: naming the condition has been shown to alter the value of health states (e.g. naming cancer lowered the values).
- Preference interactions: excluded dimensions can have consequences for the coefficients in the health state classification due to preference dependence between dimensions.

Summary of using CSPBMs: greater relevance and sensitivity vs reduced comparability between conditions and consistency between decisions.

used, provided that the values were obtained using the same valuation technique (and variant of the technique) with common anchors (full health and dead), and the values were obtained from the same type of respondents (such as a representative sample of the general population). This makes it possible to compare between QALYs that are estimated using different health state classification systems.

The results presented in Figure 8.4 and elsewhere show that CSPBMs are not comparable to EQ-5D, despite being valued using the same MVH TTO protocol. There are a number of explanations that have been given in the literature for differences including: focusing effects, naming and labelling, side effects and comorbidities (Brazier *et al.* 2012).

8.3.5.1 Focusing effects

Using more specific descriptions has implications for eliciting health state utility values based on preferences. The narrow descriptions used in many condition-specific measures may encourage a focusing effect, whereby respondents to elicitation tasks like TTO overemphasize the dimensions being brought to their attention and ignore other aspects of their life. A condition may affect just one or two symptoms, but other aspects of health are unaffected and had respondents been given information on these other aspects of health, they may not have given the health state such a low value. There is not much direct evidence on the importance of focusing effects in health. However, it is worth noting that evidence presented previously shows that most CSPBMs produce higher health state values than those from EQ-5D in the same patient population using the same valuation technique.

8.3.5.2 Naming and labelling

Many condition-specific measures and vignettes name the medical condition. There have been a number of studies that have looked at the effect of disease labels on health state values (Sackett and Torrance 1978; O'Connor 1989; Gerard *et al.* 1993; Rabin *et al.* 1993; Robinson and Bryan 2001; Rowen *et al.* 2012*b*). Rabin and colleagues found that the explicit labelling of mental conditions, such as mental handicap, schizophrenia, and dementia, tended to lower the valuations given. However, Gerard and colleagues (1993) found that the values of breast cancer states were not altered by naming and labelling, and O'Connor and her colleagues found no alteration in the context of alternative drug therapies for oncology. More recently, in one study cancer was associated with significant reductions of up to 0.253 in comparison to no label for the most severe state, whereas labelling the states as caused by irritable bowel syndrome had no impact (Rowen *et al.* 2012*b*).

There are sufficient studies demonstrating the impact of labelling to conclude that it can be important. Some conditions may have a special salience that is not captured in a generic measure like EQ-5D. By naming the condition, it allows the respondents to take this into account (Schwartz 2012). However, there is a concern that respondents may bring their own poorly informed assumptions about the impact of the condition and may actually be mistaken. Respondents may also bring their own fears about longer-term prognosis, which are inconsistent with the time frame set in the valuation exercise. Not all CSPBMs contain labels, but those that do run the risk of contamination by providing misleading or extraneous information.

8.3.5.3 Impact on preference function

A further complication with the CSPBMs is that they typically cover a narrower set of dimensions than generic measures. Even when there is no direct impact on other dimensions of health (e.g. from side effects), there is a concern that excluded dimensions may interact with those dimensions in the condition-specific measure. Preference interactions have been shown to exist in generic instruments. Dimensions of health have been found to be largely complementary (Dolan 1997; Brazier *et al.* 2002; Feeny *et al.* 2002), with the impact of a problem on one dimension of health being reduced by the existence of a problem on another domain. This has also been shown in the context of adding a pain dimension to an asthma CSPBM. A study comparing models of health state values with and without the pain dimension showed that while the pain dimension had a large and significant coefficient, there were substantial reductions in the coefficients for three out of the five dimensions of the original asthma measure when the pain dimension was added (Brazier *et al.* 2011). This, and other 'bolt-on' studies (described next), demonstrated that dimensions excluded from a health state classification system will have implications for the coefficients for the other dimensions. This is likely to create a bigger problem in condition-specific measures that focus on a small subset of health dimensions compared with generic measures that cover a broader range of health dimensions (though the problem will also exist for generic health measures, since they too may exclude important dimensions).

8.3.5.4 What is the solution?

It should be noted that some of the concerns with CSPBMs, such as focusing effects, side effects, and the impact of excluded dimensions, will also exist for generic measures. However, they are likely to be more important for a narrowly defined descriptive system. For use in cross-programme comparisons, it is ultimately a trade-off between having measures that are relevant and sensitive to those things that matter to patients on the one hand, and having problems due to excluding side effects and comorbidities otherwise reflected in generic measures, along with effects from labelling and focusing, on the other. The relative importance of the different arguments in this trade-off will vary between conditions and is likely to be influenced by the specificity of the condition, and the instrument. Labelling can be avoided in many cases. CSPBMs that include more generic health domains, such as the EORTC-8D, are more likely to reflect side effects and comorbidities. Equally, the larger generic health state classification systems, like the assessment of quality of life (AQoL) and 15D described in Chapter 7, are less likely to miss important consequences of a condition.

8.4 Bolting-on dimensions

Another solution would be to add or 'bolt-on' dimensions to the smaller generic measures like EQ-5D (Yang *et al.* 2011; Longworth *et al.* 2014). The aim of adding bolt-on dimensions is to improve the validity and responsiveness of the generic measure in specific conditions; also, by retaining the generic dimensions of the measure, it aims to address many of the threats to comparability discussed already, such as the impact of focusing effects, naming and labelling, side effects, and comorbidities.

Research into the development of bolt-ons has been largely exploratory to date and is only concerned with three-level EQ-5D. The earliest bolt-on study examined the consequences of removing (i.e. bolting-off) a sixth dimension from the original version of the EuroQol instrument. Using the VAS as the valuation method showed that the *energy* dimension did not improve the explanatory power of the model (Gudex 1991). A study to examine a cognition-specific bolt-on found it has a significant impact on VAS over and above the original five dimensions (Krabbe *et al.* 1999). Adding a sleep dimension (Yang *et al.* 2013), however, did not have a significant impact on TTO values. More recently, studies have examined the use of additional dimensions for vision, hearing, and tiredness (Longworth *et al.* 2014). It found that the extent and direction of the impact of the bolt-on varied according to the level of the bolt-on and the severity of the state to which it was added. In most cases, including a level 1 bolt-on (no problems) resulted in either no difference or higher values, the addition of level 2 (moderate problems) was mixed, and the addition of level 3 (extreme problems) tended to lower values but not in a state that already had a level 3. The surprising result was perhaps that a level 1 bolt-on seemed to make the state look more attractive.

The second related study estimated whole models with and without the vision dimension bolted-on (Longworth *et al.* 2014). This confirmed that vision had a significant impact, though the effect was only significant for level 3. It was also found that there was a potentially important, though not significant, impact on the coefficient for usual activities. It was insufficiently powered to reliably estimate interactions between the extra dimension and the core dimensions. These studies suggest that the impact of the bolt-on may not simply be additive, and so it is necessary to re-estimate whole scoring algorithms for each bolt-on.

Research points to the potential for bolt-ons to be a pragmatic way of overcoming the problem of 'missing' dimensions in GPBMs, without some of the problems with CSPBMs.

8.5 **Vignettes**

This approach involves constructing vignettes to describe health states of interest associated with a condition, and may include its treatment. These vignettes are valued using a standard method to obtain health state utility values for use in economic models, and they can incorporate a range of information about the impact of a condition and its treatment. Vignettes can take the form of a text narrative (see hip fracture example in Box 8.2), or a more structured format using bullet points similar to health states generated by generic or condition-specific measures (see gallstone disease example in Box 8.2). There are numerous examples of vignettes in the literature relating to a wide range of conditions, such as rheumatoid arthritis (Iqbal *et al.* 2012), schizophrenia (Briggs *et al.* 2008), diabetes (Matza *et al.* 2007), asthma (Lloyd *et al.* 2008), ADHD (Lloyd *et al.* 2011; Matza *et al.* 2005), depression (Revicki and Wood 1998), chronic pain (Eldabe *et al.* 2010), and cancer (Tolley *et al.* 2013). Researchers

Box 8.2 Vignette examples

Narrative format: following hip fracture

Scenario A: moderate

Jean lives in her own home and cares for herself. Before her fall, Jean was out and about quite a bit with her church group. She swam on a regular basis and occasionally looked after her grandchildren. Jean broke her hip when she fell. She is finding it difficult to do everything at home now that she walks with a stick. She needs help with shopping as she no longer drives or feels confident to shop alone. She can prepare only simple meals and is missing being able to bake for her friends. Jean can no longer manage the housework by herself. She misses her church activities but finds it too painful and tiring to be out for long periods. Jean experiences feelings of frustration and anger. Jean gets tearful thinking about all the things she can't do.

Scenario B: severe

Until her recent fall, Elizabeth lived in her own home and managed to care for herself. She was active in her local community. Elizabeth broke her hip when she fell. She is now unable to live alone as she requires a great deal of help to do most things. Elizabeth now lives in a nursing home near to her family but away from her friends. She is limited in where she can walk because of the frame and is unable to walk for long distances. She is unable to shower or dress without help from the nurse. She is unable to pursue her gardening or community work. Her leg aches sometimes at night. She has become anxious and is easily upset.

Structured format: symptomatic gallstone disease

- *Imagine you have gallstones over the rest of your life and you experience the following:*
- *You have no special procedures*
- *You are not in hospital*
- *Once a week you have an episode of severe stomach pain that lasts for three hours*
- *You do not feel like eating on the days you have pain*
- *You are able to walk after the pain is gone*
- *You do not feel like doing your usual activities on the days you have pain*
- *You have no scar*

have explored alternative narrative formats, including simulator spectacles to replicate vision states (Aballéa and Tsuchiya 2007) and videos of actors describing what it is like to live with schizophrenia (Lenert *et al.* 2004). Vignettes may be valued by either general population respondents, or by patients with a medical condition relevant to the vignettes under examination. The use of vignettes provides a convenient way to obtain utility values for a limited number of health states for use in cost-effectiveness models, and vignette-based utilities have been commonly used in submissions to agencies like NICE (Tosh *et al.* 2011).

In Box 8.3 some suggestions for good practice are made, taking into account the previous discussion of the development of CSPBMs. The suggested good practice guidelines should help to reduce biases and enhance the validity of vignette-based methods. In an effort to provide better empirical basis for vignettes, methods have been developed for constructing vignettes based on HRQL data from clinical studies.

Box 8.3 Good practice suggestions for the construction and valuation of health state vignettes

- The number of states should adequately reflect the severity distribution of the relevant patient group.

- The vignettes should be clear and comprehensible to respondents valuing them.

- The descriptions should be based on the best available evidence from multiple sources, which may include clinician interviews, patient interviews, clinical trial data, and published literature. When conducting qualitative research with patients and/or clinicians for this purpose, interviews should be conducted until consensus and saturation are reached (i.e. the point at which new interviews are not yielding new information).

- Patient-level quantitative data from patient-reported measures should be used where possible to inform statements about intensity or frequency. Examples of how to do this can be found in the literature (Lloyd *et al.* 2011; Matza *et al.* 2014*b*).

- Condition labelling and attribution should be avoided in most situations as they may introduce extraneous information and yield biased responses (Rowen *et al.* 2012*b*), although there are situations when the label may be necessary for clarity (Matza *et al.* 2014*b*).

- Vignettes should avoid statements involving uncertainty (e.g. 'you may have symptoms'), which presents difficulty for respondents in the valuation task.

- If vignettes describe change over time (i.e. path states), the amount of time in the vignette (e.g. the time horizon of the valuation task) must be considered when using the resulting utility values in a model (Matza *et al.* 2014*a*).

- Value the vignettes using methods and populations recognized by the intended audience (e.g. NICE, SMC, CVZ, or some other agency).

This has been done more formally using cluster analysis or Rasch (see examples in Sugar *et al.* 1998; Young *et al.* 2011; Mavranezouli *et al.* 2013), though these may not generate the states being used in the cost-effectiveness model. Less formal methods can use the average level across key items indicated by patients in the state of interest (Lloyd *et al.* 2011; Matza *et al.* 2014b). Finally, it is recommended that researchers carefully consider vignette characteristics, such as: whether to include the disease label; the use of statements implying risk or uncertainty; length or level of detail of the vignette; and any change over time described in the vignette (Matza *et al.* 2015; Matza *et al.* 2014a; Rowen *et al.* 2012b). Each of these factors can have a substantial impact on potential biases, the resulting utility values, and the usefulness of the values in models.

The major limitations of this methodology arise from the poor quality of the evidence and the lack of comparability between studies. There are no formal guidelines regarding the format of the vignettes or the methods for developing them, which tend to be ad hoc and based on groups of experts. GPBMs or CSPBMs are patient-reported measures of health that capture the full distribution of outcomes in a given sample of patients, vignettes are drafted to describe a small number of 'typical' patients, and therefore the vignettes are not able to represent the varied distribution of patient symptoms and impact (Peasgood *et al.* 2010). The comparability of the vignette-based utility values between studies in the same condition is limited because their content is often tied to the specific outcomes of a treatment, including different treatment outcomes and side effects.

Despite these limitations, the vignette-based approach may be useful for estimating utilities in situations when it is not feasible to derive utilities via existing GPBM, due to rarity or the severity of the condition making it difficult to obtain patient-reported outcome measures (PROMs) data (though proxies could be used). Vignettes have been used when it is argued that GPBMs are not sensitive to specific symptoms (though CSPBMs may be a better solution), certain major adverse events, or some important processes of treatment. Vignettes can be designed to isolate the utility impact of these factors (Boye *et al.* 2011; Matza *et al.* 2014a; Matza *et al.* 2013, Matza *et al.* 2007). The vignette-based approach is a convenient, easy, and quick method to implement relative to developing CSPBMs and collecting PROMs data.

8.6 **Direct utility assessment**

Direct utility measurement is when the patient is asked to value his or her own health using a preference elicitation technique such as TTO or SG, where the upper anchor is full health. It differs fundamentally from the other approaches reviewed so far, where respondents (whether or not they have the condition) are asked to value hypothetical states selected by the researcher. Using the patient's valuation of his or her own state avoids the need to describe a state of health or well-being as the patient is experiencing it. Furthermore, it generates a value on the full health–dead scale required for QALYs. However, this raises important practical problems and the normative debate about the appropriateness of using patient values for policy making, instead of those of the general public (see Chapter 4).

8.7 **Well-being**

It can be argued that the impact of health on well-being is captured by GPBMs through the preference elicitation techniques. When respondents are valuing health states using TTO (see Chapter 4), for example, they are being asked how many years of their life in full health they are willing to trade for improvements in the health-related quality of their life; they are being asked to trade all aspects of their life, and not just health (though it may not be in full or best imaginable well-being). There are a number of criticisms for using preferences of health to reflect well-being. One is focusing, because respondents are being asked to pay attention to health and so may ignore the impact on other aspects of their life. For example, there is evidence that most people in the United Kingdom and Netherlands do not think about the impact on income when valuing health states using techniques like TTO (Tilling *et al.* 2012). It assumes that individuals are able to predict the impact of health on their future experience, but this has been shown not to be the case (Dolan and Kahneman 2008). General population respondents may not take account of their adaptation to the condition, for example. As a result, Dolan and Kahneman (2008) and others have advocated a more direct measurement of 'experienced utilities' to capture subjective well-being for informing public policy, rather than relying on the preferences (based often on the guesses) of the general population. This argument relates partly to the issue of whose values, but it also has implications for the way we describe what it is we want to value.

8.7.1 **What is well-being?**

Well-being is broadly conceived as how well an individual's life is going. As a subjective construct, well-being has been described under three headings: hedonism (well-being increases when an individual experience more pleasure and/or less pain); flourishing theories (well-being increases when an individual fulfils their nature as a human being, or 'flourishes', which has been assessed using concepts of psychological well-being, such as autonomy, personal growth, self-acceptance, purpose in life, environmental mastery, and positive relations) (Ryff 1995); and life evaluation or life satisfaction (well-being increases when an individual positively assesses his or her life) (Haybron 2008). Traditionally there are also objective list accounts of well-being including items such as literacy and accommodation, and may include health (e.g. ability to see, lack of pain), accounts based on preferences (Parfit 1984) and Sen's capabilities approach (Sen 1985).

Some literature has developed around trying to measure Sen's notion of a capability set. Capability sets are made up of those things you can do or be. He advocated the use of capability sets as a measure of individual advantage in response to concerns about an overreliance on outcomes and utilities in economics. Sen argued for a concern with what you *can* do or be, rather than what you actually choose (or happen) to do or be. This contrasts with conventional consequentialist measures like EQ-5D. Although Sen remains reluctant to set out a definitive list of things that constitute desirable capabilities, there have been several attempts (Nussbaum 1999; Anand *et al.* 2009; Al-Janabi *et al.* 2012); though it is doubtful whether capability sets can be measured using questionnaires (see Burchardt 2005). An attempt to measure capabilities in health and social care is the ICECAP (Al-Janabi *et al.* 2012), which tries to achieve this by asking respondents whether they 'can have . . .' or 'are able to . . .'. The ICECAP will be described further later in the chapter (section 8.7.5.1).

There are a number of tools available to measure subjective well-being (SWB), including simple self-reported items on happiness (e.g. 'how happy have you been . . .') and life satisfaction (on the whole, are you . . . satisfied with the life you lead'? 4 very satisfied, 3 fairly satisfied, 2 not very satisfied, 1 not satisfied at all, Eurobarometer). There are also multi-item measures of psychological and mental well-being, such as the Warwick-Edinburgh Mental Well-being Scale (WEMWBS) which contains 14 positively worded items to measure concepts around feelings and psychological flourishing (Tennant *et al.* 2007; Stewart-Brown *et al.* 2009).

8.7.2 Health vs well-being—how do they compare?

There is an important question about the conceptual differences between health and well-being. Existing GPBMs of health, for example, have dimensions such as role functioning (e.g. work) and social activities captured in EQ-5D or SF-6D, that are arguably nearer to notions of psychological well-being than health; some measures even have items concerning happiness (HUI3) or feeling low (e.g. SF-6D) that were intended to assess mental health. While the dimensions of these health measures do not cover all aspects of well-being, they extend beyond what many would regard as health. However, the World Health Organization's definition of health as ' . . . a state of complete physical, mental and social wellbeing . . .' has been very influential in the development of health status measures (Ware and Sherbourne 1992), although it has also been criticized for being indistinguishable from the concept of well-being itself (Evans and Wolfson 1980).

A comparison of health and SWB scales by Richardson and colleagues (2014) found that some GPBMs account for a large proportion of variation in SWB, notably AQoL and SF-6D, while EQ-5D accounted for the least (Richardson *et al.* 2015). The descriptive systems of AQoL and SF-6D contain concepts of well-being, including simple affect statements like 'downhearted and low' and 'full of life', and AQoL also covers self-worth, social isolation, and control. However, these well-being concepts are to some extent 'diluted' by physical health dimensions like pain, mobility, and the senses. A recent comparison of health (EQ-5D) and well-being measures (including WEMWBS and the ICECAP measure of capabilities) found that they are significantly correlated, but the effect sizes associated with physical health conditions (like musculaskeletal diseases) are much larger for EQ-5D than the well-being measures (Mukuria *et al.* 2015). By contrast, well-being measures in the same study produced comparable effects sizes for mental health and had larger effect sizes associated with non-health states like employment, education, and marital status. This research is consistent with findings from studies that have tried to map EQ-5D and SF-6D onto SWB measures of happiness and life satisfaction. These have shown that the physical dimensions of mobility and physical functioning have little or no impact on SWB, and the largest coefficients are for mental health, with the coefficients of other dimensions in between (Mukuria and Brazier 2012; Dolan *et al.* 2012).

8.7.3 **Using well-being measures in economic evaluation**

There is no reason why the concept of a QALY needs to be limited strictly to health; indeed its very name indicates a rather broader view of benefits in quality of life than just health.

One way of using well-being scales in economic evaluation could be to re-weight generic measures like EQ-5D or SF-6D (O'Donnell *et al.* 2014), by replacing preferences (like those obtained from TTO and SG data) with measures of experience from SWB data. These studies have used regression techniques to estimate unanchored weights for EQ-5D and SF-6D, by using self-reported happiness and satisfaction data from members of the public or patients (Dolan *et al.* 2012; Mukuria and Brazier *et al.* 2012). This involves mapping between health as the source variable and well-being as the target variable. The methods for doing this have been described in the mapping section. The result of this mapping is that mental health gets a much larger weight than the other dimensions compared to preference-based weighting using TTO or SG. There are a number of criticisms with this approach. The cross-sectional analyses undertaken to date are limited by assuming a causal relationship from health to SWB. This limitation could be partly addressed by modelling causality using longitudinal data containing the measures of interest. There is also a concern, as with mapping studies in general (see Chapter 7), that these analyses ignore measurement error and the role of background characteristics which may result in an artificial correlation between the way self-reported health and well-being items are completed.

The use of SWB measures in economic evaluation is also limited by the fact that they are often single items that are scored assuming the response choices have equal intervals, or where there are multiple items, they are simply summed together. This makes interpretation of the predicted well-being scores problematic, since these may not reflect their cardinal value to people in the various states. Econometric techniques that avoid the assumption of cardinality do not provide weights that can be readily used in economic evaluation. Finally, well-being scales are not anchored on the zero to one scale required to calculate QALYs. This limits the application in health where mortality is a key outcome.

8.7.4 **Anchoring well-being measures**

There are two principal approaches to addressing the problems of a lack of anchoring onto a common metric that could be used in economic evaluation. One approach is to estimate the relationship between health and other outcomes in terms of income (i.e. to monetize them). This approach also uses SWB as the dependent variable, and models this in terms of a broad set of determinants including health, income, and other outcomes; then it estimates exchange rates, or marginal rates of substitution, between income and health (or other outcomes) (Ferrer-i-Carbonell and Van Praag 2002). The health descriptions to date have been in terms of disease labels alone, and so only provide values for complete cure, and not changes in health states that can be used in most health care contexts. Furthermore, monetary equivalent values change depending on the well-being measure used, though theoretically they should not (Powdthavee and van den Berg 2011). There is scope for exploring this method further.

Another approach is to develop a well-being QALY or well-being-adjusted life years (WELBY) with a classification system based around well-being rather than health-related quality of life. A multidimensional well-being classification system like EQ-5D could be formed from a measure like WEMWBS and valued using TTO, for example. The disadvantage is that a general well-being measure is less specific to any single sector, and so may have less sensitivity than more sector specific measures such as EQ-5D and ASCOT (see section 8.7.5). A criticism from those who want to use experience-based utility assessments is that this approach has re-introduced preferences into the equation in order to achieve the quantity–quality trade-off. However, a responding argument is that at least the classification system would provide a better description of the impact on people's lives than a health classification system like the EQ-5D. Ultimately, the use of well-being measures rather than health measures in determining resource allocation for health care depends on the objectives of policy makers, but it is an area requiring significant research.

8.7.5 **Preference-based measures beyond health—two examples**

There has been work to develop measures beyond more traditional notions of health, though they have not been exclusively concerned with well-being. The AQoL-8D described here already is one example of a GPBM that has explicitly attempted to incorporate more 'psychosocial' concerns. Two other examples are the ICECAP capability measures, and the ASCOT measure of social care quality of life.

8.7.5.1 **ICECAP**

The ICECAP-A (or Investigating Choice Experiments Capability Measure for Adults; Al-Janabi *et al.* 2012) is a capability well-being measure for adults that aimed to draw upon Sen's capability theory. An earlier version (ICECAP-O) was developed for use in older populations (Grewal *et al.* 2006). The ICECAP-A has five items that can take one of four levels: *stability* (being able to feel settled and secure); *attachment* (being able to have love, friendship, and support); *autonomy* (being able to be independent); *achievement* (being able to achieve and progress); and *enjoyment* (being able to have enjoyment and pleasure).

The authors claim that it measures capability, which is achieved by prefixing items with the words 'able to' or 'can', for example, 'can have a lot/quite a bit/a little/ or cannot have any'. The dimensions cover aspects of flourishing or psychological well-being along with a more hedonic item (enjoyment). The content was developed from in-depth interviews with a sample of the general adult population to define conceptual attributes of quality of life and the capabilities that are important to people in their lives (Al-Janabi *et al.* 2012).

The instrument has been scored from a survey of the general population using best–worst scaling (BWS), a technique like DCE that is rooted in a choice paradigm called random utility theory (Flynn *et al.* 2015). The values have not been anchored on the scale where zero is equivalent to being dead, but on a 0–1 scale where zero is the worst state (i.e. no capability on any dimension) and one the best state (full capability on all dimensions) defined by the measure. Anchoring zero at no-capabilities is not the same as being equivalent to dead, and the authors of the scale accept that 'although death implies no capability, the reverse is not necessarily true' (Flynn *et al.* 2015).

There is published evidence of its construct validity in the general population (Al-Janabi *et al.* 2012) and it is being used in clinical trials where more may be learnt about its properties in due course. It is comparatively untested and the wording used to design the items assesses capabilities, such as 'I can have a lot of love, friendship, and support', 'I can have a lot of enjoyment and pleasure', and need to be examined more closely. A 'think aloud' study on the ICECAP-A identified that some individuals have problems with interpreting the wording of the instrument (Al-Janabi *et al.* 2013). Another concern regards the exclusive use of positive items, which may mean that it is inappropriate for severely ill populations. More independent testing of this measure is required (see Box 8.4).

Box 8.4 ICECAP-A

About your overall quality of life

Please indicate which statements best describe your overall quality of life at the moment by placing a tick in ONE box for each of the five groups listed here.

1. **Feeling settled and secure**

   I am able to feel settled and secure in all areas of my life

   I am able to feel settled and secure in many areas of my life

   I am able to feel settled and secure in a few areas of my life

   I am unable to feel settled and secure in any areas of my life

2. **Love, friendship, and support**

   I can have a lot of love, friendship, and support

   I can have quite a lot of love, friendship, and support

   I can have a little love, friendship, and support

   I cannot have any love, friendship, and support

3. **Being independent**

   I am able to be completely independent

   I am able to be independent in many things

   I am able to be independent in a few things

   I am unable to be at all independent

4. **Achievement and progress**

   I can achieve and progress in all aspects of my life

   I can achieve and progress in many aspects of my life

I can achieve and progress in a few aspects of my life

I cannot achieve and progress in any aspects of my life

5. Enjoyment and pleasure

I can have a lot of enjoyment and pleasure

I can have quite a lot of enjoyment and pleasure

I can have a little enjoyment and pleasure

I cannot have any enjoyment and pleasure

8.7.5.2 The Adult Social Care Outcomes Toolkit

The Adult Social Care Outcomes Toolkit (ASCOT) is a measure of social care-related quality of life that is designed to assess the extent to which an individual's social care needs and wants are being met. It also draws upon Sen's theory of capabilities, with the level of met need in a domain being disaggregated into having needs met and an 'ideal' state, in which the level of functioning in the domain is consistent with individual preferences. This suggests that while capabilities matter, the individual with low levels of functioning can be judged by society as having an unacceptable level of need, regardless of whether they recognize this to be the case (Netten *et al.* 2012).

The descriptive system was developed using qualitative work with social care service users, carers, and staff. It has eight dimensions: five reflecting basic social care-related needs (*accommodation, cleanliness/comfort and safety, food and drink, personal care, being treated with dignity*), and three reflecting higher order concerns (*control over daily life, social participation*, and *involvement/occupation*). For each item the level of met need is assessed across four levels: *ideal, no unmet needs, some unmet needs* and *high unmet needs* (e.g. 'My home is: as clean and comfortable as I want, is adequately clean and comfortable, not quite clean or comfortable enough, or not at all clean or comfortable').

There are two methods of scoring the instrument. One is to use scores developed from a general population survey using BWS; another is to anchor these BWS scores onto the QALY scale, where zero is for states equivalent to being dead, chained by using TTO values for a sample of states (Netten *et al.* 2012).

It can be used in the community or in nursing/residential homes. It has been used in the Adult Social Care Survey in England and has been adopted by NICE in its methods for economic evaluation of social care (NICE 2013*b*). Evidence for its construct validity is starting to emerge (Malley *et al.* 2012), but has not been subject to any independent testing at the time of writing (see Box 8.5).

Box 8.5 The Adult Social Care Outcome Toolkit (ASCOT)

Domain level

Accommodation cleanliness and comfort

1. My home is as clean and comfortable as I want
2. My home is adequately clean and comfortable
3. My home is not quite clean or comfortable enough
4. My home is not at all clean or comfortable

Safety

1. I feel as safe as I want
2. Generally I feel adequately safe, but not as safe as I would like
3. I feel less than adequately safe
4. I don't feel at all safe

Food and drink

1. I get all the food and drink I like when I want
2. I get adequate food and drink at OK times
3. I don't always get adequate or timely food and drink
4. I don't always get adequate or timely food and drink, and I think there is a risk to my health

Personal care

1. I feel clean and am able to present myself the way I like
2. I feel adequately clean and presentable
3. I feel less than adequately clean or presentable
4. I don't feel at all clean or presentable

Control over daily life

1. I have as much control over my daily life as I want
2. I have adequate control over my daily life
3. I have some control over my daily life, but not enough
4. I have no control over my daily life

Social participation and involvement

1. I have as much social contact as I want with people I like
2. I have adequate social contact with people
3. I have some social contact with people, but not enough
4. I have little social contact with people and feel socially isolated

Dignity

1. The way I'm helped and treated makes me think and feel better about myself
2. The way I'm helped and treated does not affect the way I think or feel about myself
3. The way I'm helped and treated sometimes undermines the way I think and feel about myself
4. The way I'm helped and treated completely undermines the way I think and feel about myself

Occupation and employment

1. I'm able to spend my time as I want, doing things I value or enjoy
2. I'm able do enough of the things I value or enjoy with my time
3. I do some of the things I value or enjoy with my time, but not enough
4. I don't do anything I value or enjoy with my time

Reproduced with permission from Netten A *et al.*, 'Outcomes of Social Care for Adults: Developing a Preference Weighted Measure', *Health Technology Assessment*, Volume 16, Issue 16, pp. 1–166, Copyright © 2012.

8.8 **Conclusions**

This chapter has examined alternative methods for generating health state utility including developing and using CSPBMs, 'bolting-on' dimensions to generic measures, health vignettes (or scenarios), direct valuation by patients and the use of broader well-being measures. The methods for applying these approaches have been described in some detail, but readers wishing to develop their own measures are also recommended to go to specific publications on developing condition-specific measures and 'bolting-on' (e.g. Brazier *et al.* 2012; Longworth *et al.* 2014).

The main threat identified with using these alternatives is the potential loss of comparability between QALYs generated by different measures. However, it could be argued that using an inadequate generic measure only achieves consistency at the expense of not reflecting what matters to patients and/or the general public. For use in cross-programme comparison, the decision to use different GPBMs or CSPBMs is ultimately a trade-off between having measures that are relevant and sensitive to those things that matter to a specific condition, and its treatment against the consequences of treatment side effects, existing comorbidities, and any preference interactions between those dimensions included and those excluded in the measures. These will vary by condition, by patient group, and/or by treatment, and jurisdictions differ on the relative importance they ascribe to these issues.

This chapter has also reviewed the use of measures of well-being. Measures of well-being have been shown to overlap considerably with the descriptive systems of some of the GPBMs of health like SF-6D and AQoL (Richardson *et al.* 2014). Health economists have also used TTO or other techniques directly in people suffering ill health. Measures of SWB or direct utility reflect the way people adapt to health, particularly to physical health problems. The policy question is whether or not giving less weight to physical health would be consistent with the social objectives of a health care system like the NHS. This returns to the normative argument discussed in Chapter 4, regarding whose values should count.

Acknowledgements

Text extracts reprinted from *Value in Health,* Volume 16, Issue 1, Longworth L and Rowen D, 'Mapping to obtain EQ-5D health utility values for use in NICE HTAs', pp. 202–10, Copyright © 2013 Elsevier, with permission from Elsevier, http://www.sciencedirect.com/science/journal/10983015

References

Aballéa S, Tsuchiya A (2007). Seeing for yourself: feasibility study towards valuing visual impairment using simulation spectacles. *Health Economics* **16**:537–43.

All-Party Parliamentary Group on Well-being Economics (2014). Report by the APPG on Well-being and Economics, New Economics Foundation. Available at: http://b.3cdn.net/nefoundation/ccdf9782b6d8700f7c_lcm6i2ed7.pdf

Al-Janabi H, Flynn T, Coast J (2012). Development of a self-report measure of capability wellbeing for adults: the ICECAP-A. *Quality of Life Research* **21**:167–76.

Al-Janabi H, Keeley T, Mitchell P, Coast J (2013). Can capabilities be self-reported? A think aloud study. *Social Science and Medicine* **87**:116–22.

Anand P, Hunter G, Carter I, Dowding K, Guala F, van Hees M (2009). The development of capability indicators. *Journal of Human Development and Capabilities* **10**:125–52.

Ara R, Brazier J (2008). Deriving an algorithm to convert the eight mean SF-36 dimension scores into a mean EQ-5D preference-based score from published studies (where patient level data are not available). *Value in Health* **11**:1131–43.

Barton GR, Bankart J, Davis AC, Summerfield QA (2004). Comparing utility scores before and after hearing-aid provision. *Applied Health and Economic Health Policy* **3**:103–5.

Bass EB, Steinberg EP, Pitt HA, Griffiths RI, Lillemoe KD, Saba GP, Johns C (1994). Comparison of the rating scale and the standard gamble in measuring patient preferences for outcomes of gallstone disease. *Medical Decision Making* **14**:307–14.

Boye KS, Matza LS, Walter KN, Van Brunt K, Palsgrove AC, Tynan A (2011). Utilities and disutilities for attributes of injectable treatments for type 2 diabetes. *European Journal of Health Economics* **12**:219–30.

Brazier JE, Roberts J, Deverill M (2002). The estimation of a preference-based single index measure for health from the SF-36. *Journal of Health Economics* **21**:271–92.

Brazier JE, Yang Y, Tsuchiya A, Rowen (2010). A review of studies mapping (or cross walking) non-preference based measures of health to generic preference-based measures. *European Journal of Health Economics* **11**:215–25.

Brazier JE, Rowen D, Tsuchiya A, Yang Y, Young T (2011). The impact of adding a generic dimension to a condition-specific preference-based measure. *Social Science and Medicine* **73**:245–53.

Brazier J, Rowen D, Mavranezouli I, Tsuchiya A, Young T, Yang Y (2012). Developing and testing methods for deriving preference-based measures of health from condition specific measures (and other patient based measures of outcome). *Health Technology Assessment* **16**:1–114.

Briggs A, Wild D, Lees M, Reaney M, Dursun S, Parry D, Mukherjee J (2008). Impact of schizophrenia and schizophrenia treatment-related adverse events on quality of life: direct utility elicitation. *Health and Quality of Life Outcomes* **6**:105.

Brooks R, & the EuroQol Group (1996). EuroQol: The current state of play. *Health Policy* **37**:53–72.

Burchardt T (2005). Incomes, functionings and capabilities: the well-being of disabled people in Britain. *PhD thesis, The London School of Economics and Political Science (LSE)*.

Burr JM, Kilonzo M, Vale L, Ryan M (2007). Developing a preference-based glaucoma utility index using a discrete choice experiment. *Optometry and Vision Science* **84**:E797–809.

Cadman D, Goldsmith C, Torrance G, Boyle M, Furlong W (1986). *Development of a health status index for Ontario children: final report to the Ontario Ministry of Health.* Grant Research DM648 (00633), McMaster University, Hamilton, Ontario, Canada.

Chuang LH, Kind P, Chuang LH, Kind P (2009). Converting the SF-12 into the EQ-5D: an empirical comparison of methodologies. *Pharmacoeconomics* **27**:491–505.

Coast J (1992). Reprocessing data to form QALYs. *British Medical Journal* **305**:87–90.

Coast J, Flynn T, Grewal I, Lewis J, Natarajan L, Sproston K, Peters T (2006). *Developing an index of capability for health and social policy evaluation for older people: theoretical and methodological challenges.* HESG, University of Sheffield, UK.

Dakin H, Petrou S, Haggard M, Benge S, Williamson I (2010). Mapping analyses to estimate health utilities based on responses to the OM8-30 Otitis Media Questionnaire. *Quality of Life Research* **19**:65–80.

Dolan P (1997). Modelling valuations for EuroQol health states. *Medical Care* **35**:1095–108.

Dolan P, Gudex C, Kind P, Williams, A (1996). Valuing health states: a comparison of methods. *Journal of Health Economics* **2**:209–32.

Dolan P, Kahneman D (2008). Interpretations of utility and their implications for the valuation of health. *The Economic Journal* **118**:215–34.

Dolan P, Lee H, Peasgood T (2012). Losing sight of the wood for the trees: some issues in describing and valuing health, and another possible approach. *Pharmacoeconomics* **30**:1035–49.

Drummond MF, Sculpher M, Claxton K, O'Brien B, Stoddart GL, Torrance GW (2015). *Methods for the economic evaluation of health care programmes.* Oxford Medical Publications, Oxford, UK.

Eldabe S, Lloyd A, Verdian L, Meguro M, Maclaine G, Dewilde S (2010). Eliciting health state utilities from the general public for severe chronic pain. *European Journal of Health Economics* **11**:323–30.

Espallargues M, Czoski-Murray C, Bansback N, Carlton J, Lewis G, Hughes L, et al. (2006). The impact of age related macular degeneration on health state utility values. *Investigative Ophthalmology and Vision Science* **46**:4016–23.

Feeny DH, Furlong WJ, Torrance GW, Goldsmith CH, Zenglong Z, Depauw S, et al. (2002). Multi-attribute and single-attribute utility function the health utility index mark 3 system. *Medical Care* **40**:113–28.

Evans RG, Wolfson AD (1980). *Faith, hope and charity: health care in the utility function.* Department of Economics, University of British Columbia and Department of Health Administration, University of Toronto, unpublished paper.

Ferrer-i-Carbonell A, van Praag BM (2002). The subjective costs of health losses due to chronic diseases. An alternative model for monetary appraisal. *Health Economics* **11**:709–22.

Flynn TN, Huynh E, Peters TJ, Al-Janabi H, Moody A, Clemens S, Coast J (2015). Scoring the ICECAP-A capability instrument. Estimation of a UK general population tariff. *Health Economics* **24**:258–69.

Gerard K, Dobson M, Hall K (1993). Framing and labelling effects in health descriptions: quality adjusted life years for treatment of breast cancer. *Journal of Clinical Epidemiology* **46**:77–84.

Gerard K, Johnstone K, Brown J (1999). The role of a pre-scored multiattribute health state classification in validating condition specific health state descriptions. *Health Economics* **8**:685–99.

Gudex C (1991). *Are we lacking a dimension of energy in the Euroqol instrument?* Paper presented at the 8th Pleanary Meeting of the EuroQol Group, Lund, Sweden.

Iqbal I, Dasgupta B, Taylor P, Heron L, Pilling C (2012). Elicitation of health state utilities associated with differing durations of morning stiffness in rheumatoid arthritis. *Journal of Medical Economics* **15**:1192–200.

Gold MR, Siegel JE, Russell LB, Weinstein MC (1996). *Cost-effectiveness in health and medicine*. Oxford University Press, Oxford, UK.

Gray AM, Rivero-Arias O, Clarke PM (2006). Estimating the association between SF-12 responses and EQ-5D utility values by response mapping. *Medical Decision Making* **26**:18–29.

Grewal I, Lewis J, Flynn TN, Brown J, Bond J, Coast J (2006). Developing attributes for a generic quality of life measure for older people: preferences or capabilities? *Social Science & Medicine* **62**:1891–901.

Haybron DM (2008). *The pursuit of unhappiness: the elusive psychology of well-being*. Oxford University Press, Oxford, UK.

Hernández Alava M, Brazier J, Rowen D, Tsuchiya A (2013). Common scale valuations across different preference-based measures: estimation using rank data. *Medical Decision Making* **33**:839–52.

Hernández Alava M, Wailoo A, Ara R (2012). Tails from the peak district: adjusted limited dependent variable mixture models of EQ-5D health state utility values. *Value in Health* **15**:550–61.

Juniper EF, Guyatt GH, Ferrie PJ, Griffith LE (1993). Measuring quality of life in asthma. *American Review of Respiratory Disease* **147**:832–8.

Krabbe PF, Stouthard ME, Essink-Bot ML, Bonsel GJ (1999). The effect of adding a cognitive dimension to the EuroQol multiattribute health-status classification system. *Journal of Clinical Epidemiology* **52**:293–301.

Lenert L, Sturley AP, Rapaport MH, Chavez S, Mohr PE, Rupnow M (2004). Public preferences for health states with schizophrenia and a mapping function to estimate utilities from positive and negative scale scores. *Schizophrenia Research* **71**:83–95.

Lloyd A (2003). Threats to the estimation of benefit: are preference estimation methods accurate? *Health Economics* **12**:393–402.

Lloyd A, Doyle S, Dewilde S, Turk F (2008). Preferences and utilities for the symptoms of moderate to severe allergic asthma. *European Journal of Health Economics* **9**:275–84.

Lloyd A, Hodgkins P, Sasane R, Akehurst R, Sonuga-Barke EJS, Fitzgerald P, *et al.* (2011). Estimation of utilities in attention-deficit hyperactivity disorder for economic evaluations. *Patient* **4**:247–57.

Longworth L, Rowen D (2013). Mapping to obtain EQ-5D health utility values for use in NICE HTAs. Value in Health **16**(1):202–10.

Longworth L, Yang Y, Young T, Mulhern B, Hernández Alava M, Mukuria C, *et al.* (2014). Use of generic and condition specific measures of health-related quality of life in NICE decision-making. *Health Technology Assessment* **18**:1–224.

Lu, G, Brazier, JE, Ades, AE (2013). Mapping from disease-specific to generic health-related quality-of-life scales: a common factor model. *Value in Health* **16**:177–84.

Malley J, Towers A, Netten A, Brazier J, Forder J, Flynn T (2012). An assessment of the construct validity of the ASCOT measure of social care-related quality of life with older people. *Health and Quality of Life Outcomes* **10**:21.

Matza LS, Boye KS, Yurgin N, Brewster-Jordan J, Mannix S, Shorr JM, Barber BL (2007). Utilities and disutilities for type 2 diabetes treatment-related attributes. *Quality of Life Research* **16**:1251–65.

Matza LS, Chung K, Van Brunt K, Brazier JE, Braun A, Currie B, *et al.* (2014*a*). Health state utilities for skeletal-related events secondary to bone metastases. *European Journal of Health Economics* **15**:7–18.

Matza LS, Cong Z, Chung K, Stopeck A, Tonkin K, Brown J, *et al.* (2013). Utilities associated with subcutaneous injections and intravenous infusions for treatment of patients with bone metastases. *Patient Prefer Adherence* **7**:855–65.

Matza LS, Devine MK, Haynes VS, Davies EW, Kostilec JM, Televantou F, Jordan JB (2014*b*). Health state utilities associated with adult attention-deficit/hyperactivity disorder. *Patient Prefer Adherence* **8**:997–1006.

Matza LS, Dillon JF, Kalsekar A, Davies EW, Devine MK, Jordon JB, *et al.* (2015). Health state utilities associated with attributes of treatments for hepatitis C. *European Journal of Health Economics* **16**:1005–18.

Matza LS, Secnik K, Rentz AM, Mannix S, Sallee FR, Gilbert D, Revicki DA (2005). Assessment of health state utilities for attention-deficit/hyperactivity disorder in children using parent proxy report. *Quality of Life Research* **14**:735–47.

Mavranezouli I, Brazier JE, Young TA, Barkham M (2011). Using Rasch analysis to form plausible health states amenable to valuation: the development of the CORE-6D from a measure of common mental health problems (CORE-OM). *Quality of Life Research* **20**:321–33.

Mavranezouli I, Brazier JE, Rowen D, Barkham M (2013). Estimating a preference-based index from the clinical outcomes in routine evaluation—outcome measure (CORE-OM): valuation of CORE-6D. *Medical Decision Making* **33**:381–95.

McKenna SP, Ratcliffe J, Meads DM, Brazier JE (2008). Development and validation of a preference based measure derived from the Cambridge Pulmonary Hypertension Outcome Review (CAMPHOR) for use in cost utility analyses. *Health and Quality of Life Outcomes* **6**:65

Miller GA (1956). The magical number seven, plus or minus two: some limits on our capacity for processing information. *The Psychological Review* **63**:81–97.

Mukuria C, Brazier J (2012). Valuing the EQ-5D and the SF-6D health states using subjective well-being: a secondary analysis of patient data. *Social Science and Medicine* **77**:97–105.

Mukuria C, Peasgood T, Brazier J (2015). *An empirical comparison of wellbeing measures used in the UK.* Policy Research Unit in Economic Evaluation of Health and Care Interventions. EEPRU Report 027, Universities of Sheffield and York, UK.

Mulhern B, Smith SC, Rowen D, Brazier JE, Knapp M, Lamping DL, *et al.* (2012) Improving the measurement of QALYs in Dementia: Developing patient- and carer-reported health state classification systems using Rasch analysis. *Value in Health* **15**:346–56.

Mulhern B, Rowen D, Snape D, Jacoby A, Marson T, Hughes D, *et al.* (2014). Valuations of epilepsy-specific health states: a comparison of patients with epilepsy and the general population. *Epilepsy Behaviour* **36C**:12–17.

National Institute for Health and Clinical Excellence (NICE) (2013*a*). *NICE guide to the methods of technology appraisal.* NICE, London, UK.

National Institute of Health and Care Excellence (NICE) (2013*b*) *The social care guidance manual.* NICE, London, UK. Available at: https://www.nice.org.uk/article/pmg10/chapter/1%20Introduction

Netten A, Burge P, Malley J, Potoglou D, Towers A, Brazier J, *et al.* (2012). Outcomes of social care for adults: developing a preference weighted measure. *Health Technology Assessment* **16**:1–165.

Nussbaum MC (1999). *Sex and social justice.* Oxford University Press, Oxford, UK.

O'Connor A (1989). Effects of framing and level of probability on patient preferences for cancer chemotherapy. *Journal of Clinical Epidemiology* **42**:119.

O'Donnell G, Deaton A, Durand A, Halpern D, Layard R (2014). *Well-being and policy, Legatum Institute.* Available at: http://www.li.com/programmes/the-commission-on-wellbeing-and-policy

OECD (2013). *OECD Guidelines on Measuring Subjective Well-being*, OECD Publishing. Available at: *http://dx.doi.org/10.1787/9789264191655-en*

Papaionnou D, Brazier J, Parry G (2011). How valid and responsive are generic health status measures, such as the EQ-5D and SF-36, in schizophrenia? A systematic review. *Value in Health* **14**:907–20.

Parfit D (1984). *Reasons and persons.* Oxford University Press, Oxford, UK.

Payakachat N, Summers KH, Pleil AM, Murawski MM, Thomas III J, Jennings K, *et al.* (2009) Predicting EQ-5D utility scores from the 25-item National Eye Institute Vision Function Questionnaire (NEI-VFQ 25) in patients with age-related macular degeneration. *Quality of Life Research* **18**:801–13.

Peasgood T, Ward SE, Brazier J (2010). Health-state utility values in breast cancer. *Expert Review of Pharmacoeconomics and Outcomes Research* **10**:553–66.

Powdthavee N, van den Berg B (2011). Putting different price tags on the same health problem: Re-evaluating the well-being valuation. *Journal of Health Economics* **30**:1032.

Rabin R, Rosser RM, Butler C (1993). Impact of diagnosis on utilities assigned to states of illness. *Journal of the Royal Society of Medicine* **86**:444.

Rentz AM, Kowalski JW, Walt JG, Hays RD, Brazier JE, Yu-Ren, Lee P, Bressler N, Revicki DA (2014). Development of a preference-based index from the national eye institute visual function questionnaire-25. *JAMA Ophthalmology* **132**:310–18.

Revicki DA, Wood M (1998). Patient-assigned health state utilities for depression-related outcomes: differences by depression severity and antidepressant medications. *Journal of Affective Disorders* **48**:25–36.

Richardson J, McKie J, Bariola E (2014). Multiattribute utility instruments and their use. In: Anthony J. Culyer (ed.), *Encyclopedia of health economics*, Vol **2**. Elsevier, San Diego, CA, pp. 341–65.

Richardson JRJ, Chen G, Khan MA, Iezzi AA (2015). Can multi-attribute utility instruments adequately account for subjective well-being? *Medical Decision Making* **353**:292–304.

Rivero-Arias O, Ouellet M, Gray A, Wolstenholme J, Rothwell PM, Luengo-Fernandez R (2010). Mapping the modified Rankin scale (mRS) measurement into the generic EQ-5D health outcome. *Medical Decision Making* **30**:341–54.

Robinson S, Bryan S (2001). 'Naming and framing': an investigation of the effect of disease labels on health state valuations. Health Economics Study Group Meeting, University of Oxford, UK.

Rowen D, Brazier J, Roberts J (2009). Mapping SF-36 onto the EQ-5D index: how reliable is the relationship? *Health and Quality of Life Outcomes* **7**:27.

Rowen D, Brazier J, Young T, Gaugris S, Craig BM, King MT, Velikova G (2011). Deriving a preference-based measure for cancer using the EORTC QLQ-C30. *Value in Health* **14**:721–31.

Rowen D, Brazier J, Tsuchiya A, Young T, Ibbotson R (2012*a*). It's all in the name, or is it? The impact of labeling on health state values. *Medical Decision Making* **32**:31–40.

Rowen D, Brazier JE, Tsuchiya A, Hernández M (2012*b*). Valuing states from multiple measures on the same VAS: A feasibility study. *Health Economics* **21**:715–29.

Rowen D, Brazier J (2014). Multi-attribute utility instruments: condition-specific versions. In: Anthony J. Culyer (ed.). *Encyclopedia of health economics*, Vol **2**. Elsevier, San Diego, CA, pp. 358–65.

Ryan M, Gerard K (2003). Using discrete choice experiments to value health care programmes: current practice and future research. *Applied Health Economics and Health Policy* **2**:55–64.

Ryff CD (1995). Psychological well-being in adult life. *Current Directions in Psychological Science* **4**:99–104.

Sackett DL, Torrance GW (1978). The utility of different health states as perceived by the general public. *Journal of Chronic Diseases* **31**:697–704.

Salkeld G, Cameron ID, Cumming RG, Easter S, Seymour J, Kurrle SE, Quine S. (2000). Quality of life related to fear of falling and hip fracture in older women: a time trade-off study. *British Medical Journal* **320**:241–46.

Schwartz A (2012). Measuring health-related quality of life: new findings and new questions. *Medical Decision Making* **32**:9.

Sen A (1985). *Commodities and capabilities*. North-Holland, Amsterdam, the Netherlands.

Stewart-Brown S, Tennant A, Tennant R, Platt S, Parkinson J, Weich S (2009). Internal construct validity of the Warwick-Edinburgh Mental Well-being Scale (WEMWBS): a Rasch analysis using data from the Scottish Health Education Population Survey. *Health and Quality of Life Outcomes* **7**:15.

Stevens KJ (2009). Developing a descriptive system for a new preference-based measure of health-related quality of life for children. *Quality of Life Research* **18**:1105–13.

Stevens K, Brazier J (2016). *Estimating the exchange rate between ASCOT and EQ-5D using preference-based mapping*. EEPRU Research Report, University of Sheffield, UK.

Stiglitz JE, Sen A, Fitoussi J-P (2009). *Report by the commission on the measurement of economic performance and social progess*. Available at: http://www.stiglitz-sen-fitoussi.fr/en/index.htm

Sugar CA, Sturm R, Lee TT, Sherbourne CD, Olshen RA, Wells KB, Lenert LA (1998). Empirically defined health states for depression from the SF-12. *Health Services Research* **33**:911–28.

Sullivan PW, Ghushchyan V (2006). Mapping the EQ-5D index from the SF-12: US general population preferences in a nationally representative sample. *Medical Decision Making* **26**:401–9.

Sundaram M, Smith MJ, Revicki DA, Elswick B, Miller LA (2009). Rasch analysis informed the development of a classification system for a diabetes-specific preference-based measure of health. *Journal of Clinical Epidemiology* **62**:845–56.

Tennant R, Hiller L, Fishwick R, Platt S, Joseph S, Weich S, *et al.* (2007). The Warwick-Edinburgh Mental Well-being Scale (WEMWBS): development and UK validation. *Health and Quality of Life Outcomes* **5**:63.

Tilling C, Krol M, Tsuchiya, Brazier J, van Exel J, Brouwer W (2012). Does the EQ-5D reflect lost earnings? *Pharmacoeconomics* **30**:47–61.

Tolley K, Goad C, Yi Y, Maroudas P, Haiderali A, Thompson G (2013). Utility elicitation study in the UK general public for late-stage chronic lymphocytic leukaemia. *European Journal of Health Economics* **14**:749–59.

Tosh JC, Longworth LJ, George E (2011). Utility values in National Institute for Health and Clinical Excellence (NICE) technology appraisals. *Value in Health* **14**:102–9.

Tosh J, Brazier J, Evans P, Longworth L (2012). A review of generic preference-based measures of health-related quality of life in visual disorders. *Value in Health* **15**:118–27.

Versteegh MM, Rowen D, Brazier J, Stolk EA (2010). Mapping onto EQ-5D for patients in poor health. *Health and Quality of Life Outcomes* **8**:1–13.

Ware JE, Sherbourne CD (1992). The MOS 36-item Short-Form Health Survey (SF-36): I. Conceptual framework and item selection. *Medical Care* **30**:473–83.

Yang Y, Brazier J, Tsuchiya A, Coyne K (2009). Estimating a preference-based single index from the overactive bladder questionnaire. *Value in Health* **12**:159–66.

Yang Y, Brazier J, Tsuchiya A, Young T (2011). Estimating a preference-based index for a 5-dimensional health state classification for asthma (AQL-5D) derived from the Asthma Quality of Life Questionnaire (AQLQ). *Medical Decision Making* **31**:281–91.

Yang Y, Brazier J, Tsuchiya A (2013). The effect of adding a sleep dimension to theEQ-5D. *Medical Decision Making* **34**:422–53.

Young T, Yang Y, Brazier JE, Tsuchiya A, Coyne K (2009). The first stage of developing preference-based measures: constructing a health state classification using Rasch analysis. *Quality in Life Research* **18**:253–65.

Young T, Rowen D, Norquist J, Brazier J (2010). Developing preference-based health measures: using Rasch analysis to generate health state values. *Quality of Life Research* **19**:907–17.

Young T, Yang Y, Brazier J, Tsuchyia A (2011). Use of Rasch analysis in reducing a large condition specific instrument for preference valuation: The case of moving from AQLQ to AQL-5D. *Medical Decision Making* **31**:195–210.

Chapter 9

Design and analysis of health state valuation data for model-based economic evaluations and for economic evaluations alongside clinical trials

9.1 Introduction to design and analysis of health state valuation data

The primary purpose of collecting and analysing health state valuation data is to use the data in an economic evaluation (Chapter 2). There are two main vehicles for undertaking economic evaluation: one is to use a cost-effectiveness model, and the other is to perform economic evaluation alongside a clinical trial. In practice, these two approaches are often not mutually exclusive as decision analytic models may incorporate health state values generated from economic evaluation(s) conducted alongside a clinical trial, and limitations in the length and scope of clinical trials usually mean that some form of modelling is needed to progress from the within-trial results to the economic result of interest (Briggs 2000). It is for this reason that decision analytic models have become a standard way to conduct an economic evaluation for submissions to regulatory authorities including the National Institute for Health and Clinical Excellence (NICE).

The main methodological issues associated with decision analytic models and undertaking an economic evaluation alongside a clinical trial have been described in Drummond *et al.* (2005). This chapter focuses on the needs of these two approaches in terms of the collection and analysis of health state values for use in economic evaluation.

As described in Chapters 7 and 8, there are three main methods for the collection and analysis of health state valuation data. The first, indirect, method involves the application of generic or condition-specific preference-based measures that use a standardized health state classification system and an existing set of preference weights. The second, also indirect, method involves the valuation of bespoke vignettes or hypothetical scenarios by public or patient samples, and the third, direct, method involves the direct elicitation of preferences from patients of their current state. For standardized instruments, there are a set of issues relating to the administration of the self-reporting descriptive system including who should be asked, the relevant question/s to ask, time points for administration, mode of administration, and sample size (sections 9.2.2 and 9.2.3). There are similar design issues around the direct elicitation of preferences including whom to ask, technique, time points, and sample size. This chapter deals with the practical issues of implementing these direct and indirect approaches. The construction of hypothetical scenarios or vignettes was examined in Chapter 8, and the design of studies to value health states has been described in Chapter 4 (including whom to ask, technique of valuation, and sample size).

Collecting and analysing data for decision analytic models raises additional issues. Models can be populated from a range of sources and often involve using data from studies that may not always be reported in an ideal form. Hence the data may need modification for use in an economic model. There are also other issues specific to economic models including what health state values should be used to represent normal populations and how to handle comorbidities. Standardized generic preference-based measures and valuation techniques are often administered on patients in clinical trials and may allow the extraction of health state values for use in economic models. Such secondary use of data generated by standardized generic preference-based measures and valuation techniques raises a host of analytical questions about how to summarize such data, and how to handle missing data and uncertainty. These questions are also examined in this chapter.

The first section presents requirements which are likely to be common to any study in which health state values are collected from patients and/or members of the general population. The second section considers issues specific to trial-based economic evaluations, and the final section considers issues specific to the design and analysis of health state valuation data for economic models.

9.2 Common issues for health state valuation studies

The basic method of data collection is assumed to have been selected, along with the specific instrumentation using the criteria set out in Chapter 7, such as a standardized generic (or condition-specific) preference-based measure, or the direct use of a valuation technique. Having made this choice, the researcher then has to consider a range of design issues: whom to ask; mode of administration; when to administer the instrument or valuation technique; and sample size.

9.2.1 Whom to ask

For economic evaluations of interventions in health care, it has become common practice to obtain health status data directly from patients where possible (Bowling 2004). Patients are usually in the best position to know how their health has affected their functioning and well-being. There is evidence from a range of sources that proxies do not tend to give the same response patterns to standardized generic preference-based or non-preference-based measures of health as patients themselves (Coucill *et al.* 2001; Eiser and Morse 2001; Brunner *et al.* 2005; Bryan *et al.* 2005; Sloane *et al.* 2005; Gabbe *et al.* 2012; Dinglas *et al.* 2013). Therefore, it seems appropriate to obtain patient responses in cases where patients are able and willing to provide such data. However, it is not always possible to ask patients questions about their own health, such as people with severe mental health problems, severe dementia, or patients who are simply too ill. In such instances, proxy measures may be obtained from family members or carers or from parents in the case of young children (see Box. 9.1).

Box 9.1 Patient versus proxy measurement of health-related quality of life? The cases of dementia and children

Dementia

In a study of patients with dementia, Coucill *et al.* (2001) found that patients' carers reported higher levels of disability across all five dimensions of the EQ-5D than patients themselves, whereas clinicians reported fewer problems on the 'pain/discomfort' and 'anxiety/depression' dimensions. Overall, the level of agreement was only fair (using a statistical measure of agreement known as the weighted kappa score). A study by Makai *et al.* (2014) investigated the influence of proxy characteristics on responses to the ICECAP-O capability well-being measure's German translation in older people with dementia living in a nursing home. It was found that work experience and gender influenced proxy responses. The findings from both of these studies raise important questions regarding which is the most appropriate proxy. Currently, it is also unclear as to the level of dementia severity at which patients are able to provide valid ratings of health-related quality of life using preference-based measures.

Children

In a recent review, Eiser and Varni (2013) investigated the similarities and differences between children and their parents in health status and symptom reporting. They noted three main findings from the available empirical evidence. Firstly, in relation to healthy children, parents typically rate their child's health status better than children themselves. In contrast, among children with chronic health conditions, parents typically rate their child's health status as worse than children themselves. Secondly, parents tend to be more in agreement with their children in relation to objective physical domains such as walking and running, but less so in terms of emotional or social functioning, as well as internal symptoms such as pain, fatigue, and gastrointestinal symptoms. Thirdly, parents' reporting of their children's health status is related to their reporting of their own health status. For example, mothers who are more distressed tend to rate their child's health status as worse than mothers who are less distressed. As is the case in patients with dementia, there is no general agreement as to the situations in which parent proxy-reporting should replace child self-report ratings of health-related quality of life using preference-based measures.

9.2.2 **Mode of administration**

To date, the vast majority of studies designed to generate health state values from generic preference-based measures (GPBMs) or condition-specific preference-based measures (CSPBMs) have used self-administered questionnaire formats, either in 'paper and pencil' versions, or more recently using digital and online formats. Historically, an interviewer mode of administration has been used more often for valuation techniques (where values have been elicited using health state descriptions or vignettes (Brazier *et al*. 2006; Milne *et al*. 2006) and for eliciting health state values directly from patients using an established procedure e.g. time trade-off (TTO) or standard gamble (SG) (Szabo *et al*. 2010; Wang *et al*. 2014)). More recently, digital and online formats have started to become more widely used for both the administration of generic preference-based measures with patients and general population samples, and for health state valuation exercises (Oppe *et al*. 2014; Ratcliffe *et al*. 2012; Bansback *et al*. 2012).

9.2.2.1 **Face-to-face interviews**

In a face-to-face interview, the interviewer rather than the respondent typically holds the responsibility of recording the responses. Interviewer-administered questionnaires facilitate the collection of larger amounts of information and more detailed and complex data. Response rates to interview surveys are typically much higher than for postal surveys due to their interactive and personal nature. Sample composition bias is typically reduced by ensuring that information is obtained from the target respondents. Interviews also enable responses from people with reading and writing difficulties, and from ethnic minorities whose first language is not English. The quality of the collected data may be enhanced through an interview, because the interviewer is on hand to offer clarification and reduce any misunderstandings. These advantages are particularly important in the context of both preference-based measures and health state valuation, but they are arguably more important for health valuation techniques including SG and TTO, due to their complexity.

The disadvantages of interviews include their expense and the possibility of interviewer bias due to differences in the way in which questions are posed or responses are recorded. There may also be a degree of respondents trying to please the interviewer.

9.2.2.2 **Telephone interviews**

Telephone interviews are a relatively low cost and speedy method of data collection, although the response rate may not be as high as with face-to-face interviews due to the lack of direct contact between the interviewer and the respondent. An advantage of telephone interviews is that strict control and close supervision of interviewers is possible because (with the consent of the respondent and the interviewer) interviewers can be monitored by supervisors listening in. Complex questions should be avoided in a telephone interview as it is more difficult for the respondent to answer reliably when there are a large number of possible responses. Similarly, long interviews should be avoided as respondents are more likely to terminate the call.

This approach has been used in valuation, most notably forming one component of the Oregon Medicaid experiment in the United States in the mid-1990s, where combinations of medical conditions and treatments were prioritized by members of the general public (Kaplan 1994) using a rating scale approach. It would be more difficult to operationalize in the case of more complex valuation techniques, such as SG and TTO. Furthermore, the more commonly used versions of these techniques require props or computer assistance (Brazier *et al.* 1999; Luo *et al.* 2013; Oppe *et al.* 2014).

9.2.2.3 Self-completion questionnaires

Historically, postal self-completion surveys have been the most common format for preference-based measures, although supervised self-completion questionnaires (where the respondent completes the questionnaire in the presence of a clinician or researcher who is able to offer assistance and explanation where required) have also been frequently used in assessing health status or quality of life. More recently, the internet or other electronic means have been taking over as the method of choice for the collection of health state valuation data for both preference-based measures and for patients valuing their own state. The main advantage of self-completion questionnaires is their low cost, which enables researchers to study large groups within a study population. Self-completion questionnaires are generally quicker to administer than interviewer-based surveys, and respondents may feel that they are able to respond more truthfully to sensitive questions using this approach.

The main disadvantage of self-completion questionnaires is that typically they result in lower response rates. Data collection periods may therefore extend over several months to allow for follow-ups and possibly telephone or computer-generated (e.g. email) reminders to try and boost the response rate. It is also often quite difficult to obtain a complete and accurate list of the population needed to act as a sampling frame. Responder bias, whereby respondents differ from non-respondents in terms of their socio-demographic characteristics, is also a real possibility. Such responder bias leads to a bias in the estimates obtained from a given sampling frame. Self-completion questionnaires are best suited to clear uncomplicated research questions which can be easily explained. Unfortunately, there is no opportunity to probe beyond the answer given. Respondents may be more likely to exhibit primacy effects where they select the first response which seems applicable, instead of considering the full range of alternatives.

There are self-complete paper and pen and electronic versions of all the main generic preference-based measures available, and electronic versions are increasingly becoming the most popular format. Due to their relative complexity, valuation techniques (e.g. for patients valuing their own health or imagined health states using TTO or SG approaches) are not often used in a self-completion format, though there are some notable examples (Lundberg *et al.* 1999; Ross *et al.* 2003).

9.2.2.4 Computerized technologies

Computerized technologies include traditional personal computers (e.g. desktop computers), mobile tablets and personal computers, hand-held computers, or personal digital assistants. Computerized technologies may be used for either interviewer-administered or self-completion questionnaires. In this approach, the interviewer or the respondent keys in answers to questions which appear on a computer screen.

Computer-assisted approaches may facilitate the completion of relevant questions and the skipping of irrelevant questions and branching. In addition, the results tend to be made more readily available, because the data entry process is not required. This is potentially a real advantage for valuation techniques, such as those that use 'ping-pong' and other iterative methods. Another alternative is the SmartPen technology. This is a pen-like device that is used to select responses on paper and it uniquely identifies the respondent and the assessment. While the SmartPen is a printed paper version, it also carries the advantages of electronic data capture.

There are an increasing number of studies reporting on examples of computer- and internet-based surveys to elicit health state values from patients themselves, and from members of the general public who are asked to imagine that they themselves are in the health state in question (Baron and Ubel 2001; Lenert *et al.* 2002; Prosser *et al.* 2011; Viney *et al.* 2011; Bansback *et al.* 2012; Buitinga *et al.* 2012). There are also increasing numbers of studies reporting upon the administration of preference-based measures via computer and the internet; for example, a recent study reported upon the administration of the EQ-5D-5L by mobile phone (O'Gorman *et al.* 2014). This study compared the equivalence of delivering the EQ-5D-5L across two administration modes (paper and mobile phone) using a random allocation procedure. It was found that completing the EQ-5D-5L using mobile phones produces equivalent results and response rates to more traditional pencil and paper methods, and the respondents were positive towards completing questionnaires using these methods (see Box 9.2).

Computerized technologies are becoming more prevalent for the capture of data relating to both preference-based measures and valuation techniques. The main advantages of computerized technologies include the ability to reach a large number of potential respondents at relatively low cost and the ease of data capture. However these advantages need to be considered alongside the potential drawbacks in relation to respondent understanding, completion rates, and the quality of the data obtained. Overall the choice of administration depends upon the particular study question, the resources available to complete the study, the complexity of the task, and the innate abilities of the respondents. These factors all interact to affect the reliability and validity of responses. Ultimately, the researcher needs to make the necessary judgements about the relevance of each mode of administration to their own study.

9.2.3 Timing of assessments

The timing of quality of life assessments is an important design consideration for all studies where standardized generic preference-based intruments are being applied. In a review of methodological considerations for the systematic identification of health state values for incorporation into economic models, Papaioannou and colleagues (Papaioannou *et al.* 2013) highlight that it is important at the outset to determine the distinct health states for a disease or condition pathway that require health state valuation data. It is also important to assess how the disease or condition pathway relates to key clinical events (e.g exacerbations) or treatments.

Additional considerations are the time horizon adopted for the economic evaluation and the need to reflect population subgroups. Economic evaluations conducted alongside clinical trials typically adopt the same time horizon as that specified for the

Box 9.2 Example of an internet-based survey to elicit health state preferences

Study: Prosser LA, Payne K, Rusinak D, Shi P, Uyeki T, Messonnier M (2011). Valuing health across the lifespan: Health state preferences for seasonal influenza illnesses in patients of different ages. *Value in Health* 14:135–143.

This study sought to assess whether public values for health states vary according to the age of the individual affected. A survey was developed for administration via the internet comprising descriptions of hypothetical health states for an uncomplicated episode of influenza illness, an influenza-related hospitalization, a severe allergic reaction (anaphylaxis) after vaccination, and Guillain–Barré syndrome after vaccination. The health state descriptions included hypothetical individuals of different ages (1-year-old, 8-year-old, 35-year-old, and 85-year-old). The only differences in the health state descriptions (apart from age) related to usual activities which were defined as work, leisure, or volunteer activities for adults and older people, or as playing and attending daycare or school for children. The survey included descriptions of each health state and measured values for those states using a time trade-off (TTO) exercise and a willingness to pay (WTP) approach. The TTO exercise asked respondents to value a state of health by trading time from the end of their life. The WTP asked respondents to value health states using dollars as a metric. Both types of valuation questions used two dichotomous-choice questions followed by an open-ended question to ascertain the maximum willingness to trade time or maximum WTP. In order to minimize anchoring bias (whereby respondents' values are influenced by the initial and follow-up TTO or WTP amounts included in the survey), respondents were randomized to four different survey versions that included different initial and follow-up TTO or WTP amounts. The survey was completed by 1,012 members of the general population. While the internet-based survey performed well in obtaining plausible utilities for seasonal influenza illnesses in patients of different ages, there may be certain inherent biases in the administration of an internet-based research study relating to the quality of the data obtained, the characteristics of the sample, and the need to facilitate access to the internet to view and complete the online survey.

Source: data from Prosser LA *et al.*, 'Valuing health across the lifespan: Health state preferences for seasonal influenza illnesses in patients of different ages', *Value in Health*, Volume 14, Issue 1, pp. 135–43, Copyright © 2011 International Society for Pharmacoeconomics and Outcomes Research (ISPOR).

trial, whereas decision models consider what happens to patients over a longer period of time (typically a lifetime). A series of health state values are required to reflect the changes in patients' health states over the relevant time period. When considering the values required for health states, it may also be important to capture subgroup level health state valuation data, for example, relating to different stage of disease, the presence or absence of comorbidities, age group, or ethnic group.

Regardless of the approach adopted, to be useful in the context of economic evaluation, all health state valuation studies should include an assessment of health status at baseline. This provides useful pre-treatment/pre-intervention data that can be compared with any post-treatment/post-intervention data obtained. It also allows a characterization, in health status terms, of the population under consideration.

9.2.4 Sample size

Once a decision has been made as to what to measure, from whom and when, the next stage is to determine how many individuals are required to be sampled. Ultimately, the sample size of any study seeking to provide estimates of health state values should be based on careful weighing up of the marginal value of additional information against the marginal cost of collecting such data. The most rigorous approach to addressing this would be through value of information analysis. This requires that an economic model is populated with distributions around parameter inputs that reflects the extent of current uncertainty, and then to explore the impact of reducing uncertainty around mean health state values. Value of information analysis explicitly considers the uncertainty surrounding the currently available evidence to guide health care decisions (Claxton *et al.* 2005: Siebert *et al.* 2013). In making a decision to adopt or reject a new health care technology, Siebert *et al.* note that there are two fundamental questions to address. Firstly, what decision should be made now given the best available evidence? Secondly, subsequent to the current decision and given the magnitude of the remaining uncertainty, should further evidence be gathered (i.e. should additional studies be performed), and if yes, which studies should be undertaken (e.g. relating to efficacy, side effects, health status, costs), and what sample sizes are needed? Hence, by using this approach, it is clear that a sample calculation for a health state valuation study should be based upon the impact or added value to the decision maker of reducing uncertainty around mean health state values.

In practice, where instruments to measure health from the patient's perspective (e.g. EQ-5D and SF-36) are used as primary outcome measures, it is common to determine a minimally important difference between treatments, and then use existing data on variation and assumed levels of power (e.g. 80 per cent) and significance (e.g. 95 per cent) to calculate the required sample size (Walters and Brazier 2005; Gerhards *et al.* 2011). The key variables in this calculation are the minimally important difference, power, and level of significance. The former has been developed in the quality of life literature, since its meaning is not obvious from the conventional and often arbitrary scoring rules of non-preference-based measures. To date, two broad strategies have been used to interpret changes in health status and quality of life measures in health care: distribution-based approaches using the effects size; and anchor-based measures that use the concept of a minimum clinically important difference (Norman *et al.* 2001; Guyatt *et al.* 2002).

Distribution-based approaches relate the difference in health between treatment and control groups within the context of an economic model, clinical trial, or other experimental design to some measure of variability. Cohen's standardized effect size is the most commonly utilized distribution-based approach (Cohen 1998). This estimates the mean change in health-related quality of life for treatment and control groups divided by the standard deviation of the change to produce an effect size index, which can then be used for sample size estimation. Cohen has suggested that standardized effect sizes of 0.2–0.5 should be regarded as 'small', 0.5–0.8 as 'moderate', and those above 0.8 as 'large'. Cohen's effect size may be influenced by the degree of homogeneity or heterogeneity in the sample. Distribution-based methods express an effect in terms of the underlying distribution of the results.

Anchor-based methods examine the relationship between a measure of health and an independent measure to determine the significance of a particular degree of change. Therefore, anchor-based methods require an independent standard or anchor that can be easily interpreted and which has some overlapping elements with the instrument being assessed. One item that has been used to provide an independent anchor has been the self-reported global rating of change scale that contains responses from 'much better' through to 'much worse' (Guyatt et al. 2002; Walters and Brazier 2003; Walters and Brazier 2005). What is a minimally important change on such a scale may be open to some debate, with some arguing a half-point change on a seven-point scale.

There has been some interest in the economics literature in applying the concept of minimally important difference. It has been suggested that differences of 0.03 may be important, and there is some empirical evidence to support this using the methods outlined here (Walters and Brazier 2003; Gerhards et al. 2011). However, in a comparison of the minimally important difference for the EQ-5D and the SF-6D, Walters and Brazier (2005) found that the mean minimally important difference for the EQ-5D (0.074) was almost double that of the SF-6D (0.041). It is noted that the minimally important difference estimates appear to be proportionally equivalent, if not equal, in the context of the range of utility scores for each scale (the EQ-5D scale having approximately twice the range of the SF-6D scale). Walter and Brazier recommend that further empirical work is undertaken to see whether or not this finding holds true for other utility measures, patient groups, and populations. In addition, Drummond et al. (2005) suggest that if the ultimate objective is to influence resource allocation decisions, as is the case within economic evaluation of health care, then it is the difference in cost-effectiveness between alternative treatments that is important and not the change in health-related quality of life. Therefore, changes in health alone may not be of interest without also considering the cost of bringing about such changes. This requires a value of information approach.

9.2.5 Linking quality-adjusted life years gained and costs

Typically the mean costs and quality-adjusted life years (QALYs) gained associated with an intervention are combined to form incremental cost-effectiveness ratios (ICERs) that estimate the additional cost per QALY gained associated with a new intervention relative to other interventions and/or standard treatment. The cost-effectiveness plane (CE plane) is often employed to show how decisions can be related to both costs and QALYs (see Chapter 2). The plane is divided into four quadrants indicating four possible situations relating to the additional costs and additional QALYs associated with a new therapy, compared with a standard therapy. When one therapy is clearly less costly

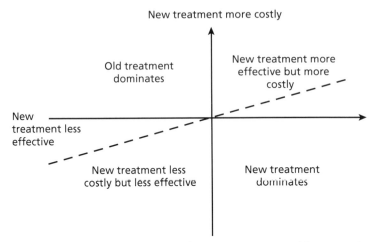

Fig. 9.1 The cost-effectiveness plane comparing a new treatment with a currently provided control treatment.

and more effective than the other (quadrants II and IV of the CE plane: see Fig. 9.1), then it is said to be dominant and it is obvious which of the therapies should be chosen over the other. However, the more common situation is where one intervention (typically the new intervention) is both more costly and more effective in terms of additional QALYs generated, and hence the decision as to its possible adoption is no longer clear. A decision has to be made as to whether the additional costs are justified by the additional QALYs that would be generated should the new intervention be adopted.

If it is possible to define a maximum willingness to pay (WTP) for a QALY, then this ceiling value can be used to judge whether the intervention under consideration is cost-effective. The ceiling value of the ICER can be represented by the slope of the dashed line on the CE plane. All incremental costs and QALYs plotted to the right of this line may be considered cost-effective, while points to the left of the line represent cost-ineffective interventions. The steeper the gradient of the dashed line, the higher the cost per QALY threshold.

The aim of an economic evaluation is to estimate the expected value of the incremental cost per QALY. In the context of any model or trial-based economic evaluation, there will inevitably be a degree of uncertainty surrounding the costs and QALY data, and this uncertainty needs to be represented.

9.2.6 **Handling uncertainty**

In a review of the use of health state values in decision analytic models for economic evaluation, Ara and Wailoo recommend handling uncertainty in health state values for preference-based measures and mapping functions by incorporating the variance-covariance matrices within probabilistic sensitivity analysis (Ara and Wailoo 2011). Probabilistic sensitivity analysis is a method for handling stochastic uncertainty, which produces a confidence interval estimate around the mean cost per QALY to represent uncertainty due to sampling variation (methods for handling other forms of uncertainty are discussed in Drummond *et al.* 2005). Due to the unknown nature of the ICER's sampling distribution, commentators have suggested the non-parametric approach of bootstrapping as an appropriate method of estimating confidence limits for the ICER (Briggs and Fenn 1998). This approach has since been employed in a large number of studies using clinical trial data and in economic models (see Dijkgraaf *et al.* 2005; Ratcliffe *et al.* 2006; Jowett *et al.* 2011; Manning *et al.* 2015). The bootstrap method uses the original data to provide an empirical estimate of the sampling distribution through repeated re-sampling from the observed data (Polsky *et al.* 1997).

In the case of the ICER, where data on costs and QALYs exist for two groups of patients, with sample sizes n_a and n_b receiving treatments **a** and **b**, respectively, the bootstrap method involves three key stages (Briggs and Fenn 1998):

1. Sample with replacement n_a cost/QALY pairs from the sample of patients who received treatment **a** and calculate the mean of the bootstrapped estimate of costs and QALYs for the bootstrap sample.

2. Sample with replacement n_b cost/QALY pairs from the sample of patients who received treatment **b** and calculate the mean of the bootstrapped estimate of costs and QALYs for the bootstrap sample.

3. Calculate the bootstrap replicate of the ICER generated by the ratio of the bootstrapped incremental costs divided by the bootstrapped incremental QALYs.

This three-stage process is repeated many times to produce a vector of bootstrapped estimates, which provide an empirical estimate of the sampling distribution of the ICER. The percentile method, which employs the $(\acute{a}/2)90$ and $(1-\acute{a}/2)90$ percentiles of the empirical sampling distribution, then offers the most straightforward method for estimating confidence limits around the ICER.

An alternative approach to estimating confidence intervals around ICERs to represent the uncertainty surrounding the cost-effectiveness of a health care intervention in the case of decision making involving two interventions is to estimate cost-effectiveness acceptability curves (CEACs). A CEAC represents the probability that an intervention is cost-effective at each value of WTP for a QALY (or whatever measure of effect is used).

The methods for deriving CEACs for decisions involving two or multiple interventions are broadly similar. Firstly, stochastic analysis is applied to generate a distribution of costs and QALYs for each intervention. For clinical trial-based data analyses, these estimates are estimated by bootstrapping. The cost and effect distributions for each intervention are then combined to form a series of distributions, one for each intervention and each level of λ. The probability that the intervention of interest is optimal is quantified and plotted graphically for every conceivably possible value of λ.

Where two interventions are being considered, the analysis can be undertaken using incremental net benefits (INBs). For any particular simulation, the intervention of interest is considered to be optimal compared with the alternative intervention when the INB is positive. Hence, for each value of λ, the technique involves determining the proportion of iterations in which the intervention of interest has a positive INB. Figure 9.2 illustrates a standard CEAC curve for an intervention that has a single comparator.

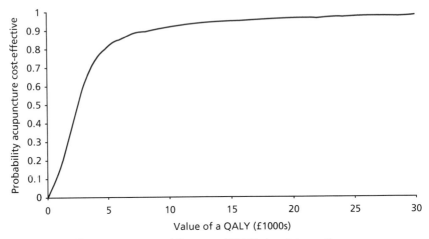

Fig. 9.2 Cost-effectiveness acceptability curve (CEAC): two interventions.

The vertical axis represents the probability that the intervention (in this case, acupuncture for low back pain relative to standard treatment) is cost-effective, and the horizontal axis represents alternative values of λ or WTP for a QALY. Assuming an implicit threshold maximum WTP value of £20,000 for a QALY, Figure 9.2 illustrates that the probability of the cost per QALY of the intervention of interest falling below this threshold value is close to 90 per cent. CEACs provide a geographical representation of the probability that a particular intervention is cost-effective over a range of maximum WTP for a QALY values (Fenwick *et al.* 2001; Maiwen 2013). They can be constructed for decisions involving any number of interventions, although the literature has largely concentrated upon the scenario of two interventions being compared with each other. CEACs indicate the probability that an intervention is optimal for any externally set limit (λ) or maximum WTP for a QALY. This threshold is currently set at between £20,000 and £30,000 per QALY for England (National Institute for Health and Care Excellence 2013). However, recent research by Claxton and colleagues (2013) to develop methods to estimate the NICE CE threshold, making use of routinely available data for England, indicates that the central or 'best' threshold value is somewhat lower than this at £12,936 per QALY. In practice, the central or 'best' threshold value is likely to vary from country to country.

CEACs may be considered as a more flexible approach to representing uncertainty than estimation of confidence limits around the ICER, since they directly address the decision problem relating to the probability that the intervention is cost-effective for all potential values of the ceiling ratio, and CEACs avoid the issue of negative values for the ICER, which convey no useful meaning.

9.3 Additional issues in estimating health state values from clinical trials

Designing a rigorous economic evaluation to be conducted alongside a clinical trial requires close collaboration between trialists and health economists (Petrou and Gray 2011).

While pragmatic clinical trials provide a vehicle for estimating health state values and assessing the cost-effectiveness of a new technology under real-world conditions, less naturalistic trial designs are often more restrictive since they tend to focus primarily on issues relating to safety and efficacy. In practice, even with pragmatic trials, the health state values generated may not offer the best representation of the condition of interest due to strict inclusion and exclusion criteria and restrictive trial protocols. In addition, the health state values obtained within the limited time horizon of a clinical trial may be quite different to those reflecting the longer time (and often lifetime) perspective adopted within a decision analytic model.

9.3.1 Timing of baseline assessment

Where health state valuation data at baseline is being elicited from a clinical trial, this assessment should preferably be made prior to randomization (if this is being done). This is because there is some evidence to suggest that patients who complete their baseline assessment prior to randomization tend to have better health-related quality of life scores than patients who have already been randomly assigned and are aware of their treatment allocation (Brooks *et al.* 1998).

9.3.2 Intention to treat

In common with clinical data, QALY data within clinical trials should be analysed on the basis of intention-to-treat analysis. This form of data analysis provides a strategy for analysing data in which all participants are included in the treatment group to which they were originally assigned at randomization, whether or not they completed the intervention given to the group. Intention-to-treat analysis prevents bias caused by the loss of participants over the period of the trial, which may disrupt the baseline equivalence established by random assignment, and may reflect non-adherence to the clinical trial treatment protocol.

9.3.3 QALY estimation

When using preference-based measures (e.g. EQ-5D) or valuation techniques (e.g. SG or TTO) within a clinical trial, there will be health state values for each patient at each time point capturing particular health states (when completed). These health state values can be most easily converted into QALYs by using a well-established method for assessing repeated measures, known as the area under the curve method (Mathews *et al.* 1990). A simple QALY calculation for a treatment versus control therapy for patients in a 12-month clinical trial using the EQ-5D is illustrated in Figure 9.3. A patient in the treatment group has a baseline EQ-5D health state of 22322, a 6-month EQ-5D health state of 21222, and a 12-month EQ-5D health state of 12211. A patient in the control group has a baseline EQ-5D health state of 22322, a 6-month EQ-5D health state of 22222, and a 12-month EQ-5D health state of 21122 (see Table 9.1). An assumption is made that health status changes between measurements are smooth and gradual over time, so that changes in utility scores can be approximated by a straight line. The area under the curve for each of the treatment and control profiles is then estimated using the trapezium rule (Appendix 9.1).

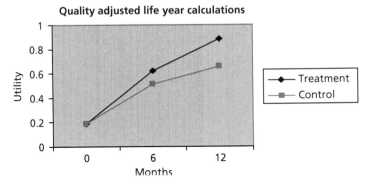

Fig. 9.3 Quality-adjusted life years profile treatment versus control group.

The beauty of applying the area under the curve methods to health state values is that provided the duration is expressed in years or a fraction of a year, the product will be the number of QALYs experienced during the period of the clinical trial (or a longer time horizon when an economic model is employed). For the treatment group patient, the QALY gain is 1.981 {[0.5(0.189 + 0.620)6 + 0.5(0.620 + 0.883]6)/12}, and for the patient in the control group it is 0.998 {[0.5(0.189 + 0.516)6 + 0.5(0.516 + 0.656)6]/12}.

Although in this simple example the baseline EQ-5D health state of patients in the treatment and control group are equivalent, Manca and colleagues (2005) point out that in practice it is quite common for baseline mean utility values to be imbalanced between treatment arms. They argue that this imbalance in baseline utility needs to be taken into account in the estimation of QALY differences between treatment arms,

Table 9.1 EQ5D health states and corresponding tariff scores at each time point

Time	Health state	EQ-5D score
Treatment		
0 months	22322	0.189
6 months	21222	0.62
12 months	11211	0.883
Control		
0 months	22322	0.189
6 months	22222	0.516
12 months	21122	0.656

Reproduced from Mathews JNS et al., 'Analysis of serial measurements in medical research', *British Medical Journal*, Volume 300, Issue 6719, pp. 230–35, Copyright © 1990, with permission from the BMJ Publishing Group Ltd.

because it typically contributes to the QALY calculation. This is because a patient's baseline utility is likely to be highly correlated with their QALYs over the follow-up period. A review of methodology and transparency in the calculation of QALYs in the published literature found that most economic evaluations estimating QALYs had failed to recognize the need to adjust for imbalance in baseline utility (Richardson and Manca 2004). Manca and colleagues (2005) use a practical example from a large clinical trial comparing lapararoscopic-assisted hysterectomy with standard methods to illustrate how multiple regression methods can be utilized to generate appropriate estimates of QALY differences between treatment arms and an associated measure of sampling variability, while simultaneously controlling for differences in baseline mean utility between treatment arms. Controlling for baseline utility in estimating QALY differences between treatment arms is now becoming standard practice for economic evaluations that use patient-level data (Briggs *et al.* 2006; Jowett *et al.* 2011; Manning *et al.* 2015).

9.3.4 Handling missing data

The majority of economic evaluations conducted alongside clinical trials relate to extended time periods and, as such, therefore patients' health-related quality of life may need to be assessed at several time points, often by means of a self-completion questionnaire. In such studies, it is common for a proportion of health-related quality of life data to be missing at one or more time points. Responses missing at a particular time point (t) can be categorized in three main ways (Little and Rubin 2002). First, responses may be missing completely at random, where the probability of response at time point t is independent of both the previously observed value and the unobserved value at time t and other variables collected at this, or previous, time points—for example, measures of disease severity. An extension of responses being missing completely at random is covariate-dependent missingness, whereby the probability of response at time point t may depend on observed baseline covariates (e.g. age and gender), but is independent of the missing and observed values (Faria *et al.* 2014). This distinction is useful for studies with multiple data collection points; for example, economic evaluations conducted alongside randomized controlled trials where the probability that data are missing may depend on individuals' baseline characteristics, but not on the previously observed value or the unobserved value at time t (Faria *et al.* 2014). Secondly, responses may be missing at random, where the probability of response at time t depends on the previously observed value or other variables collected during the study, but not on the unobserved values at time t. The third category of missing response is non-ignorable non-response, when the probability of response at time t depends on the unobserved values at time t and possibly also on the previously observed values.

Where the intervention being considered involves treatment for a severe condition, patients may be very ill before receiving the intervention and it is common for a proportion of participants to fail to complete questionnaires because of death or the severity of their illness at any time point. Such data represent non-ignorable non-response because the missing data are directly dependent on the health status of the patient; hence this type of data is often referred to as representing 'informative drop-out'.

Approaches for handling missing data may be classified into simple and more sophisticated imputation approaches.

9.3.4.1 Simple approaches

Simple approaches for handling missing data include complete case analysis and available case analysis. Complete case analysis is the default approach for handling missing data utilized by the vast majority of statistical software packages. This approach involves deletion of those patients where data is incomplete. The advantages of this approach are its simplicity and the fact that it allows analysis of the same sample of patients for all analyses. However, this approach is inefficient, because some potentially informative data are discarded. Alternatively, available case analysis avoids the inefficiency of complete case analysis by estimating the mean for the complete cases for each variable. However, the main problem with this approach is that different samples of patients will contribute to the estimation of different variables, leading to problems in comparability between variables.

9.3.4.2 Imputation-based approaches

Imputation methods for handling missing data attempt to overcome the disadvantages of complete and available case analyses. Imputation is where the missing data can be replaced with statistical estimates of the missing values. A complete data set is therefore made available, which can be analysed using statistical methods for complete data. Imputation methods include regression-based approaches, last value carried forward, maximum likelihood approaches, and multiple imputation.

1. *Regression imputation*. Regression analysis can be used to provide estimates of the missing data, conditional upon the complete cases for the variable under consideration within the data analysis. Missing data are usually multivariate, and it is possible to extend the procedure of regression-based imputation to deal with multivariate missing data. It is possible to fit a model for each missing value within the data set using the complete cases for all the other variables (Buck 1960). Alternatively, an iterative regression approach can be adopted (Holt and Benfer 2000; Brick and Kalton 1996), whereby missing values in a given variable are predicted from a regression of that variable on the complete cases of all other variables in the data set. This process is repeated for all variables with missing values using complete cases of the other variables (including previously imputed values) until a completed rectangular data set has been generated. The imputation of missing values for each variable is then re-estimated in turn using the complete set of data, and the process continues until the imputed values stop changing (Briggs *et al.* 2003).

2. *Last value carried forward/backward*. This approach is widely used in the calculation of QALY data, where health status data at particular time point(s) are missing for individual patients while still being available at other relevant time points. This approach is quite simple to employ, hence its popularity. It involves carrying forward the last observed health status value for an individual in order to complete the data set. The main disadvantage of this approach is that, in practice, it is unlikely that the health status of a patient in a clinical trial remains at exactly the same point over a period of time. It is far more likely to fluctuate. Hence, extensive use of the

last value carried forward/backward may lead to a situation whereby the actual variability in health state values across patient groups is lost.

3. ***Maximum likelihood approaches***. The maximum likelihood (ML) approach involves formulating a statistical model and basing inference on the likelihood function of the incomplete data (Briggs *et al.* 2003). For multivariate missingness, the expectation maximization (EM) algorithm can be applied. This involves iterating between an estimation step (E) and a maximization step (M). The E step involves estimating the missing data by averaging the complete data likelihood over the predictive distribution of the missing data, given the parameters of the model to be estimated. The M step involves providing updated estimates of the parameters through maximization of the likelihood given the complete data set. Following convergence (Wu 1983), predicted values for the missing data can be obtained directly by using the parameters.

4. ***Multiple imputation***. This method is a Monte Carlo simulation technique where each missing data case is replaced by a set of plausible estimates, which are drawn from the predictive distribution of the missing data given the observed data. In contrast to the more naïve approaches previously highlighted, multiple imputation has the advantage that it includes a random component to reflect the fact that imputed values are estimated, rather than treating the imputed values as if they are known with certainty. As such, it is likely to produce more accurate estimates of the standard errors (SE) and variances of mean health state values at each time point than other methods of imputation (Manca and Palmer 2005).

There are three main stages to multiple imputation. First, a number of imputed data sets are produced by estimating missing values for incomplete observations based upon values generated from their predictive distributions. The number of imputed data sets required is determined by the rate of missing information for the variable being estimated (Rubin 1987; Schafer 1999). Secondly, these data sets are analysed using standard statistical methods. Thirdly, the results from each of these analyses are pooled to provide estimates and confidence intervals, which incorporate the uncertainty relating to the missing data (see Box 9.3).

Joint modelling and chained equations represent the two main approaches to implementing multiple imputation and are available in standard statistical software packages (Faria *et al.* 2014). Joint modelling is a parametric approach where the variables to be imputed are assumed to follow a multivariate normal distribution. Chained equations specify one imputation model for each variable. Imputed values in one variable are then used to predict missing values in other variables in an iterative way, until the model converges to achieve a stable solution. Faria *et al.* highlight that the chained equations approach should accommodate non-normal variables (e.g. QALYs that are typically bimodal, left skewed, and with a spike at 1) better than joint modelling, because the model for each variable can be specified separately. An additional advantage of chained equations is their ability to allow for interactions and non-linear terms, and incorporate variables that are functions of imputed variables. In addition, the fully conditional specification of chained equations makes it easier to handle data sets with a large number of missing data variables, which is often the case in economic evaluations alongside clinical trials.

Box 9.3 A practical example of the impact of imputing values for EQ-5D health states

Study: Ratcliffe J, Longworth L, Young T, Buxton M (2005). An assessment of the impact of informative drop-out and non-response in measuring the health-related quality of life of liver transplant recipients using the EQ-5D descriptive system. *Value in Health* 8:53–8

This study investigated the impact of imputing EQ-5D values to allow for informative drop-out and non-response in a longitudinal assessment of the health-related quality of life of liver transplant recipients. The EQ-5D was administered at defined time intervals pre- and post-transplantation to all adults who were listed to receive a liver transplant at each of the Department of Health-designated treatment centres in England and Wales over a time period of 36 months. During the course of the study, missing data arose due to informative drop-out and non-response. Informative drop-out was accounted for by giving those patients who died an EQ-5D score of zero, and those patients who were too ill to respond an EQ-5D score equivalent to the fifth percentile of respondents for each time point pre-transplantation. Non-response was accounted for using relatively naïve approaches (last value carried forward and upper/lower 95 per cent confidence interval around the mean) and contrasted with a more sophisticated multiple imputation method based upon the approach described by Schafer (1999).

Of the 400 patients surveyed, 31 patients became too ill to participate at some point during the course of the study, and 81 patients dropped out due to death. Within the non-response group, 114 individuals chose not to respond to the questionnaire at one or more time point, and 16 individuals' responses were unusable as they were incomplete. Adjusting for informative drop-out in isolation resulted in a marked deterioration in mean scores over time pre-transplant relative to the base case situation in which no such adjustments were made. Post-transplant data indicated highly statistically significant improvements in quality of life over time for the base case ($P < 0.001$), whereas no statistically significant improvements over time were found when informative drop-out was allowed for in isolation ($P = 0.402$), or when informative drop-out and non-response were allowed for simultaneously ($P = 0.95–0.185$).

The authors conclude by recommending that future studies which purport to assess the health-related quality of life over time of patients, such as those with end-stage liver disease, include an allowance for informative drop-out and non-response within the analysis.

Source: data from Ratcliffe J et al., 'An assessment of the impact of informative drop out and non-response in measuring the health-related quality of life of liver transplant recipients using the EQ-5D descriptive system', *Value in Health*, Volume 8, Issue 1, pp. 53–8, Copyright © 2005 International Society for Pharmacoeconomics and Outcomes Research (ISPOR).

A review of missing data methodology in economic evaluations conducted alongside randomized controlled trials conducted by Noble and colleagues in 2012 revealed that despite the introduction of more sophisticated methods, including multiple imputation approaches, for handling missing data, complete case analysis is still the most popular approach to handling missing data, and its use has actually increased with time. Noble *et al.* found that missing data in cost-effectiveness analyses remains a much overlooked issue, which is often poorly reported and the methodologies utilized to handle missing data in published studies are often unclear. It is noted that the best way to handle missing data is to make concerted efforts not to have it at all. In practice, however, given that economic evaluations are typically conducted over extended time periods, some degree of missing data is inevitable. Good practice in the conduct of economic evaluations requires the routine reporting of the number of complete cases in the cost-effectiveness analysis, a justification of the methodology used to handle missing data (including an examination of why the data might be missing), and an assessment of the impact upon the results of using different approaches to missing data through appropriate sensitivity analysis.

9.4 Additional issues in populating an economic model

It is increasingly being recognized that the aim of economic evaluation is to inform decisions, and that it is unlikely that a single trial will be able to collect all the relevant data for informing such a decision. Trials are often not aimed at a particular resource allocation decision, and, furthermore, there may be other important sources of evidence on efficacy, cost, and health status. The purpose of modelling is to synthesize evidence from a range of sources in order to determine the relative cost-effectiveness of different uses of resources in order to inform decisions. Such evidence may come from several clinical trials and other observational data on clinical efficacy, as well as specific studies on costs, quality of life, and health state valuations.

An example of a simple decision analytic model has been reproduced in Figure 9.4, which compares surgical and medical interventions for some undefined medical condition. A patient may be categorized with the assumption of ending up in one of three states following treatment—either a good, intermediate, or bad outcome—but it is not known in advance which of these states the patient will ultimately be in. A decision analytic model will have probabilities associated with the different outcomes, as indicated in Figure 9.4, and these will differ between treatments. Each outcome is associated with a cost and a certain number of QALYs. The expected cost of each intervention is the cost of the respective interventions plus the therapy-specific sum of the cost associated with each of the three outcomes, weighted by the probability of the outcome occurring. The expected QALY of each treatment is then estimated in the same way.

In practice, economic models for economic evaluation tend to be considerably more complex and may have many more branches than the simple model presented in Figure 9.4. An alternative structure is the Markov model, which assumes that a patient is always in one of a finite number of health states. Probabilities are used to determine the movement between these states, and only designated transitions are allowed. The overall time duration of patients in each state, along with their associated cost and

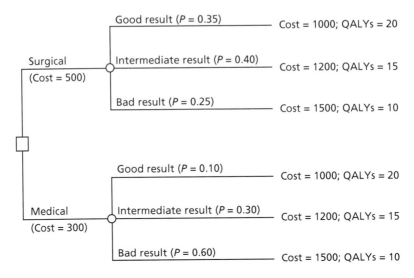

Expected cost of surgery: 500 + (0.35 × 1000) + (0.40 × 1200) + (0.25 × 1500) = 1705
Expected QALYs of surgery: (0.35 × 20) + (0.40 × 15) + (0.25 × 10) = 15.5
Expected cost of medicine: 300 + (0.10 × 1000) + (0.30 × 1200) + (0.60 × 1500) = 1660
Expected QALYs of medicine: (0.10 × 20) + (0.30 × 15) + (0.60 × 10) = 12.5

Incremental cost per QALY gained of surgery: (1705–1660)/(15.5–12.5) = 15

Fig. 9.4 Simple decision analytic model.
Reproduced from Michael F Drummond *et al. Methods for the Economic Evaluation of Health Care Programmes*, Third Edition, Oxford University Press, Oxford, UK, Copyright © Oxford University Press 2005., with permission from Oxford University Press.

health state values, is used to estimate the expected costs and QALYs associated with each treatment.

These types of model require mean values for each health state in the model in order to be able to estimate QALYs. In addition, there needs to be some account taken of the uncertainties surrounding these values. Conventional deterministic sensitivity analysis would need at least a range to reflect any underlying uncertainty in order to explore the consequences of varying the mean estimate. More sophisticated probabilistic methods of sensitivity analysis require distributions over the likely range of values. This is explored in section 9.4.2.

9.4.1 **Model structure**

A model-based economic evaluation requires health state values in order to estimate the incremental QALY gains from multiple interventions. Indeed the values given to health states in a model may form driving variables in determining the cost-effectiveness of a new intervention (Siebert *et al.* 2012).

The needs of a model are determined by its structure, since this differentiates the number and definition of the health states to be valued. Economic models require mean values (and their distributions) for a number of health states. Health states may be distinguished according to clinical events, for example, myocardial infarction or angina in coronary heart disease (Lindgren *et al.* 2004; Barton *et al.* 2011), or according to the severity of symptoms, for example, normal, mild, moderate, and severe depression (Kaltenthaler *et al.* 2002), or an acute depressive episode and a chronic course of depression (Afzali *et al.* 2012).

However, it is important to note that reducing the large range of health state values typically found in observational studies or clinical trials to a few health states for incorporation into an economic model may result in a loss of information, thereby reducing the sensitivity of the model to detect confirmed differences between interventions. If this loss of information is important, then the structure of the model needs to be modified to take this into account by expanding the number of states represented in the model. The structure of a model needs to take into account not just the patient care pathway, but also the appropriateness of the health states as a summary of the resource use and costs, and the associated utilities experienced by patients over time (Caro and Möller 2014; Roberts *et al.* 2012).

An important issue arises for patients who present with comorbidities, for example a stroke alongside arthritis. Recent research has highlighted a number of different methods, although there is currently no consensus on the most appropriate method to estimate health state values for comorbid health conditions (See Box 9.4).

9.4.2 **Estimating distributions**

For a model it is necessary to specify a mean health state value and its associated distribution. For this, it is necessary to specify a shape to the distribution. For health states which are very unlikely to be associated with utility values of less than zero, the most pragmatic approach is to fit a beta distribution, a flexible class of parametric distributions. A standard beta distribution is supported on the interval $(0, 1)$ and is specified by its mean and variance (Karnon and Brown 2002; Briggs *et al.* 2012).

For health states that may have utility values of less than zero, various alternative approaches have been suggested. The simplest approach is to use the triangular distribution, the parameters for which are the most likely value, a minimum value, and a maximum value (Karnon *et al.* 2005; Briggs *et al.* 2006). However, the triangular distribution draws straight lines from the mode down to the minimum and maximum values that assign too much probability to values near the furthest extreme, and as such overemphasizes the tail of the distribution. An alternative to the triangular distribution is the PERT distribution, which is related to the beta distribution. The PERT distribution has the same three parameters as the triangular distribution, but interprets them with a smooth curve that places less emphasis on the furthest extreme (Oscar 2004).

Alternatively, utility values can be described as decrements from perfect health, that is, as a simple transformation of $X = 1 - U$ where U is the utility decrement. If a lower constraint is placed on possible utility value, for example, the worst EQ-5D health state where a patient has severe problems associated with each dimension of the scale has a tariff value of -0.6, a scaled beta distribution may be used where the standard beta distribution is scaled upwards by a height parameter (λ), so that the distribution is

Box 9.4 A comparison of methods for estimating health state values for comorbid health conditions

Study: Ara R and Brazier J (2012). Comparing EQ-5D scores for comorbid health conditions estimated using five different methods. *Medical Care* 50:452–59.

This study assessed the accuracy of estimated health state values for comorbid health conditions by applying five different methods to an EQ-5D data set. EQ-5D data (n = 41,174) from the Health Survey for England were used to compare actual and estimated health state values for individuals living with comorbid conditions. Three conventional methods (additive, multiplicative, and minimum methods) were applied alongside two relatively new approaches: the adjusted decrement estimator and a linear regression model. A comparison of the three conventional methods, in terms of average errors and the proportions of estimated health state values accurate to within a given magnitude, indicated that the additive method was the least accurate and the multiplicative method was the most accurate. When using an age-adjusted baseline, the accuracy of both the additive and multiplicative methods increased with the multiplicative method remaining the most accurate. The additive and multiplicative methods underestimated the majority of health state values and the magnitude of the errors increased as the actual health state values increased. In contrast, the minimum and adjusted decrement estimator methods overestimated the majority of health state values, and the magnitude of errors increased as the actual health state values decreased. The simple linear model produced the most accurate results. However, there was a tendency for the simple linear model to underpredict higher health state values and overpredict lower health state values. The simple linear model also requires validating in external data obtained from the EQ-5D and other preference-based measures. Based on the current evidence base, Ara and Brazier recommend that the multiplicative method is used to combine health state values using EQ-5D data. It is also recommended that a range of univariate sensitivity analyses are performed to test the sensitivity of the model to changes in the health state values used.

Source: data from Ara R and Brazier J, 'Comparing EQ-5D scores for comorbid health conditions estimated using five different methods', *Medical Care*, Volume 50, pp. 452–59, Copyright © 2012 International Society for Pharmacoeconomics and Outcomes Research (ISPOR).

supported on a $(0, \lambda)$ scale. If no lower constraint is assumed, a log normal or gamma distribution can be applied to the utility decrement, such that the utility decrement is on an interval between zero and positive infinity.

9.4.3 Source of values

Models are able to take their values from a variety of sources. As reported in Chapter 8, an increasingly important source of health state value data is the literature. For many health states, there are already multiple values. A model needs a central value with a distribution to reflect the uncertainty around that value. The first problem is selecting an appropriate value from the literature, or perhaps in the future synthesizing values, in order to obtain the best estimates for health states in a model. As demonstrated in Chapter 8, the basis for selection is partly determined by the requirements of the policy maker who will be using the results of the model, but also by the appropriateness of the descriptions and methods of valuation. The problems are made even more difficult by the fact that published sources may not have values for the same patient group as the one in your model. Adjustments will need to be made for the background characteristics of the patients in the trial, and some methods for doing this were described in Chapter 8.

A recent study by Papaioannou and colleagues (2013) used a case study to demonstrate and provide guidance in relation to the systematic searching and selection of health state values from the literature. Prior to this publication little guidance was available on how to identify health state value evidence systematically for the health states used in economic models. The guidance is summarized in Box 9.5. It is recommended that, subject to resource limitations, a sensitive approach is adopted to searching for relevant health state values by searching a variety of sources, including multiple electronic databases, reference list checking, and citation searching. In practice, resources may be constrained for this component of model building, and as such, the searching process may need to adopt a less comprehensive strategy based around the extraction of key papers including relevant health state values. Reviews included as part of health technology assessment submissions to NICE or other regulatory bodies may also provide a useful mechanism for the efficient extraction of health state values for incorporation within an economic model.

For health state value reviews the quality of included studies is more difficult to assess than for reviews of clinical effects as there are no agreed reporting standards for these types of studies. However, the quality assessment process may usefully focus upon respondent selection and recruitment, inclusion and exclusion criteria, the background characteristics of the population, response rates, and any loss to follow-up, particularly where values are collected over a period of time.

In common with clinical effectiveness reviews, Papaioannou *et al.* (2013) also recommend that the process of data extraction is undertaken by two independent reviewers using a pre-piloted data extraction form which specifies exactly what data is required to be extracted.

A common error in economic models is to assume that the baseline health state for a person without the condition of interest is perfect health and therefore is assigned a value of 1.0 on the QALY scale. Recent research has indicated that the realism of baseline health state values within economic models may be improved by using baselines adjusted to reflect the health state values associated with the age, gender, and relevant health condition(s) of the population under consideration, rather than baselines that assume perfect health (Ara and Brazier 2010). In a study using a cardiovascular disease model to generate cost per QALY thresholds, Ara and Brazier assessed the consequences of using different baseline health state utility profiles (perfect health, no history of cardiovascular disease, general population) in conjunction with models (minimum, additive, multiplicative) frequently used to approximate scores for health states with multiple health conditions. It was found that assuming a baseline of perfect

Box 9.5 Recommendations for undertaking health state utility value reviews (the scope and identification of the evidence for health state utility reviews needs to be kept broad initially)

Searching

◆ Ideally use a variety of resources and methods to identify relevant studies, for example, electronic database searching, reference list checking, and contacts with experts. The scope of the review and inclusion/exclusion criteria will be refined during the stage of evidence selection according to the nature of the evidence base.

Selecting

◆ Selecting evidence for health state utility value reviews is an iterative process and may involve preliminary data extraction of key characteristics (population details, approach used to describe the health state, elicitation technique). Based on that data, decisions can be made on how to amend and develop inclusion criteria further.

Reviewing

◆ Criteria for quality and relevance need to be carefully considered.

Pooling

◆ Where there is more than one set of values meeting the requirements of the reimbursement agency and that are relevant to the model, the final selection needs to be justified with sensitivity analyses using alternative values, and consideration given to pooling to improve the precision of the estimates.

health ignores the natural decline in quality of life associated with age, overestimating the benefits of treatment. It was found that the results generated using baselines from the general population were comparable to those obtained using baselines from individuals with no history of cardiovascular disease.

A second study utilized pooled EQ-5D data from four consecutive Health Surveys for England obtained from the general population (N = 41,174). This was stratified by self-reported history of prevalent health condition(s) and age to assess whether data from the general population may be used to approximate baselines in decision analytic models when condition-specific data are not available (Ara and Brazier 2011). The results suggest that data from the general population irrespective of health status could be used in place of condition-specific data to represent the health state values associated with not having a particular health condition in some analyses, but not all. In particular, the findings indicated that health state values from the general population would not be appropriate for cohorts who have just one health condition. If the condition-specific data are not available, it is suggested that age-stratified mean health state values from respondents who report they have none of the prevalent health conditions form a better approximation of baseline health state values for cohorts who have just one health condition. Ara and Brazier note that the study findings require validation in additional data sets, and also highlight that further research of a similar nature should be conducted to examine subgroups of patients with precisely defined health conditions.

9.5 **Conclusions**

This chapter has considered the issue of how to value the quality adjustment weight component of QALYs for use within the methodology of economic evaluation. The requirements of clinical trial and model-based economic evaluations were considered. In a clinical trial context, it has become common practice to obtain quality of life data directly from patients wherever possible, since patients are often most aware of how their health has impacted upon their functioning and well-being. Generic preference-based measures, for example EQ-5D and SF-6D, have tended to be used most often in a clinical trial setting. Typically these instruments have been administered for self-completion using a pen and paper format, (although the use of online formats is now increasing). Model-based economic evaluations are increasingly being used and many of the issues relating to trial-based economic evaluations also apply to model-based economic evaluations. A typical economic model requires mean values for each health state in the model in order to be able to estimate QALYs. It is also necessary to specify a distribution around the mean health state value. There are various distribution types which can be applied, although the most pragmatic approach (a standard beta distribution) is not suitable for health states that may have values of less than zero.

It is important to note that for the purpose of conducting an economic evaluation, clinical trials may not be the best source of effectiveness data for the estimation of QALYs. Health state values extracted from the literature or observational data may provide more relevant sources, but this raises concerns about the realism of health state values for individuals without the condition and for capturing the impact of co-morbidities. We have made recommendations on the basis of best available evidence, however this is an evolving field. In addition, if the ultimate objective of economic evaluation is to influence resource allocation decisions, then sample size calculations based upon expected differences in health status between alternative treatment groups may not be sufficient. It will also be necessary to consider the costs of bringing about such changes. Techniques such as value of information analysis offer a promising way forward in this area.

References

Afzali H, Karnon J, Gray J (2012). A proposed model for economic evaluations of major depressive disorder. *European Journal of Health Economics* **13**:501–10.

Ara R, Brazier J (2010). Populating an economic model with health state utility values: moving toward better practice. *Value in Health* **13**:509–18.

Ara R, Brazier J (2011). Using health state utility values from the general population to approximate baselines in decision analytic models when condition-specific data are not available. *Value in Health* **14**:539–45.

Ara R, Brazier J (2012). Comparing EQ-5D scores for comorbid health conditions estimated using 5 different methods. *Medical Care* **50**:452–9.

Ara R, Wailoo A (2011). *The use of health state utility values in decision models*. NICE decision support unit technical support document No 12. University of Sheffield, UK.

Bansback N, Tsuchiya A, Brazier J, Anis A (2012). Canadian valuation of EQ-5D health states: preliminary value set and considerations for future valuation studies. *PLoS One* **7**:e31115.

Baron J, Ubel PA (2001). Revising a priority list based on cost-effectiveness: the role of the prominence effect and distorted utility judgments. *Medical Decision Making* **21**:278–87.

Barton P, Andronis L, Briggs A, McPherson K, Capewell S (2011). Effectiveness and cost effectiveness of cardiovascular disease prevention in whole populations: modelling study. *British Medical Journal* **28**;343:d4044. doi: 10.1136/bmj.d4044.

Bowling A (2004). *Measuring Health: a review of quality of life measurement scales*. Open University Press, Oxford, UK.

Brazier J, Deverill M, Green C, Harper R, Booth A (1999). A review of the use of health status measures in economic evaluation. *Health Technology Assessment* **3**:1–164.

Brazier J, Dolan P, Karampela K Towers I (2006). Does the whole equal the sum of the parts? Patient assigned utility scores for IBS-related health states and profiles. *Health Economics* **15**:543–1.

Brick JM, Kalton G (1996). Handling missing data in survey research. *Statistical Methods in Medical Research* **5**:215–38.

Briggs A (2000). Handling uncertainty in cost-effectiveness models. *Pharmacoeconomics* **17**:479–500.

Briggs A, Clark T, Wolstenholme J, Clarke P (2003). Missing presumed at random: cost analysis of incomplete data. *Health Economics* **12**:377–92.

Briggs A, Fenn P (1998). Confidence intervals or surfaces? Uncertainty on the cost-effectiveness plane. *Health Economics* **7**:723–40.

Briggs A, Sculpher M, Claxton K (2006). *Decision modelling for health economic evaluation*. Oxford University Press, Oxford, UK.

Briggs AH, Weinstein MC, Fenwick EA, Karnon J, Sculpher MJ, Paltiel AD (2012). Model parameter estimation and uncertainty analysis: a report of the ISPOR-SMDM modelling good research practices task force working group-6. *Medical Decision Making* **32**:722–32.

Brooks MM, Jenkins LS, Schron EB, Steinberg JS, Cross JA, Paeth DS for the AVID investigators (1998). Quality of life at baseline: is assessment after randomization valid? *Medical Care* **36**:1515–9.

Brunner HI, Johnson AL, Barron AC, Passo MH, Griffin TA, Graham TB, Lovell DJ (2005). Gastrointestinal symptoms and their association with health related quality of life of children with juvenile rheumatoid arthritis: validation of a gastrointestinal symptom questionnaire. *Journal of Clinical Rheumatology* **11**:194–204.

Bryan S, Hardyman W, Bentham P, Buckley A, Laight A (2005). Proxy completion of EQ-5D in patients with dementia. *Quality of Life Research* **14**:97–118.

Buck SF (1960). A method of estimation of missing values in multivariate data suitable for use with an electronic computer. *Journal of the Royal Statistical Society Series B* **22**:302–6.

Buitinga L, Braakman-Jansen LM, Taal E, van de Laar MA (2012). Construct validity of the interview time trade-off and computer time trade-off in patients with rheumatoid arthritis: a cross-sectional observational pilot study. *BMC Musculoskeletal Disorders* **13**:112.

Caro JJ, Möller J (2014). Decision-analytic models: current methodological challenges. *Pharmacoeconomics* **32**:943–50.

Claxton K, Cohen JT, Neumann PJ (2005). When is evidence sufficient? *Health Affairs* **24**:93–101.

Claxton K, Martin S, Soares M, Rice N, Spackman E, Hinde S, *et al.* (2013). *Methods for the Estimation of the NICE Cost Effectiveness Threshold.* Centre for Health Economics Research Report no 81. University of York, York, UK.

Cohen J (1998). *Statistical power analysis for the behavioural sciences.* Lawrence Erlbaum, Mahwah, New Jersey.

Coucill W, Bryan S, Bentham P, Buckley A, Laight A (2001). EQ-5D in patients with dementia: an investigation of inter-rater agreement. *Medical Care* **39**:760–1.

Dijkgraaf MG, van der Zanden BP, de Borgie CA, Balnken P, van Ree JM, van den Brink W (2005). Cost utility analysis of co-prescribed heroin compared with methadone maintenance treatment in heroin addicts in two randomised trials. *British Medical Journal* **330**:1297.

Dinglas VD, Gifford JM, Husain N, Colantuoni E, Needham DM (2013). Quality of life before intensive care using EQ-5D: patient versus proxy responses. *Critical Care Medicine* **41**:9–14.

Drummond MF, Sculpher MJ, Torrance GW, O'Brien BJ, Stoddart GL (2005). *Methods for the economic evaluation of health care programmes.* Oxford University Press, Oxford, UK.

Eiser C, Morse R (2001). Quality of life measures in chronic diseases of childhood. *Health Technology Assessment* **5**:1–157.

Eiser C, Varni JW (2013). Health-related quality of life and symptom reporting: similarities and differences between children and their parents. *European Journal of Pediatrics* **172**:1299–304.

Faria R, Gomes M, Epstein D, White IR (2014). A guide to handling missing data in cost-effectiveness analysis conducted within randomised controlled trials. *Pharmacoeconomics* **32**:1157–70.

Fenwick E, Claxton K, Sculpher M (2001). Representing uncertainty: the role of cost-effectiveness acceptability curves. *Health Economics* **9**:779–87.

Gabbe BJ, Lyons RA, Sutherland AM, Hart MJ, Cameron PA (2012). Level of agreement between patient and proxy responses to the EQ-5D health questionnaire 12 months after injury. *Journal of Trauma and Acute Care Surgery* **72**:1102–5.

Gerhards SA, Huibers MJ, Theunissen KA, de Graaf LE, Widdershoven GA, Evers SM (2011). The responsiveness of quality of life utilities to change in depression: a comparison of instruments (SF-6D, EQ-5D, and DFD). *Value in Health* **14**:732–9.

Guyatt GH, Osoba D, Wu AW, Wyrwich KW, Norman GR and the Clinical Signficance Consensus Meeting Group (2002). Methods to explain the clinical significance of health status measures. *Mayo Clinic Proceedings* **77**:371–83. *Health Affairs (Millwood)* **24**:93–101.

Holt B, Benfer RA (2000). Estimating missing data: an iterative regression approach. *Journal of Human Evolution* **39**:289–96.

Jowett S, Bryan S, Mant J, Fletcher K, Roalfe A, Fitzmaurice D, *et al.* (2011) Cost effectiveness of warfarin versus aspirin in patients older than 75 years with atrial fibrillation. *Stroke* **42**:1717–21.

Kaltenthaler E, Shackley P, Stevens K, Beverley C, Parry G, Chilcott J (2002). A systematic review and economic evaluation of computerised cognitive behaviour therapy for depression and anxiety. *Health Technology Assessment* **22**:1–89.

Kaplan RM (1994). Value judgements in the Oregon Medicaid experiment. *Medical Care* **32**:975–88.

Karnon J (2002). Planning the efficient allocation of research funds: an adapted application of a non-parametric Bayesian value of information analysis. *Health Policy* **61**:329–47.

Karnon J, Brennan A, Pandor A, Fowkes G, Lee A, Gray D, *et al.* (2005). Modelling the long term cost effectiveness of clopidogrel for the secondary prevention of occlusive vascular events in the UK. *Current Medical Research and Opinion* **21**:91–12.

Karnon J, Brown J (2002). Tamoxifen plus chemotherapy versus tamoxifen alone as adjuvant therapies for node-positive postmenopausal women with early breast cancer—a stochastic economic evaluation. *Pharmacoeconomics* **20**:119–37.

Lenert LA, Sturley A, Watson ME (2002). iMPACT3: Internet-based development and administration of utility elicitation protocols. *Medical Decision Making* **22**:464–74.

Lindgren P, Jonsson B, Yusuf S (2004). Cost-effectiveness of clopidogrel in acute coronary syndromes in Sweden: a long-term model based on the cure trial. *Journal of Internal Medicine* **255**:562–70.

Little DB, Rubin RJA (2002). *Statistical analysis with missing data*, 2nd edn. Wiley Series on probability and statistics. John Wiley and Sons Inc., New York, NY.

Lundberg L, Johannesson M, Isacson DG, Borquist L (1999). The relationship between health state utilities and the SF-12 in a general population. *Medical Decision Making* **19**:128–40.

Luo N, Li M, Stolk EA, Devlin NJ (2013). The effects of lead-time and visual aids in TTO valuation: a study of the EQ-VT framework. *European Journal of Health Economics* 14 Suppl **1**:S15–24.

Maiwen MJ (2013).Cost-effectiveness acceptability curves revisited. *Pharmacoeconomics* **31**:93–100.

Makai P, Beckebans F, van Exel J, Brouwer WB (2014). Quality of life of nursing home residents with dementia: validation of the German version of the ICECAP-O. *PLoS ONE* **9**:e92016.

Manca A, Hawkins N, Sculpher MJ (2005). Estimating mean QALYs in trial-based cost-effectiveness analysis: the importance of controlling for baseline utility. *Health Economics* **14**:487–96.

Manca A, Palmer S (2005). Handling missing data in patient-level cost-effectiveness analysis alongside randomized clinical trials. *Applied Health Economics and Health Policy* **4**:65–75.

Manning VL, Kaambwa B, Ratcliffe J, Scott DL, Choy E, Hurley MV, Bearne LM (2015). Economic evaluation of a brief education, self-management and upper limb exercise training in people with rheumatoid arthritis (EXTRA) programme: a trial-based analysis. *Rheumatology (Oxford)* **54**:302–9.

Mathews JNS, Altman D, Campbell MJ (1990). Analysis of serial measurements in medical research. *British Medical Journal* **300**:230–5.

Milne RJ, Heaton-Brown KH, Hansen P, Thomas D, Harvey V, Cubitt A (2006). Quality of life valuations of advanced breast cancer by New Zealand women. *Pharmacoeconomics* **24**:281–92.

National Institute for Health and Care Excellence (NICE) (2013). *Guide to the methods of technology appraisal*. National Institute of Care Excellence, London, UK.

Noble SM, Hollingworth W, Tilling K (2012). Missing data in trial-based cost-effectiveness analysis: the current state of play. *Health Economics* **21**:187–200.

Norman GR, Sridhar FG, Guyatt GH, Walter SD (2001). Relation of distribution- and anchor-based approaches in interpretation of changes in health-related quality of life. *Medical Care* **39**:1039–47.

O'Gorman H, Mulhern B, Rotherham N, Brazier J (2014). Comparing the equivalence of EQ-5D-5L across different modes of administration. *Value in Health* **17**: A517.

Oppe M, Devlin NJ, van Hout B, Krabbe PF, de Charro F (2014). A program of methodological research to arrive at the new international EQ-5D-5L valuation protocol. *Value in Health* **17**:445–53.

Oscar T (2004). Dosenresponse model for thirteen strains of salmonella. *Risk Analysis* **24**:41–9.

Papaioannou D, Brazier J, Paisley S (2013). Systematic searching and selection of health state utility values from the literature. *Value in Health* **16**:686–695.

Petrou S, Gray A (2011). Economic evaluation alongside randomised controlled trials: design, conduct, analysis and reporting. *British Medical Journal* **342**:d1548 doi: 10.1136/bmj.d1548.

Polsky D, Glick HA, Wilke R, Schulman K (1997). Confidence intervals for cost-effectiveness ratios: a comparison of four methods. *Health Economics* **6**:243–52.

Prosser LA, Payne K, Rusinak D, Shi P, Uyeki T, Messonnier M (2011).Valuing health across the lifespan: health state preferences for seasonal influenza illnesses in patients of different ages. *Value in Health* **14**:135–43.

Ratcliffe J, Brazier JE, Campbell WB, Palfreyman S, MacIntyre JB, Michaels JA (2006). Cost-effectiveness analysis of surgery versus conservative treatment for uncomplicated varicose veins in a randomized clinical trial. *British Journal of Surgery* **93**:182–6.

Ratcliffe J, Stevens K, Flynn T, Brazier J, Sawyer M (2012). Whose values in health? An empirical comparison of the application of adolescent and adult values for the CHU9D and AQOL-6D in the Australian adolescent general population. *Value in Health* **15**(5):730–6.

Richardson G, Manca A (2004). Calculation of quality adjusted life years in the published literature: a review of methodology and transparency. *Health Economics* **13**:1203–10.

Roberts M, Russell LB, Paltiel AD, Chambers M, McEwan P, Krahn M (2012). Conceptualizing a model: a report of the ISPOR-SMDM modeling good research practices task force—2. *Value in Health* **15**:804–11.

Ross PL, Littenberg B, Fearn P, Scardino PT, Karakiewicz PI, Kattan MW (2003). Paper standard gamble: a paper-based measure of standard gamble utility for current health. *International Journal of Technology Assessment in Health Care* **19**:135–47.

Rubin DB (1987). *Multiple imputation for non-response in surveys*. Wiley, New York, NY.

Schafer JL (1999). Multiple imputation: a primer. *Statistical Methods in Medical Research* **8**:3–16.

Siebert U, Alagoz O, Bayoumi AM, Jahn B, Owens DK, Cohen DJ, Kuntz KM (2012). State-transition modeling: a report of the ISPOR-SMDM Modeling Good Research Practices Task Force-3. *Medical Decision Making* **32**:690–700.

Siebert U, Rochau U, Claxton K (2013). When is enough evidence enough?—Using systematic decision analysis and value-of-information analysis to determine the need for further evidence. *Evid Fortbild Qual Gesundhwes* **107**:578–84.

Sloane PD, Zimmerman S, Williams CS, Reed PS, Gill KS, Preisser JS (2005). Evaluating the quality of life of long term care residents with dementia. *Gerontologist* Special issue **1**:37–49.

Szabo SM, Beusterien KM, Pleil AM, Wirostko B, Potter MJ, Tildesley H, *et al.* (2010). Patient preferences for diabetic retinopathy health states. *Investigative Ophthalmology and Vision Science* **51**:3387–94.

Viney R, Norman R, King MT, Cronin P, Street DJ, Knox S, Ratcliffe J (2011). Time trade-off derived EQ-5D weights for Australia. *Value in Health* **14**:928–36.

Walters S, Brazier J (2003). What is the relationship between the minimally important difference and health state utility values? The case of the SF-6D. *Health and Quality of Life Outcomes* **11**:1–4.

Walters S, Brazier J (2005). Comparison of the minimally important difference for two health state utility measures: EQ-5D and SF-6D. *Quality of Life Research* **14**:1523–32.

Wang P, Tai ES, Thumboo J, Vrijhoef HJ, Luo N (2014). Does diabetes have an impact on health-state utility? a study of Asians in Singapore. *Patient* **7**:329–37.

Appendix 9.1 The trapezium rule

The trapezium rule is a way of estimating the area under a curve. The area under a curve is calculated using a mathematical technique known as integration, and so the trapezium rule gives a method of estimating integrals. The trapezium rule works by splitting the area under a curve into a number of trapeziums.

If we want to find the area under a curve between the points x_0 and x_n, we divide this interval up into smaller intervals, each of which has length h (see Fig 9.3).

Then we find that:

$$\int_{x_0}^{x_n} f(x)dx = \frac{1}{2}h\left[(y_0 + y_n) + 2(y_1 + y_2 + \cdots + y_{n-1})\right]$$

where $y_0 = f(x_0)$ and $y_1 = f(x_1)$, etc.

If the original interval was split up into n smaller intervals, then h is given by: $h = (x_n - x_0)/n$.

Chapter 10

A QALY is a QALY is a QALY—or is it not?

10.1 Do all QALYs have the same social value?

So far, we have assumed that a unit of health improvement is of the same social value regardless of whom the health gain goes to, or what the circumstances are—and therefore, 'a QALY is a QALY is a QALY' (QALY = quality-adjusted life year). This chapter will present a theoretical framework for a diversion from it and examine different ways in which the value of a QALY may not be constant, so that a cost per *weighted* QALY analysis becomes more appropriate. For example, welfarists may want to weight QALYs to reflect the different monetary values that people give to their own health (a richer person may be willing to pay more for an additional QALY for themselves than a poorer person); or, welfarists (and possibly non-welfarists) may want to weight QALYs to reflect the different non-health benefits that a unit of health improvement generates to wider society, depending on who the patient is. On the other hand, non-welfarists may ask whether it is egalitarian enough to assign constant social value to a unit of health gain regardless of context. The chapter will then take a brief look at the challenges associated with the elicitation of public preferences, the empirical findings, and the practical issues involved in weighting QALYs.

10.2 Theory of weighted cost per QALY analyses

10.2.1 The health-related social welfare function and weighted QALYs

Cost per QALY analysis with a fixed budget assumes a health-related social welfare function, which abstracts away from anything else that may affect peoples' lives (e.g. economic productivity, or social capital), and assumes that health-related social welfare (W) is a simple sum of the health (H) of different individuals ($i = 1, 2, \ldots, N$) that can be achieved given a fixed health care budget:

$$W^0 = H_1 + H_2 + \cdots + H_N. \qquad \text{Eq. 0}$$

The health (H) of different individuals (and thus social welfare) is measured in QALYs over the relevant time period. This is a function of health alone with no reference to costs, because under a fixed budget, the opportunity cost of improving the health of one person is the foregone health improvement of another person. No weights are applied, which in effect means each *unit* of health is given the same weight, regardless of whose health it is or how healthy they are—in other words, equal and constant marginal social value of a QALY holds:

$$\partial W^0 / \partial H_i = 1.$$

Each unit of improvement in anybody's health increases social welfare by one unit—'a QALY is a QALY is a QALY'. The idea of relaxing this so that a unit of health may have different impacts on societal welfare can be operationalized in two distinct approaches: one is by reconsidering the arguments (whether to make any adjustments to *H*) and the other is by reconsidering the functional form (how to aggregate). Let us look at two simple examples.

The first approach (reconsidering adjustments to *H*) might take the following form:

$$W^1 = a_1 H_1 + a_2 H_2 + \cdots + a_N H_N. \qquad \text{Eq. 1a}$$

This introduces a set of parameters ($a_i > 0$) so that it is not the raw level of individual health that enters the social welfare function, but its weighted value. Eq. 0 is a special case of Eq. 1a, where $a_i = a_j = 1$ ($i \neq j$). The weights vary *depending on whose health it is* (but not by their level of health). Marginal social value of individual health is:

$$\partial W^1 / \partial H_i = a_i.$$

Thus, each unit improvement in individual *i*'s health improves social welfare by a_i units. The weight given to one unit health gain to one individual (*i*) relative to a reference individual (*r*) is:

$$\partial H_r / \partial H_i = a_i / a_r. \qquad \text{Eq. 1b}$$

On the other hand, the second approach (reconsidering how to aggregate) might take the following form:

$$W^2 = \left[H_1^{-b} + H_2^{-b} + \cdots + H_N^{-b} \right]^{-\frac{1}{b}}. \qquad \text{Eq. 2a}$$

This introduces a parameter ($b \geq -1$; $b \neq 0$), so that social welfare is no longer a simple function of the levels of individual health, but a non-linear function of their exponents. Eq. 0 is a special case of Eq. 2a, where $b = 1$. Marginal social value of individual health is:

$$\partial W^2 / \partial H_i = -b H_i^{-b-1} \left[H_1^{-b} + H_2^{-b} + \cdots + H_N^{-b} \right]^{-\frac{1}{b}-1}.$$

The advantage of the formulation of Eq. 2a is that the weight given to one unit health gain to individual *i* relative to a reference individual *r* takes a very simple form:

$$\partial H_r / \partial H_i = \left[H_i / H_r \right]^{-b-1}. \qquad \text{Eq. 2b}$$

The relative impact of a unit improvement in individual i's health on social welfare depends on the size of H_i relative to the size of H_r (but not on whose health it is, because the parameter b is the same for everybody).

Combinations of these, and more complex specifications are possible, but these two examples will suffice for the purposes here. In the following section, some of the considerations for weighting QALYs will be examined under four headings using these two formulations. In the following section, adjustments to the functional form (Eq. 2) will be addressed before adjustments to the arguments (Eq. 1).

10.2.2 **Different reasons for weighting QALYs**

A key question to ask is: suppose there are two patient groups of the same size, with the same expected QALY gain, at the same cost, but the groups differed in one aspect—what would that aspect be if the two groups are to be treated differently legitimately? And why? Table 10.1 is loosely based on considerations that may lead to weighting QALYs differently that have been raised in the literature in some form or other; some come from the theoretical literature, and others from more observational sources.

Table 10.1 Candidate considerations for weighted QALYs

Candidate considerations for weighted QALYs	Eff[1]	Eq[2]
Non-health benefits to patients	√	
Health and non-health benefits to close family and informal care givers	√	
Non-health benefits to the wider society	√	
The nature of the intervention (e.g. curative or palliative; innovative technology; no other curative alternative available) or of the health benefit (e.g. life-saving or HRQoL improving)	√	
Patients are at the 'end of life'	√	
Age and life stage of patients	√	√
Socio-economic background of patients	√	√
Expected lifetime health of patients—or the 'fair innings argument'		√
Severity of pre-treatment health prospects—or the 'burden of illness'		√
Severity of pre-treatment health status		?
The number of patients with the condition and whether or not they are 'identifiable'– or the rule of rescue		?
How long patients have had the condition for		√
NHS treatments that the patient has received in the past		√
Whether patients brought the ill health on to themselves		√
Whether the NHS has caused the ill health		√

(1): a tick in the column indicates an efficiency-based consideration.

(2): a tick in the column indicates an equity-based consideration.

Some considerations are primarily efficiency-based: for example, weighting health gains by non-health benefits to wider society. There are also a number of considerations that could have both efficiency and equity justifications. For example, giving higher priority to health gains to young adults over the elderly could be efficient (because young adults are more productive) or equitable (because the elderly have already enjoyed being young adults). The two reasons could go in opposite directions: it might be more efficient to give higher priority to professionals than low skill workers (because of wider social benefits), but it might be more equitable to give the professionals lower priority (because they tend to have better lifetime health prospects). The expected lifetime health of patients as an equity-based criterion is generic and could cover many specific variations (age, severity, socio-economic background).

Arguments put forward to support different considerations are examined using four distinct categories:

A. due to diminishing marginal social value of health, as the level of health increases, corresponding to Eq. 2a;

B. due to variation in the social value of health for *efficiency* reasons depending on whose health it is, corresponding to Eq. 1a;

C. due to variation in the social value of health for *equity* reasons depending on whose health it is, also corresponding to Eq. 1a; and

D. due to other considerations beyond consequentialist cost-effectiveness.

A. Considerations due to diminishing marginal social value of health, as the level of individual health increases

Marginal social value of individual health ($\partial W/\partial H_i$) is the social value resulting from one extra unit of health to different people. Eq. 2a means that if $b < 1$ then the social value of one extra unit of health diminishes in the level of health of the recipient; other things being equal, an extra QALY contributes the most to social welfare when it is given to the person with the lowest level of health (H_i). So this would represent the ethical concern for the worst-off and prioritarianism (Parfit 1997). If each additional unit of health was always given to the person with the worst health at the time of each decision, inequality in health will reduce over time, and therefore, diminishing marginal social value of health can be characterized as being 'inequality averse'. The concern here is entirely around the social value of individual health and equity, and not the individual utility of own health and efficiency—in other words, this consideration is non-welfarist. (Also see Box 3.2.) Prioritarianism can be adapted to the health sector by focusing on disadvantages in lifetime expected health, prospective health, or health-related quality of life (HRQoL) alone.

The fair innings argument (Williams 1997; also see Harris 1985) offers a theoretical foundation for the operatinalization of prioritarianism, using lifetime expected QALYs as the measure of health. This is made up of past QALYs (which has already taken place and is now fixed) and future QALYs (which yet to happen and is uncertain). The level of the fair innings will be the reference H_r. Since lifetime expected QALYs increase in age, provided $b < 1$, the fair innings weights given in Eq. 2b will be decreasing in age. The fair innings argument can also serve as a theoretical basis for giving higher priority to those with more severe health problems, or poorer socio-economic backgrounds, to the extent that their lifetime expected QALYs are lower than the others.

Some have questioned the use of lifetime QALYs, and argued in favour of focusing entirely on prospective health (Nord 2005). This would mean ignoring past health, and thus, age. While in most countries there are legislations against discrimination by age, arguably treating people of different ages the same with respect to prospective health may be unethical. For example, if two patients aged 20 and 70 years faced identical future prospects in terms of baseline prognosis and capacity to benefit, arguably it is unfair to treat them the same, because the 50 extra years of life already lived by the 70-year-old should also be a relevant consideration (see Daniels 1988; Lockwood 1988; Tsuchiya 2000).

Prioritarianism could also be operationalized by focusing on the severity of HRQoL over a fixed or unspecified duration (Nord 1993). This, too, ignores age. In addition, it only addresses one type of disadvantage, namely having a large HRQoL loss for the fixed duration (e.g. acute illness), but not having a smaller HRQoL loss for a longer duration (e.g. permanent disability).

B. Considerations due to variation in the social value of health for *efficiency* reasons, depending on whose health it is

This category of considerations appeals to benefits beyond what is captured in QALY gains to patients (and informal carers, where relevant). So it may include non-health benefits to the patient, to close family, or informal care givers, and to wider society (see Box 10.1). In terms of the social welfare function, it means applying different weights to people's health (a_i), as in Eq. 1a. The assumption is that health gain to different patients generates more or less social welfare compared to a reference patient ($a_i \neq a_r$), in proportion to the size of the health gain, and independently of their level of health (Eq. 1b). If the motivation is to make the QALY measure better reflect

Box 10.1 Extending the QALY beyond health

A large proportion of non-health benefits from health care comes from productivity gains, which are generated when patients increase their (paid and unpaid) activities as a result of improved health. At the same time, a patient living longer will consume more (health care, and other goods and services). Therefore, it is possible to quantify the net impact to the wider society arising from health care treatment. One attempt to capture such effects was the age weighting used in an early version of the disability-adjusted life year (DALY) measure (see Chapter 11). In another attempt, Roberts (2016) estimates wider social impact at the individual level by patient age, gender, disease (ICD code), and HRQoL level, so that the average net non-health benefit of treatment can be modelled for a marginal QALY gain by disease. This can then be used to adjust QALY gains in economic evaluations to reflect wider social benefit from health care.

variation in the amounts of money people are willing to pay for their own health (e.g. by ability to pay), for different kinds of health gain for themselves (e.g. HRQoL improvement vs life extension), and/or for different kinds of health care interventions for themselves (e.g. prevention vs cure), then these are more welfarist.

An example of efficiency-based consideration is age: young people and very old people rely on others to support them—not just on an individual basis, but in terms of sustaining a community, an economy, and a legal system. In this respect, if somebody's HRQoL could be improved by a fixed amount for one year, treating an adult will, on average, be more efficient than a child or a very old person (see Box 10.1). However, there are two considerations. First, if the reason the very old are not as productive is because their health is poorer, then this would be double counting and inappropriate. Second, children may be less productive than adults now, but their health can have investment value (being healthy now may facilitate development and lead to higher returns in the future), so that efficiency considerations focusing entirely on the present may be too myopic.

Another example of an efficiency-based consideration is to give higher weight to those at the end of their lives. Faced with the prospect of imminent death, the impact to the overall welfare of the person and their immediate family of having a modest health gain may well be much larger than the same number of QALYs gained at an earlier stage of life of the same person (Coast *et al.* 2008). There may also be wider benefits to people in society for knowing that one's welfare or that of their loved ones will be given higher priority when their time comes. Welfarism provides a straightforward justification for weighting QALYs for such reasons. On the other hand, the issue for non-welfarists is whether the calculus of social value should reflect such personal wants, and recognize a unit of health gain to a person at the end of their life (i) has more *social* value than the same unit of health gain to the reference person at an earlier stage of life (r). If yes, then individual weights ($a_i > a_r$) can accommodate this. Again, this would be independently of their level of health.

C. Considerations due to variation in the social value of health for *equity* reasons depending on whose health it is

If one is disadvantaged because of factors beyond one's control, many will regard that as unfair (Dworkin 1981*a*, 1981*b*; Fleurbaey and Schokkaert 2009). Of course, in practice, it may not be easy to determine the cause of ill health, *and* to judge the patient's responsibility for it: but in theory, ill health can be caused by, for instance, family background, genetics, pollution, accidents, medical negligence or malpractice, and so on. Diminished lifetime expected QALYs itself is accounted for by the fair innings argument already mentioned above, and the aim here is to compensate for the unfairness itself. In other words, should alleviating such ill health be given larger priority than attending to ill health of the same magnitude arising as a result of deliberate choice by informed and competent individuals themselves (such as sports injuries in adults)? If yes, the a_i weights in Eq. 2b can accommodate the role of individual responsibility so that improving the health of some people are given larger or smaller weights, as determined by their responsibility status, independently of their levels of health. This would have the effect of using the health care system as a means to achieve some social justice beyond fairness in health.

A further type of equity-based consideration draws on the principle of equality of opportunity. Equality of opportunities to life and health is addressed by the fair innings argument through diminishing social value of a QALY. The social value of a QALY may further vary by the opportunity of receiving health care. An example of this is geographical access. If there are 'economies of scale' in the way hospitals operate, so that larger hospitals were more efficient than smaller ones, this will be an efficiency-based justification for having a smaller number of larger hospitals across the country. However, if this is going to compromise access to health care for people living in remote areas, then there is scope to consider a trade-off between securing equal geographical access and achieving maximum health improvements, to be represented in Eq. 2b.

D. Considerations beyond consequentialist cost-effectiveness

It is possible to conceive of further considerations that do not fall within the consequentialist cost-effectiveness paradigm. For example, the rule of rescue supports giving priority to identified individuals in immediate peril, and in effect, to suspend cost-effectiveness (Jonsen 1986). While such moral codes of individual behaviour may be of relevance at the clinical bedside level, it is arguably of limited relevance in the paradigm of economic evaluation and policy level decision making (Cookson *et al.* 2008).

10.3 Who should weigh the different QALYs, from which perspective?

While theory can inform the ways in which weights may be applied to QALYs, it cannot determine the magnitudes of such weights. If the reason why a unit of health gain to people should be valued differently by society is because of efficiency, then once that normative judgement is made, the magnitude of the weight should be based on the actual size of the benefit in question, which (provided the QALY measure holds) is a factual matter (see Box 10.1). However, if the reason is equity, then the magnitude of the weight itself is a matter of value judgement.

Most empirical studies exploring the relative value of a QALY aim to survey a representative sample of the general public. For instance, the Citizens' Council convened by the National Institute for Health and Care Excellence (NICE) is a body that aims to elicit the views of exactly such a group of people (Rawlins and Culyer 2004). Parallel to the health valuation literature, the two alternative groups to survey might be stakeholders such as patients and carers, and health care professionals. The obvious immediate shortcoming of surveying stakeholders is that they are stakeholders. The notion of the relative value of QALYs requires comparing the societal value of a health gain to one group relative to the same health gain in another group. Although surveying patients in the context of health valuations has its attractions because this is the group that knows best about a given health problem, the same reason makes them less attractive for the present context. The neutrality aspect of procedural justice requires that the relative values across different groups of patients should be obtained from those who can be expected to be detached and unbiased judges (Dolan *et al.* 2007).

The justification of not surveying health care experts also comes from procedural justice: since the issue is about how to allocate publicly funded health care resources, the voice of those who are paying should be reflected, not the views of health care managers or professionals that are not democratically elected representatives. There is some empirical evidence to suggest that the views on weighted QALYs held by members of the general public and the views of health care policy makers may differ (Dolan and Tsuchiya 2007; although Whitty *et al* 2011 have found them to be similar).

A representative sample can be surveyed from two distinct perspectives: one is the perspective of a private consumer, and the other is the perspective of a societal citizen (Dolan *et al.* 2003). For example, a survey question using the private perspective will ask respondents to choose on the basis of how they might choose for themselves, or for their family. A survey question using the societal perspective will ask them to imagine themselves as a health care policy maker or public health representative, and to choose on the basis of how they think such an official ought to choose. If the objective of the health care system is to mimic a private insurance system, then the former perspective may be appropriate; however, a publicly funded health care system may have other objectives, and it may be more appropriate to use the societal perspective.

10.4 How to weigh the relative value of different QALYs

This can be broken down into two parts: the valuation method and the mode of administration. Regarding the former, since the objective is to quantify the relative value of a QALY so that weights can be derived, the method needs to generate quantitative results—in other words, to involve trade-offs. Most methods involve respondents being presented with hypothetical scenarios involving multiple patient groups (typically, two) described in terms of the relevant characteristics, and being asked to choose which group to treat first, or how to split a fixed budget between them (or to rank, if there are three or more groups). Box 10.2 gives two examples.

The issues concerning the mode of administration in health state valuation discussed in Chapter 4 are also applicable here: the survey can take the form of individual face-to-face interviews, telephone surveys, postal surveys, internet (online) surveys, or discussion sessions in small groups. The issues are arguably more complex in the context of equity, so there should be ample time to hear and to understand the various opinions and their implications. This makes telephone, postal, and online surveys less attractive compared to face-to-face methods. On the other hand, face-to-face methods have their own problems. In particular, the more evidence and the more opportunity for deliberation participants are given, the farther away they become from the average voter on the street. There is the danger that their participation in the survey transforms them into mini-experts, undermining the objective of eliciting the views held by a representative sample of the general public. Furthermore, if the existence of an interviewer or fellow study participants is going to make people react in ways that they think, rightly or wrongly, are more socially acceptable and politically correct than ways that reflect their genuine opinions, then there may be some merit in study designs with no face-to-face contact.

Box 10.2 Presenting multidimensional scenarios across two patient groups

The first example here uses an entirely verbal presentation in a budget pie exercise. Schwappach (2003) posed priority setting scenarios, in which respondents were asked to allocate percentages of a fixed budget across two patient groups of equal size, described using six attributes (see Fig. 10.1). The survey was conducted online, and respondents could find more detailed explanations by clicking on the underlined text. Similar presentations can be used for binary choice (where the respondent simply chooses one or the other group) as in discrete choice experiments, or for person trade-off exercises.

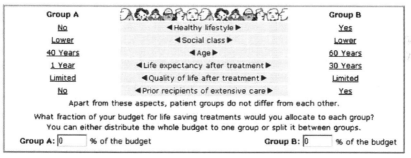

Fig. 10.1 An example of a verbal presentation of a multidimensional choice exercise. Reproduced with permission from Schwappach DL, 'Does it matter who you are or what you gain? An experimental study of preferences for resource allocation', *Health Economics*, Volume 12, Issue 4, pp. 255–67, Copyright © 2003 John Wiley and Sons Ltd.

The second example, shown in Figure 10.2, uses a visual aid. Rowen *et al.* (2016) operationalized severity as 'burden of illness', or the decrement in one's future health prospects due to a particular illness, and is operationalized as the difference between one's 'normal' quality-adjusted life expectancy and current quality-adjusted life expectancy given the illness. The two rectangles represent two patient groups, A and B, of equal size. All patients are of the same age. For each rectangle, the width represents length of time in years from 'today' and covers the patients' life expectancy given current age. The height represents HRQoL, with zero per cent equivalent to being dead and 100 per cent corresponding to full health. The full rectangle represents the patients' normal quality-adjusted life expectancy at current age. The dark smaller rectangle corresponds to the patients' quality-adjusted life expectancy given the illness, while the L-shape represents health gain from treatment. The same information is presented verbally in the box in the lower part of Figure 10.2.

Respondents were asked which patient group should be given priority over the other. Rowen *et al.* (2016) used a discrete choice experiment, where the shape and

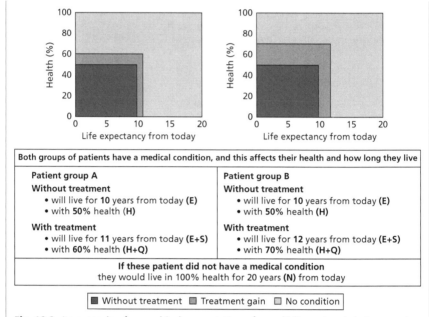

Fig. 10.2 An example of a graphical presentation of a multidimensional choice exercise. Reproduced from Rowen D et al., 'Eliciting societal preferences for weighting QALYs for burden of illness and end of life', *Medical Decision Making*, Volume 36, Number 2, pp. 210–22, Copyright © The Author(s) 2016, with permission from Sage.

sizes of the dark rectangle and the L-shaped areas varied from choice task to choice task. A similar presentation can be used for budget pie and person trade-off exercises.

As with health state valuation tasks discussed in Chapter 4, some methods are 'iterative'—the numeraire attribute is changed systematically until indifference between the groups is achieved. The numeraire can be the number of patients (person trade-off), the size of the health gain (benefit trade-off), or the split of the budget allocated to each group (budget pie). The existence of a numeraire attribute may introduce focusing bias, and the procedure of iteration can introduce ordering bias. Alternatively, the method can be non-iterative—each respondent only gives ordinal responses to each pair (set) of scenarios. This can be a pairwise discrete choice experiment, ranking, or best–worst scaling, all of which can be analysed using random utility theory (see Chapter 6).

10.5 The empirical evidence: people's views on the relative value of QALYs

The empirical literature on the relative societal value of a QALY is rapidly growing, and for instance, a recent review (Gu *et al.* 2015) has identified 22 empirical studies on the social value of health published between 1993 and 2014. Of these, six were published in the 1990s, another six prior to 2010, and a further ten between 2011 and 2014. Patient age and severity of the condition (including end of life) were the two most frequently examined characteristics, while other studies addressed the socio-economic status of the patients, the nature of the health gain, and costs of treatment.

Overall, there is enough evidence to suggest that public preferences are largely consistent with a health-related social welfare function that is increasing in individual health, but at the same time, with limited support for simple QALY gain maximization and constant marginal social value of a QALY across different considerations. For example, there is a tendency to prefer giving higher priority to treat patients who are: young (Charny *et al.* 1989; Busschbach *et al.* 1993; Cropper *et al.* 1994; Nord *et al.* 1996; Johannesson and Johansson 1997; Rodriguez and Pinto 2000; Eisenberg *et al.* 2011; Petrou *et al.* 2013); in worse health (including notions of burden of illness) or health status (Nord 1993; Ubel and Loewenstien 1995; Cookson and Dolan 1999; Ubel 1999; Schwappach 2003; Abásolo and Tsuchiya 2004, 2013; Green 2009; Whitty *et al.* 2011; Diederich *et al.* 2011; Linley and Hughes 2013; Rowen *et al.* 2016); at the end of their lives (Shah *et al.* 2014; Rowen *et al.* 2016), although not always (Linley and Hughes 2013; Shah *et al.* 2015); and those who are not responsible for their ill health (Lewis and Charny 1989; Nord *et al.* 1995; Ubel *et al.* 1999; Ratcliffe 2000; Dolan and Tsuchiya 2009; Edlin *et al.* 2012; Norman *et al.* 2013), although not always (Diederich 2011; Lim *et al.* 2012). There are a number of systematic literature reviews in this area that the reader is directed to: Sassi *et al.* (2001), Schwappach (2002), Dolan *et al.* (2005), Shah (2009), Green (2011), Johri and Norheim (2012), Cleemput *et al.* (2014), and Gu *et al.* (2015).

10.6 Practical concerns for cost per weighted QALY analyses

For cost per weighted QALY analyses actually to succeed, both theoretical arguments and empirical evidence need to be in place. On the one hand, theory can be useful in formulating the different ways in which the marginal social value of a QALY may vary, and in identifying the legitimate considerations, but on its own, it cannot be used to identify what size the relative weights should be. On the other hand, simply because people seem to support certain types of priorities, if this cannot be underwritten by a theoretical justification then it should not form the basis of policy making. For example, in modern liberal societies, it is unacceptable to give different weights to the health of people according to their ethnicity, religious beliefs, or sexual orientation.

Studies have typically examined one characteristic at a time (e.g. the effect of age, or the effect of severity, on its own), which had two implications. First, the results may have been susceptible to focusing bias (see Chapter 4). Second, it was not clear how the results could be combined to generate weights across the characteristics (i.e. for combinations of different age and severity): should the overall weights be multiplicative, additive, or some other combination of the two characteristics? Some more recent studies have looked at multiple characteristics at the same time (e.g. socio-economic background of patients, alongside severity of baseline health, rarity of condition, and size of health gain). Furthermore, studies are emerging that analyse the results in a way that generate weights that correspond to Eq. 1b or Eq. 2b (Norman *et al.* 2013; Abásolo and Tsuchiya 2004; Rowen *et al.* 2016).

The final issue to be addressed is how to reflect the resulting weights in policy decision making (Johri and Norheim 2012). It is clear that if weights are to be used in health care resource allocation, they will be used at the macro, central planning level; to some extent, meso level (i.e. the regional, or institution level) decisions could also be expected to reflect the weights.

10.7 Conclusion

This chapter has looked at a theoretical framework for diversions from the assumption that all units of health gain have equal social value, and examined different ways in which welfarists and non-welfarists may call for cost per *weighted* QALY analyses, for efficiency-based reasons, and equity-motivated reasons. A distinction was drawn between the value of health to individuals (which is a matter of preferences) and the value of health of different people to society (which is a matter of normative judgement). Another distinction was drawn between weighting QALYs across different people because of who they are (the a_i parameter) and weighting QALYs across different people because of the level of their baseline health (the b parameter). The chapter also presented a brief look at the challenges associated with empirical research in the topic, their findings, and the practicalities of cost per weighted QALYs.

References

Abásolo I, Tsuchiya A (2004). Exploring social welfare functions and violation of monotonicity: an example from inequalities in health. *Journal of Health Economics* **23**:313–29.

Abásolo I, Tsuchiya A (2013). Is more health always better for society? Exploring public preferences that violate monotonicity. *Theory and Decision* **74**:539–63.

Busschbach JJV, Hessing DJ, Decharro FT (1993). The utility of health at different stages in life—a quantitative approach. *Social Science and Medicine* **37**:153–8.

Charny MC, Lewis PA, Farrow SC (1989). Choosing who shall not be treated in the NHS. *Social Science and Medicine* **28**:1331–8.

Cookson R, Dolan P (1999). Public views on health care rationing: a group discussion study. *Health Policy* **49**:63–74.

Coast J, Flynn T, Sutton E, Al-Janabi H, Vosper J, Lavender S, *et al.* (2008). Investigating choice experiments for preferences of older people (ICEPOP): evaluative spaces in health economics. *Journal of Health Services Research & Policy* **13**(suppl 3):31–7.

Cookson R, Dolan P (1999). Public views on health care rationing: a group discussion study. *Health Policy* **49**:63–74.

Cookson R, McCabe C, Tsuchiya A (2008). Public health care resource allocation and the rule of rescue. *Journal of Medical Ethics* **34**:540–4.

Cleemput I, Devriese S, Kohn L, Devos C, Van Til J, Groothuis-Oudshoorn K, *et al.* (2014). *Incorporating societal preferences in reimbursement decisions*. Good Clinical Practice (GCP) Belgian Health Care Knowledge Centre (KCE), Brussels, Belgium. KCE Reports 234; 22/12/ 2014. Available from: https://kce.fgov.be/node/2633

Cropper ML, Aydede SK, Portney PR (1994). Preferences for life saving programs—how the public discounts time and age. *Journal of Risk and Uncertainty* **8**:243–65.

Daniels N (1988). *Am I my parents' keeper? An essay on justice between the young and the old.* Oxford University Press, London, UK.

Diederich A, Winkelhage J, Wirsik N (2011). Age as a criterion for setting priorities in health care? A survey of the German public view. *Plos One* **6**:e23930.

Dolan P, Edlin R, Tsuchiya A, Wailoo A (2007). It ain't what you do, it's the way that you do it: Characteristics of procedural justice and their importance in social decision-making, *Journal of Economic Behavior and Organization* **64**:157–70.

Dolan P, Olsen JA, Menzel P, Richardson J (2003). An inquiry into the different perspectives that can be used when eliciting preferences in health, *Health Economics* **12**:545–51.

Dolan P, Shaw R, Tsuchiya A, Williams A (2005). QALY maximisation and people's preferences: a methodological review of the literature. *Health Economics* **14**:197–208.

Dolan P, Tsuchiya A (2007). Do NHS staff and members of the public share the same views about how to distribute health benefits? *Social Science & Medicine* **64**:2499–503.

Dolan P, Tsuchiya A (2009). The social welfare function and individual responsibility: Some theoretical issues and empirical evidence from health: *Journal of Health Economics* **28**:210–20.

Dworkin R (1981*a*). What is equality? Part 1: equality of welfare. *Philosophy and Public Affairs* **10**:185–246.

Dworkin R (1981*b*). What is equality? Part 2: equality of resources. *Philosophy and Public Affairs* **10**:283–345.

Edlin R, Tsuchiya A, Dolan P (2012). Public preferences for responsibility versus public preferences for reducing inequalities. *Health Economics* **21**:1416–26.

Eisenberg D, Freed GL, Davis MM, Singer D, Prosser LA (2011). Valuing health at different ages: evidence from a nationally representative survey in the US. *Applied Health Economics and Health Policy* **9**:149–56.

Fleurbaey M, Schokkaert E (2009). Unfair inequalities in health and health care. *Journal of Health Economics* **28**:73–90.

Green C (2009). Investigating public preferences on 'severity of health' as a relevant condition for setting healthcare priorities. *Social Science and Medicine* **68**: 2247–55.

Green C (2011). *Looking for the 'values' to inform value-based pricing: a review of the empirical ethics (equity) evidence!*, paper presented at the Health Economists' Study Group meeting, Bangor, UK.

Gu Y, Lancsar E, Ghijben P, Butler JRG, Donaldson C (2015). Attributes and weights in health care priority setting: A systematic review of what counts and to what extent. *Social Science and Medicine* **146**:41–52.

Harris J (1985). *The value of life: an introduction to medical ethics.* Routledge, London, UK.

Johannesson M, Johansson P-O (1997). Is the valuation of a QALY gained independent of age? Some empirical evidence. *Journal of Health Economics* **16**:589–99.

Johri M, Norheim OF (2012). Can cost-effectiveness analysis integrate concerns for equity? Systematic review, *International Journal of Technology Assessment in Health Care* **28**:125–32.

Jonsen AR (1986). Bentham in a box: technology assessmsment and health care allocation. *Law, Medicine and Health Care* **14**:172–4.

Lewis PA, Charny M (1989). Which of two individuals do you treat when only their ages are different and you can't treat both? *Journal of Medical Ethics* **15**:28–32.

Lim MK, Bae EY, Choi SE, Lee EK, Lee TJ (2012). Eliciting public preference for health-care resource allocation in South Korea. *Value in Health* **15**:S91–4.

Linley WG, Hughes DA (2013). Societal views on NICE, cancer drugs fund and value-based pricing criteria for prioritising medicines: A cross-sectional survey of 4118 adults in Great Britain. *Health Economics* **22**:948–64.

Lockwood M (1988). Quality of life and resource allocation. In: Bell JM and Mendus S (eds.). *Philosophy and medical welfare*. Royal Institute of Philosophy Lecture Series 23, Cambridge University Press, Cambridge.

Nord E (1993). The trade-off between severity of illness and treatment effect in cost-value analysis of health-care. *Health Policy* **24**:227–38.

Nord E (2005). Concerns for the worse off: fair innings versus severity. *Social Science and Medicine* **60**:257–63.

Nord E, Richardson J, Street A, Kuhse H, Singer P (1995). Maximizing health benefits vs egalitarianism—an Australian survey of health issues. *Social Science and Medicine* **41**:1429–37.

Nord E, Street A, Richardson J, Kuhse H, Singer P (1996). The significance of age and duration of effect in social evaluation of health care. *Health Care Analysis* **4**:103–11.

Norman R, Hall J, Street D, Viney R (2013). Efficiency and equity: A stated preference approach, *Health Economics* **22**:568–81.

Parfit D (1997). Equality and priority. *Ratio* **10**:202–21.

Petrou S, Kandala NB, Robinson A, Baker R (2013). A person trade-off study to estimate age-related weights for health gains in economic evaluation. *Pharmacoeconomics* **31**:893–907.

Ratcliffe J (2000). Public preferences for the allocation of donor liver grafts for transplantation. *Health Economics* **9**:137–48.

Rawlins MD, Culyer AJ (2004). National Institute for Clinical Excellence and its value judgments. *British Medical Journal* **329**:224–7.

Rodriguez E, Pinto JL (2000). The social value of health programmes: is age a relevant factor? *Health Economics* **9**:611–21.

Roberts G (2016). *Methodology for estimating the net production/wider societal impact of treatments*. Policy Research Unit in Economic Evaluation of Health and Care Interventions. EEPRU Research Report 039, Universities of Sheffield and York, UK.

Rowen D, Brazier J, Mukuria C, Keetharuth A, Hole AR, Tsuchiya A, *et al.* (2016). Eliciting societal preferences for weighting QALYs for burden of illness and end of life. *Medical Decision Making* **36**:210–22.

Sassi F, Archard L, Le Grand J (2001). Equity and the economic evaluation of healthcare. *Health Technology Assessment* **5**:1–138.

Schwappach DL (2002). Resource allocation, social values and the QALY: a review of the debate and empirical evidence. *Health Expectations* **5**:210–22.

Schwappach DL (2003). Does it matter who you are or what you gain? An experimental study of preferences for resource allocation. *Health Economics* **12**:255–67.

Shah KK (2009). Severity of illness and priority setting in health care: A review of the literature. *Health Policy* **93**:77–84.

Shah KK, Tsuchiya A, Wailoo AJ (2014). Valuing health at the end of life: an empirical study of public preferences. *The European Journal of Health Economics* **15**:389–99.

Shah KK, Tsuchiya A, Wailoo AJ (2015). Valuing health at the end of life: A stated preference discrete choice experiment. *Social Science and Medicine* **124**:48–56.

Tsuchiya A (2000). QALYs and ageism: philosophical theories and age weighting. *Health Economics* **9**:57–68.

Ubel PA (1999). How stable are people's preferences for giving priority to severely ill patients? *Social Science and Medicine* **49**:895–903.

Ubel PA, Loewenstein G (1995). The efficacy and equity of retransplantation—an experimental survey of public attitudes. *Health Policy* **34**:145–51.

Ubel PA, Baron J, Asch DA (1999). Social responsibility, personal responsibility, and prognosis in public judgments about transplant allocation. *Bioethics* **13**:57–68.

Williams A (1997). Intergenerational equity: an exploration of the 'fair innings' argument. *Health Economics* **6**:117–32.

Whitty JA, Scuffham PA, Rundle-Thielee SR (2011). Public and decision maker stated preferences for pharmaceutical subsidy decisions. *Applied Health Economics and Health Policy* **9**:73–9.

Chapter 11

Measuring and valuing health: an international perspective

11.1 International perspective—an introduction

So far in this book, our primary consideration has been the measurement and valuation of health for economic evaluations in settings such as the United Kingdom, where the National Institute for Health and Care Excellence (NICE) has formalized the requirement for evidence on cost-effectiveness of interventions, expressed in terms of costs per quality-adjusted life year (QALY), as an input to national decision making on health technologies (NICE 2009). Somewhat paradoxically, the institutionalized demand for cost-effectiveness evidence in low- and middle-income countries—where this sort of information is arguably even more urgently required—has yet to gain traction to the same extent that it has in various countries in the industrialized world. On the other hand, there are several important exceptions to this general observation, and these may signal a rising interest in undertaking and applying cost-effectiveness analyses (CEAs) in developing countries. Some notable examples include the body of work from the World Health Organization's CHOICE (CHOosing Interventions that are Cost Effective) project, which developed guidelines on conducting 'generalized cost-effectiveness analysis' (Tan-Torres Edejer *et al.* 2003); periodic revisions of the Disease Control Priorities Project on cost-effectiveness for a range of interventions related to major health problems in low- and middle-income countries (Jamison *et al.* 2006; Jamison 2015); and—most recently—an initiative led by the Bill and Melinda Gates Foundation to develop guidance for conducting cost-effectiveness analyses relevant to global health programming (Bill and Melinda Gates Foundation 2014).

In this chapter, we revisit some of the key topics covered in the preceding chapters of this volume through the particular lens of the developing country perspective. We provide an introduction to the disability-adjusted life year (DALY), which is an alternative to the QALY that has been favoured in much of the cost-effectiveness work in developing countries. We will also extend the discussions of key issues in the definition, description, and valuation of health to address some of the added considerations demanded by cross-cultural applications of the methods and tools that are the focus of this book.

11.2 **The disability-adjusted life year**

The DALY was first developed for the primary purpose of quantifying the global burden of disease (Murray and Lopez 1994). In this context, it was constructed as a summary measure of population health—specifically, to be used as an indicator of the relative magnitude of losses of healthy life associated with different causes of diseases and injuries. The construction of summary measures of population health has much in common with the construction of measures of the benefits from health interventions (Box 11.1). Indeed, the developers of the DALY explicitly intended that the measure could be used as both a unit of account for the burden of disease, and a metric for health benefits in the denominator of cost-effectiveness ratios (Murray

---

Box 11.1 Summary measures of population health

Broadly, there are two families of summary measures of population health, with distinct features and uses: (i) health expectancy measures capture the overall, average level of health in a population—useful as a single summary index of population health; (ii) health gaps, typically decomposed by cause, indicate the overall loss of health associated with a given problem in reference to some defined target for healthy survivorship (Murray *et al.* 2000). Both health expectancies and health gaps can combine information on mortality with information on non-fatal health outcomes and express these outcomes in time-based units, that is, as healthy years lived, or healthy years lost. In both families of population health measures, as in measures of intervention benefits such as QALYs, health state valuations provide the critical link between the mortality and non-fatal outcomes. By quantifying health levels on a continuum from the best to the worst levels, and scaling these values in reference to optimal health and dead, extensions (or reductions) in longevity and improvements (or decrements) in health levels can be aggregated in composite measures.

The mechanics of combining information on health levels with information on longevity or premature mortality in population health measures are similar to those in the measurement of intervention benefits (see Chapter 9). For cost-effectiveness analyses, the benefits of interventions are estimated by computing the difference between the estimated life expectancy with or without the intervention, weighting each life year in a way that reflects the levels of health (or utility or quality of life) associated with the sequence of health states that are experienced in either case. For the health expectancy family of population health measures, an analogous operation at the aggregate level extends the demographic measure of life expectancy to account for the levels of health experienced in the population at different ages. For health gap measures, such as the DALY, losses associated with a particular problem are measured in terms of years of life lost, reflecting premature mortality compared with some yardstick for longevity at each age, combined with years lived with disability, which reflect the severity and duration of non-fatal health decrements.

et al. 1994). The major debut of the DALY in the World Bank's *World development report 1993* introduced applications of the measure toward both ends (World Bank 1993). Subsequently, guidelines from the WHO-CHOICE project on conducting generalized CEAs included an explicit recommendation to use reductions in DALYs as the measure of benefit in these analyses (Tan-Torres Edejer *et al.* 2003). Most recently, the 'Gates Reference Case' recommended by the Bill and Melinda Gates Foundation Methods for Economic Evaluation Project (MEEP) also specifies that DALYs should be used as the outcome measure in economic evaluations in low- and middle-income countries (Bill and Melinda Gates Foundation 2014).

As discussed in this book with reference to QALYs, a key issue in the construction of DALYs is the definition and interpretation of the weights attached to non-fatal health outcomes. As described in Chapters 2 and 3, there have been a range of different interpretations of the weights that are included in QALYs, originating from alternative theoretical perspectives (welfarist versus non-welfarist) and complicated by the diversity of measures that are used to elicit these weights. In computing weights for QALYs, some researchers have explicitly defined valuations in terms of the individual utility associated with health states, while others have favoured an alternative view of QALYs as an indicator of changes in population health to be used as the maxim and in a social objective function (see Chapter 3 for a full discussion). The interpretation of the 'disability weights' used in DALYs has been more closely aligned with the latter position in the competing views of QALYs. However, the approach used to elicit these weights has evolved through successive iterations of the DALY measure, from the first detailed methodological presentation of disability weights in 1994, through a major revision of the measurement approach in 1996, and the most recent overhaul reported in 2012. We describe this evolution in the following section.

11.2.1 Development of disability weights for DALYs

11.2.1.1 Global burden of disease (GBD)—first round (1993–1994)

The development of the DALY as a metric for the GBD has required, as one input, a set of disability weights that reflect the relative severity of an array of disabling consequences that follow from the disease and injury causes included in the study. These consequences are generally organized as a set of discrete 'sequelae', with each cause typically mapped to more than one sequela by experts who are familiar with the disease or injury and its key clinical features, natural history, and epidemiology. The goal of this mapping is to define a relatively parsimonious set of outcomes that represent the spectrum of functional consequences and symptomatology that result from a particular causes. For example, diabetes mellitus is a disease cause in the study, and its sequelae include diabetic neuropathy, amputation, and blindness, among others. Disability weights are required for each sequela in the study.

As the name implies, disability weights were originally conceived in terms of a construct that resides at an intermediate point in the spectrum from impairment to handicap, as proposed in the International Classification of Impairments, Disabilities, and Handicaps (ICIDH), appearing in revised form as the International Classification of

Functioning, Disability and Health. The choice of disability rather than impairment reflects an interest in capturing the overall consequence of disease, in terms of its impact on the performance of an individual (which is how disability is conceptualized), rather than the narrower impact at the level of a particular body part or organ system (which is how impairment is conceptualized). Disability was also preferred to handicap as the relevant measure (the latter defined as overall consequences within a particular social environment), based on the argument that a focus on handicap could further exacerbate disparities by placing a greater emphasis on the impact of a particular disability among those who already have a relative advantage. As quoted in Murray (1994), one example of this thinking appeared in the ICIDH manual: 'Subnormality of intelligence is an impairment, but it may not lead to appreciable activity restriction; factors other than the impairment may determine the handicap because the disadvantage may be minimal if the individual lives in a remote rural community, whereas it could be severe in the child of university graduates living in a large city, of whom more might be expected'.

The assignment of disability weights to the range of sequelae in the initial iteration of the global burden of disease study (Murray 1994) was based on first defining six different disability classes in reference to limitations in activities of daily living such as eating and personal hygiene; instrumental activities of daily living such as meal preparation; and four other domains (procreation, occupation, education, and recreation). Weights were assigned to the different classes by a panel of public health experts using a rating scale approach, on a scale on which zero represents no disability and one represents disability equivalent to being dead, with the weight taken as the average of the values from the expert panel. For example, the least severe class, defined as 'limited ability to perform at least one activity in one of the following areas: recreation, education, procreation or occupation', had a weight of 0.096, implying a reduction of around 10 per cent from full health; the most severe class, defined as 'needs assistance with activities of daily living such as eating, personal hygiene, or toilet use', had a weight of 0.920, implying a decrement of more than 90 per cent. Given these classes and their associated weights, the disability weight for a particular sequela was estimated by distributing incident cases across the different classes—reflecting either the proportion of time an average incident case would spend in different disability classes, or the proportion of incident cases that would be characterized by different severity levels—and computing the average weight. The distribution of cases across the severity classes was determined by disease experts. For example, sequelae of meningitis included intellectual disability and deafness. For intellectual disability, it was estimated that 50 per cent of the instances of this sequel would reflect a 'Class 2 disability' (with a weight of 0.220) and the other 50 per cent a 'Class 3 disability' (with a weight of 0.400), resulting in a weighted average disability weight of 0.31; for deafness, 100 per cent of cases were allocated to Class 3 disability, resulting in an overall disability weight of 0.400 (Murray and Lopez 1994). In this example, the overall non-fatal disease burden related to meningitis would then be computed by summing the burdens related to each of the individual sequelae, which are computed as a function of the disability weight and the number of years lived with each sequelae in a particular population of interest.

11.2.1.2 Global burden of disease—1996 revision

For the revision of the global burden of disease study published in 1996, a new approach to estimating disability weights was devised based on the person trade-off (PTO) method. The revision of the approach was inspired by some specific criticisms of the original approach: (i) that the disability classes were appropriate only for adults (e.g. since children were naturally dependent on adults for various of the referenced activities); (ii) that no formal, replicable protocol was available to guide those aspiring to undertake a national burden of disease exercise; (iii) that the class with the lowest level of disability was valued at 0.096, which produced a scale that was too blunt to capture very mild conditions; and, finally, (iv) that the valuation task itself did not allow the expert panellists to reflect on the policy implications of their values (Murray 1996).

New health state valuations were elicited from a single panel of 12 international health professionals following an explicit protocol (Murray 1996). In the protocol, a first stage focused on a set of 22 indicator conditions, evaluated through an intensive group exercise involving two variants of the PTO and incorporating a deliberative process to encourage reflection on the values that emerged during the exercise. The first type of PTO question asked participants to trade-off life extension in a population of healthy individuals versus life extension in a population of individuals having a particular condition. The second type of PTO question asked participants to trade-off life extension for healthy individuals versus health improvements in individuals with the particular condition. Participants were required to resolve inconsistencies in the numerical weights implied by the two alternative framings of the PTO. The final consistent values implied by the reconciled PTO responses, averaged across participants, defined the disability weights for the 22 indicator conditions, which were then grouped into seven different severity classes, each including at least two of the indicator conditions (Box 11.2).

To generate disability weights for the approximately 500 disabling sequelae in the study, participants were asked to estimate distributions across the seven classes for each sequela. In this second phase of the protocol, the main purpose of the indicator conditions was to serve as concrete examples of the level of severity reflected in each class, replacing the functional classifications used to describe the six disability classes in the 1993–1994 iteration of the study. As described here for the first iteration, the distributions across classes were intended to reflect either the proportion of time a typical case for a given sequela would spend in each of the disability classes, or the percentage of cases that would be categorized in each of the different classes. Distributions across disability classes were estimated separately for treated and untreated cases where relevant, and weights could also vary by age group. Box 11.2 presents a few examples of the resulting disability weights for common causes.

11.2.1.3 Global burden of disease 2010 (GBD 2010)

More recently, prompted by a more general research agenda on developing internationally comparable summary measures of population health at the World Health Organization, the use of the PTO as the basis for disability weights in DALYs has been reconsidered. The most recent thinking on DALYs reflects an effort to delineate the concept embodied in the non-fatal component of the measure more precisely, which

Box 11.2 Disability weights in the global burden of disease study, 1996 revision

Based on a deliberative protocol built around the PTO method, disability weights for 22 indicator conditions were estimated, and the conditions were then grouped into seven different classes reflecting a spectrum of severity levels:

◆ Class 1, with weights ranging from 0.00 to 0.02, included vitiligo on face; and two weight-for-height standard deviations or more below the reference median

◆ Class 2, with weights ranging from 0.02 to 0.12, included watery diarrhoea; severe sore throat; and severe anaemia

◆ Class 3, with weights ranging from 0.12 to 0.24, included radius fracture in a stiff cast; infertility; erectile dysfunction; rheumatoid arthritis; and angina

◆ Class 4, with weights ranging from 0.24 to 0.36, included below-the-knee amputation; and deafness

◆ Class 5, with weights ranging from 0.36 to 0.50, included rectovaginal fistula; mild mental retardation; and Down's syndrome

◆ Class 6, with weights ranging from 0.50 to 0.70, included unipolar major depression; blindness; and paraplegia

◆ Class 7, with weights ranging from 0.70 to 1.00, included active psychosis; dementia; severe migraine; and quadriplegia

Weights for the full range of sequelae in the study were derived by estimating the distribution of incident cases across these seven classes, using the indicator conditions in each class as illustrative benchmarks. Examples of the resulting weights include:

◆ Episodes of otitis media: 0.02

◆ Cases of asthma: 0.10 (untreated); 0.06 (treated)

◆ Episodes of malaria: 0.21 (ages 0–4 years); 0.17 (ages 15 and older)

◆ Rheumatoid arthritis cases: 0.23 (untreated); 0.17 (treated)

◆ Episodes of meningitis: 0.62

◆ Terminal cancer: 0.81

Adapted with permission from The Global Burden of Disease: A comprehensive assessment of mortality and disability from diseases, injuries, and risk factors in 1990 and projected to 2020, Christopher JL Murray and Alan D Lopez (eds.), 'The GBD's Approach to Measuring Health Status', pp. 6-13, Copyright © 1996 World Health Organization. All rights reserved. Available from http://apps.who.int/iris/bitstream/10665/41864/1/0965546608_eng.pdf (accessed April 2016).

has led to the explicit definition of disability weights as measures of overall levels of health associated with health states, rather than as measures of the utility associated with these states or the contribution of health to overall welfare (Salomon *et al.* 2003*a*). As a precursor to the disability weights measurement in GBD 2010, a series of research studies examined approaches to separate out some of the other values that combine with judgements about health levels in valuation elicitation techniques, such as the time trade-off (TTO), standard gamble (SG), and PTO, by formally modelling responses as a function of both underlying health judgements and these other values (Salomon and Murray 2004) (see Chapter 4 for a discussion of these non-health factors), and use of alternative valuation methods such as ones based on ordinal data collection strategies (Salomon 2003; see also Chapter 6). The latter strategy forms the basis of the most recent major revision of the disability weights measurement strategy in the global burden of disease study.

A significant update of the global burden of disease study 2010 (GBD 2010) was published in 2012, and one component in this revision was development of a completely new set of disability weights using a novel measurement approach applied in a large-scale multi-country empirical data collection effort (Salomon *et al.* 2012). The new study made changes to both the descriptions of consequences of diseases or injuries, and the valuation approach. The disease and injury list was expanded to 291 and their associated sequelae to 1,160. An important new feature of the study was the development of 220 health states that collectively summarized common disease sequelae across conditions. Consultations with advisory and experts groups was undertaken to develop the shorter list of health states. For example, anaemia is identified as a disease sequela of 19 diseases and is associated with three health states: mild, moderate, and severe anaemia (Salomon *et al.* 2012). For each health state, a lay description was developed for use in the valuation studies with emphasis on the main functional consequences and symptoms associated with each health state, presented with simple, non-clinical vocabulary (Salomon *et al.* 2012). The lay descriptions were also developed by consultation with experts involved in the GBD 2010 study. This process was supported by the use of existing measures, as well as with standardized worksheets describing the dimensions and symptoms of health. Resulting descriptions focused less on specific sequelae and more on functioning and symptoms; for example, the health state 'infectious disease, acute episode, mild' had a lay description 'has a low fever and mild discomfort but no difficulty with daily activities'. In this new approach, a single weight was estimated for each sequela by attempting to characterize the typical health experience of living with that seqeuela, rather than defining how cases would distribute across discrete classes of disability, as in the prior two disability weight measurement studies described here previously.

In the valuation study, the GBD 2010 study relied primarily on a paired comparison technique (see Chapter 6) in which respondents considered two hypothetical people, each with a lay description of a particular health state, and were asked to indicate which of these people they regarded as 'being healthier'. Some respondents also answered questions based on a 'population health equivalence' question, in which they were asked to select the programme with the greater overall health benefits in a comparison between two programmes: one of which was life-saving, while the other prevented limitations in functioning or symptoms that were described in lay terms. The number of lives saved was fixed at 1,000, while the number of people benefiting from prevention was randomly selected from 1,500, 2,000, 3,000, 5,000, or 10,000. The population health equivalence question resembles a person trade-off question, but is framed retrospectively, and in terms of comparisons of overall population health improvements rather than individual preferences.

A final innovation of the GBD 2010 was the collection of data from the general population rather than experts, as was done in previous GBD studies. Data were collected from more than 30,000 respondents through four household surveys (in Bangladesh, Indonesia, Peru, and Tanzania), a telephone survey in the United States, and an open access internet survey. Respondents in the household and telephone surveys completed 15 paired comparisons generated from a pool of 108 health states. Those who completed the internet survey did one of four versions, one of which was equivalent to the household survey, while others included additional health states, different framing for temporary health states, and the population health equivalence questions (Salomon *et al.* 2012).

The paired comparison responses were analysed using probit regression with indicator variables for each of the unique health states in the study, and the resulting weights were rescaled onto the 0-to-1 disability weights scale based on a transformation defined in reference to the 'population health equivalence' question using regression analysis. The study produced disability weights for 220 unique health states defining the range of outcomes across the 1,160 sequelae in the 2010 global burden of disease, and including estimation uncertainty around these, for the first time. Box 11.3 presents selected examples of disability weights estimated for the GBD 2010. An interesting empirical finding in the study was that the paired comparison responses were quite consistent across the different surveys, despite there being considerable diversity in the language, education, and cultural settings from which the samples were drawn. Following the 2012 study, a major addition of empirical data has come from

Box 11.3 Disability weights in the global burden of disease 2010 study

Examples of disability weights from the GBD 2010 study (with point estimates and 95 per cent uncertainty intervals, the latter in parentheses) include:

◆ Infectious disease: acute episode, mild: 0.005 (0.002–0.011)

◆ Stroke: long-term consequences, mild: 0.021 (0.011–0.037)

◆ Asthma, uncontrolled: 0.132 (0.087–0.190)

◆ Major depressive disorder: moderate episode: 0.159 (0.107–0.223)

◆ Distance vision: severe impairment: 0.191 (0.128–0.269)

◆ Cancer: diagnosis and primary therapy: 0.294 (0.199–0.411)

◆ Low back pain: chronic, with leg pain: 0.374 (0.252–0.506)

◆ End-stage renal disease: on dialysis: 0.573 (0.397–0.749)

◆ Multiple sclerosis: severe: 0.707 (0.522–0.857)

replication of the approach in four European countries, and these surveys have been pooled with the earlier ones in updating disability weights for the most recent round of GBD revisions, published in 2014 and 2015 (Salomon *et al.* 2015).

11.2.2 Other social value choices in DALYs

Another feature of DALYs that has received considerable attention relates to the inclusion of other social value choices, besides the valuations of health states used to construct disability weights. Many of the arguments around discounting invoked in the context of the QALY measure have also been rehearsed in the discussion of DALYs as a population health measure. For DALYs, discounting is relevant to the calculus of streams of lost life, either due to mortality (where the losses are potential years surrendered to early death) or due to non-fatal conditions (where the losses are durations of experience of lost health extending into the future). Prior to the GBD 2010, the use of a three per cent annual discount rate had become the default standard in the construction of the DALY, as in the recommended base case analysis for cost-effectiveness studies; in both cases it was generally advised that alternatives should be considered in sensitivity analyses. In the GBD 2010, as part of a broader attempt to define DALYs as measures of health as opposed to measures of well-being or representations of preferences, temporal discounting has been dropped from the measure; in other words, all future streams of life years are counted as undiscounted.

In addition to discounting, some have argued for assigning unequal weights to life years lived at different ages, and the standard DALY before the GBD 2010 included weights that gave the highest values to years lived in young adulthood. A range of arguments were considered in relation to age weighting, with reference to empirical findings on weights that people attach to years over the life course (Busschbach *et al.* 1993; Jelsma *et al.* 2002). The developers of the DALY measure previously argued for unequal age weighting based on the social roles played at different ages (Murray 1996), but age weights have been controversial (e.g. see Anand and Hansen 1997). In the GBD 2010, along with the move away from discounting, the standard DALY has also dropped age weights, such that life years are weighted equally across all ages (conditional on living in the same health state). The question of age weighting is considered more fully in Chapter 10.

In summary, for use in economic evaluations of health interventions, the DALY is best viewed as a close relative of the QALY with a few historical differences, as summarized in Box 11.4.

11.3 International comparisons of health state valuations

Stepping back from the specifics of the DALY measure in international CEA, we turn now to more general issues around measurement and valuation of health for cross-national applications. While we will refer to applications that span both developed and developing countries here, we will note in particular where work has taken place in low- and middle-income settings.

Box 11.4 DALYs and QALYs

The relationship between DALYs and QALYs has been characterized as follows by developers of the DALY: 'DALYs can be considered as a variant of QALYs which have been standardized for comparative use' (Murray and Acharya 1997).

One key distinction between DALYs and QALYs is the way that outcomes are typically presented as stimuli for valuation. For example, as described here, the latest efforts to estimate disability weights for DALYs in the global burden of disease study uses surveys that describe health states with short narrative vignettes in lay language; in contrast, the dominant approach in deriving weights for QALYs relies on health state classification systems that result in standardized descriptions of levels on different health dimensions. Other key distinctions between DALYs and QALYs include the following:

- Because the DALY is a negative measure that reflects health losses, the scale used to quantify non-fatal health outcomes in DALYs is inverted compared with the scale used in QALYs, that is, numbers near zero represent relatively good health levels (or small losses) in DALYs, while numbers near one represent relatively poor health levels (or large losses). The inverted scale means that interventions that improve health result in DALYs *averted*, whereas QALYs are *gained*.

- Disability weights in DALYs are intended to reflect the degree to which health is reduced by the presence of different conditions, whereas at least one interpretation of the weights in QALYs is based on the individual utility derived from different states.

- Another important difference in the measurement approach to derive weights for DALYs compared to the typical approach used in estimating QALY weights is that QALYs typically use health state classification systems that are defined in terms of standard dimensions and associated level structures. Estimation of disability weights for DALYs, on the other hand, is based on vignette-type lay descriptions of sequelae, as described here already.

- The standard formulation of DALYs prior to the GBD 2010 study weighed healthy life lived at different ages according to a variable function that peaks at young adult ages, while QALYs do not typically incorporate unequal age weights (although these can be added; see Chapter 10). It should be noted there has always been the option to compute DALYs with equal age weights, and in the GBD 2010 study, equal weights are standard.

- For measuring the burden of disease, years of life lost due to premature mortality at different ages are computed in reference to a standard life table. In the original GBD study, this standard was defined by the period life expectancy at birth for Japanese females. More recently, for the GBD 2010 study, the standard has been revised, based on a synthetic life table that uses the lowest observed country-level mortality rate for each age group, and thus is an amalgamation of mortality rates from different settings. For purposes of cost-effectiveness, this general distinction between QALYs and DALYs is largely inconsequential, since the standard life expectancy approximately cancels out when benefits of interventions are computed as the *change in* DALYs.

11.3.1 International adaptation of health status measures

There has been significant interest in adapting health status measurement instruments to varied cultural settings, and several reviews of these efforts are available, some of which suggesting guidelines for the process of cross-cultural adaptation (e.g. Guillemin *et al.* 1993; Anderson *et al.* 1996; Beaton *et al.* 2000). In addition to adaptation of generic instruments, one review on cross-cultural adaptation of health status measures (Sommerfeld *et al.* 2002) surveyed a range of studies on cross-cultural adaptations of condition-specific instruments for health problems ranging from epilepsy (Cramer *et al.* 1998) to genital herpes (Doward *et al.* 1998). The International Society for Pharmacoeconomics and Outcomes Research established a working group to review and consolidate guidelines for translating and adapting health measurement instruments, and in 2005 the group published a set of principles of good practice for the translation and cultural adaptation of patient-reported outcome measures (Wild *et al.* 2005). Another review has examined methods used to translate health status measurement instruments for use in multinational clinical trials (Acquadro *et al.* 2008) and identified aspects of translation protocols that evidently produce better translations, such as use of a multistep approach, and the authors developed a checklist to summarize the recommended steps. Extensive efforts to translate and adapt health measurement instruments to diverse settings have given considerable attention to issues of linguistic equivalence in translation, which has been emphasized in many of the existing guidelines (Guillemin *et al.* 1993; Sartorius and Kuyken 1994; Bullinger *et al.* 1998). However, concerns have been raised about the cultural equivalence of translations (Herdman *et al.* 1997, 1998), and a review of 58 papers reporting on the translation of eight generic instruments concluded that more attention must be given to ensuring conceptual equivalence (Bowden and Fox-Rushby 2003).

Certain generic health measurement instruments, including the SF-36 and the EQ-5D, have been the focus of large-scale efforts at adaptation and translation into a wide range of languages and settings. The International Quality of Life Assessment (IQOLA) project produced translations of the SF-36 for use in more than 60 countries (e.g. see Keller *et al.* 1998; Ware *et al.* 1995; or the IQOLA website at http://www.iqola.org). The EQ-5D instrument has been translated even more widely, with official language versions of the EQ-5D-3L instrument available for 170 countries and official language versions of the EQ-5D-5L available for 127 countries as of October 2015 (see http://www.euroqol.org). Until 2007, when the first edition of this book was published, most efforts to translate and adapt instruments—either generic or condition-specific—had focused nearly exclusively on high-income countries; examples from low- and middle-income countries were relatively rare. For the standardized instruments discussed extensively in this book, exceptions to this general rule included adaptations of the SF-36 in China (Li *et al.* 2003), Mexico (Zuniga *et al.* 1999), Bangladesh (Ahmed *et al.* 2002), Tanzania (Wagner *et al.* 1999), and several other developing countries; followed by the EQ-5D in China (Wang *et al.* 2005), Zimbabwe (Jelsma *et al.* 2003), and South Africa (Jelsma *et al.* 2004). Since the first edition, however, a significant number of translations of these instruments have accumulated from low- and middle-income countries. For example, translations of the EQ-5D in its different versions now include language versions for use in Algeria, Argentina, Bangladesh, Botswana, Brazil, Burma, Egypt,

India, India, Malaysia, Philippines, South Africa, Tanzania, Uruguay, Vietnam, among others; the SF-6D has now been translated and valued in Brazil and China.

Other large-scale examples of adapting and applying standardized health measurement instruments in developing countries include two waves of surveys conducted by the World Health Organization: the Multi-Country Survey Study on Health and Responsiveness (MCSS), conducted in 61 countries during 2000–2001 (Üstün *et al.* 2003*a*), and the World Health Surveys, conducted in 72 countries during 2002–2003 (Üstün *et al.* 2003*b*). The MCSS included a generic health status module including items with five-category response scales on six core domains (affect, cognition, mobility, pain, self-care, and usual activities). The World Health Survey included a modified health module with items on eight domains (affect, cognition, energy, interpersonal activities, mobility, pain, self-care, and vision).

11.3.2 International research on valuation approaches

To date, international research on health state valuations has been much less extensive than research on adapting existing health status instruments. The great majority of studies on valuation approaches such as the TTO, SG, and PTO have been conducted in North America, Western Europe, and Australasia. A smaller number of studies have been conducted in developing countries to consider the feasibility of administering valuation techniques where educational attainment, literacy, and numeracy are low. Application of these techniques across cultures introduces a range of additional challenges that compound the universal concerns about the abstract nature and cognitive demands of questions such as the SG. Sommerfeld *et al.* (2002) provide a concise summary of some of the considerations for cross-cultural application of these techniques, including varying notions of illness, risk and probability, and time.

The following examples illustrate some of the key findings from studies that have been conducted outside the industrialized world to compare the feasibility of different valuation techniques.

Sadana (2002) undertook a valuation study in Phnom Penh, Cambodia. In the study, pre-tests of the PTO, SG, and visual analogue scale (VAS) were conducted in a sample of women aged 18–45 years. For the PTO, conducted from the perspective of a societal decision maker, the pre-tests indicated that respondents were reluctant to answer both variants of the question used in the study, although the author concluded that comprehension problems were not a major concern. For the SG (from an individual perspective), the pre-test found that no respondents could complete the task. Of the three methods examined, only the VAS (also posed from an individual perspective) was successfully implemented in pre-test, yielding consistent orderings of the five indicator conditions in the study (blindness, infertility, below-the-knee amputation, severe headache, and unipolar major depression).

Mahapatra *et al.* (2002) conducted a valuation study in Andhra Pradesh State, India, including two components: (i) a multimethod study using ranking, VAS, TTO, and PTO among a convenience sample of more educated respondents; and (ii) a community sample survey in a rural village using ranking and VAS. The community survey included graphical depictions of domain levels for the range of hypothetical states to facilitate communication to respondents. The study found reasonable agreement between responses from the different valuation approaches in the multimethod component, with the smallest number of logically inconsistent responses on the VAS. In the community survey, while substantial measurement error appeared to characterize the VAS responses, the aggregate results were compared with VAS responses from a similar study in the Netherlands, and a high correlation was observed.

Baltussen *et al.* (2002) developed and applied a culturally adapted version of the VAS in a rural village in Burkina Faso. Considering nine hypothetical states, respondents were asked to indicate the severity of overall health decrements associated with those states using wooden blocks as physical units. The authors found that this procedure had high test–retest reliability (0.90 using Pearson's *r*) and concluded that the adapted approach to eliciting VAS responses was feasible to implement in a rural African setting.

One of the most extensive efforts to implement health state valuations in developing countries was undertaken as part of a survey programme led by the World Health Organization (Salomon *et al.* 2003*b*). Household surveys including a health state valuation module were conducted in 14 countries: China, Colombia, Egypt, Georgia, India, Iran, Lebanon, Indonesia, Mexico, Nigeria, Singapore, Slovakia, Syria, and Turkey. The surveys were nationally representative except in China, India, and Nigeria. Each country fielded both a sample survey in the general community using ranking and VAS, as well as a more detailed survey among respondents with high levels of educational attainment using ranking, VAS, TTO, SG, and PTO. The multimethod study found systematically different results by methods, with the lowest valuations from the VAS and the highest valuations from PTO. SG valuations were close to PTO valuations for most states, and TTO valuations tended to be nearer to VAS. The degree of measurement error varied widely across countries, but the broad patterns of differences across methods were consistent in the range of settings. The community survey revealed consistent orderings of the valuations for the 33 hypothetical states in the study using the VAS, although for any given state there was variation across countries in the mean VAS values.

Recently, the global burden of disease update published in 2012 (see Section 11.2.1.3) included sample surveys in Bangladesh, Indonesia, Peru, Tanzania, and the United States, and a non-representative internet survey that included respondents from 167 different countries (Salomon *et al.* 2012). The use of a paired comparison approach to eliciting judgements about health outcomes was found to be feasible to implement, even among respondents with little or no formal schooling. After analysing the paired comparison responses using probit regression, an examination of the regression results across the household surveys revealed very high correlations across settings, which suggested an unexpectedly high degree of consistency in comparative assessments of health.

11.3.3 Estimation of valuation functions across countries

Several of the major health status descriptive systems have been linked to valuation functions estimated in multiple countries. Given the high cost of undertaking valuation surveys, early work using preference-based measures tended to use the valuation results from just one or two countries, which for the EQ-5D and SF-6D was the United Kingdom, and for the Health Utilities Index (HUI) was Canada. However, given rising interest in cross-country variation in health state valuations, and some suggestive evidence that results from one country cannot necessarily be transferred to other countries, the number of valuation studies in other countries has been growing. A recent review of health state valuation in low and middle-income countries (Kularatna *et al.* 2013) identified 17 studies, including seven that aimed to develop valuation functions for generic preference-based measures of health. We have already reported on comparative results from several of the major generic preference-based measures of health in Chapter 7, but shall recap selected examples here.

The instrument with the largest number of country-specific valuation functions is the EQ-5D, through the efforts of the EuroQol group. EQ-5D-3L valuation functions have been estimated for 13 countries, and for six European countries combined (see http://www.euroqol.org). Outside Europe, the countries include Japan, New Zealand, the United States, and Zimbabwe. For some countries including Denmark, Germany, Spain, and the United Kingdom, alternative valuation functions are available based on either VAS or TTO responses. A comparison of the valuations predicted using the country-specific EQ-5D-3L functions reveals certain differences. Figure 11.1 shows an

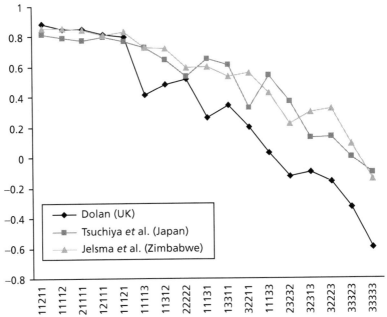

Fig. 11.1 Predicted valuations for selected EQ-5D states based on published valuation functions estimated from surveys in the United Kingdom, Japan, and Zimbabwe. Source data from Dolan P. Modelling valuations for EuroQol health states. *Medical Care*, Volume 35, Issue 11, pp. 095–108, Copyright © 1997 Lippincott-Raven Publishers; Tsuchiya A, Ikeda S, Ikegami N, Nishimura S, Sakai I, Fukuda T, *et al.* Estimating an EQ- 5D population value set: the case of Japan. *Health Economics*, Volume 11, pp. 341–53, Copyright © 2002 John Wiley and Sons; and Jelsma J, Hansen K, De Weerdt W, De Cock P, Kind P. How do Zimbabweans value health states? *Population Health Metrics*, Volume 1, Issue 1, pp. 11, Copyright © 2003 Jelsma et al.

example of predictions from published EQ-5D valuation functions that were estimated based on TTO surveys in the United Kingdom, Japan, and Zimbabwe (Dolan 1997; Tsuchiya *et al.* 2002; Jelsma *et al.* 2003). Perhaps surprisingly, the predictions from the Tsuchiya *et al.* (2002) model (based on a study in Japan), and the Jelsma *et al.* (2003) model (based on a study in Zimbabwe) are very similar, while the Dolan (1997) model (estimated from a UK study) produces predictions that diverge from both of these, particularly for severe health states. A major effort has been underway to develop valuation sets for the new five-level version of the EQ-5D system (the EQ-5D-5L), including 19 countries with valuation studies either complete or underway as of April 2015.

As reported in Chapter 7, valuations for SF-6D have been undertaken in Japan, Hong Kong, Brazil, Portugal, Spain, and Australia in addition to the United Kingdom with other countries planned for SF-6D v2, and valuations for HUI2 have been undertaken in the United Kingdom and for HUI3 in France. Along with the EQ-5D research, the findings from these studies suggest that there are often significant differences in the values given to the same states as defined by these health state classification systems.

11.4 **Summary and conclusions**

This chapter has provided a brief introduction to the DALY as an alternative to the QALY used increasingly in economic evaluations in low- and middle-income countries. We have highlighted similarities and differences in the two measures and traced the evolution of conceptual and empirical work supporting the measurement and valuation of non-fatal outcomes in DALYs.

We also have discussed the expanding interest in adapting instruments for describing and valuing health in diverse settings and reviewed some of the key developments in this area. As the number of adaptations and translations of existing instruments grows, it is important to think critically about various ways of evaluating equivalence. In the realm of valuation, it is essential to continue to examine whether prevailing modes of data collection and analysis are suitable in settings of varying educational levels and diverse cultures.

Evidence on cross-cultural variation in valuations is limited, but some of the research thus far points to possible differences. A clear understanding of the extent, direction, and substantive importance of these differences awaits further empirical research, and understanding the reasons for any variation that has been observed to date is challenging. Differences in observed valuations may reflect genuine differences in population values for health; differences in attitudes toward time (in the TTO) or risk (in the SG), or different uses of response scales (in the VAS); or differences in the interpretations of health state labels and descriptions across countries. As the evidence base on valuations across settings widens, parsing out the possible determinants of variation, and thinking carefully about the policy implications of these findings, remains a priority.

References

Acquadro C, Conway K, Hareendran A, Aaronson N, European Regulatory Issues and Quality of Life Assessment (ERIQA) Group (2008). *Value in Health* **11**:509–21.

Ahmed SM, Rana AK, Chowdhury M, Bhuiya A (2002). Measuring perceived health outcomes in non-western culture: does SF-36 have a place? *Journal of Health, Population, and Nutrition* **20**:334–42.

Anand S, Hanson K (1997). Disability-adjusted life years: a critical review. *Journal of Health Economics* **16**:685–702.

Anderson RT, Aaronson NK, Bullinger M, McBee WL (1996). A review of the progress towards developing health-related quality-of-life instruments for international clinical studies and outcomes research. *Phamacoeconomics* **10**:336–55.

Baltussen RMPM, Sanon M, Sommerfeld J, Würthwein R (2002). Obtaining disability weights in rural Burkina Faso using a culturally adapted visual analogue scale. *Health Economics* **11**:155–63.

Beaton DE, Bombardier C, Guillemin F, Ferraz MB (2000). Guidelines for the process of cross-cultural adaptation of self-report measures. *Spine* **25**:3186–91.

Bill and Melinda Gates Foundation, NICE International (2014). *Methods for Economic Evaluation Project—Final Report.*

Bowden A, Fox-Rushby JA (2003). A systematic and critical review of the process of translation and adaptation of generic health-related quality of life measures in Africa, Asia, Eastern Europe, the Middle East, South America. *Social Science and Medicine* **57**:1289–306.

Bullinger M, Alonso J, Apolone G, Leplege A, Sullivan M, Wood-Dauphinee S, *et al.* (1998). Translating health status questionnaires and evaluating their quality: the IQOLA Project approach. International Quality of Life Assessment. *Journal of Clinical Epidemiology* **51**:913–23.

Busschbach JJ, Hessing DJ, de Charro FT (1993). The utility of health at different stages in life: a quantitative approach. *Social Science and Medicine* **37**:153–8.

Cramer JA, Perrine K, Devinsky O, Bryant-Comstock L, Meador K, Hermann B (1998). Development and cross-cultural translations of a 31-item quality of life in epilepsy inventory. *Epilepsia* **39**:81–8.

Dolan P (1997). Modelling valuations for EuroQol health states. *Medical Care* **35**:1095–108.

Doward LC, McKenna SP, Kohlmann T, Niero M, Patrick D, Spencer B, Thorsen H (1998). The international development of the RGHQoL: a quality of life measure for recurrent genital herpes. *Quality of Life Research* **7**:143–53.

Guillemin F, Bombardier C, Beaton D (1993). Cross-cultural adaptation of health related quality of life measures: literature review and proposed guidelines. *Journal of Clinical Epidemiology* **46**:1417–32.

Herdman M, Fox-Rushby J, Badia X (1997). 'Equivalence' and the translation and adaptation of health-related quality of life questionnaires. *Quality of Life Research* **6**:237–47.

Herdman M, Fox-Rushby J, Badia X (1998). A model of equivalence in the cultural adaptation of HRQoL instruments: the universalist approach. *Quality of Life Research* **7**:323–35.

Jamison DT, Breman JG, Measham AR, Alleyne G, Claeson M, Evans DB (eds) (2006). *Disease control priorities in developing countries*, 2nd edn. Oxford University Press, New York, NY.

Jamison DT (2015). *Disease Control Priorities*, 3rd edn: improving health and reducing poverty. *Lancet* pii: S0140-6736(15)60097-6 (Epub ahead of print).

Jelsma J, Mkoka S, Amosun L, Nieuwveldt J (2004). The reliability and validity of the Xhosa version of the EQ-5D. *Disability and Rehabilitation* **26**:103–8.

Jelsma J, Hansen K, De Weerdt W, De Cock P, Kind P (2003). How do Zimbabweans value health states? *Population Health Metrics* **1**(1):11.

Jelsma J, Shumba D, Kristian H, De Weerdt W, De Cock P (2002). Preferences of urban Zimbabweans for health and life lived at different ages. *Bulletin of the World Health Organization* **80**:204–9.

Keller SD, Ware JE, Gandek B (1998). Testing the equivalence of translations of widely used response choice labels: results from the IQOLA project, International Quality of Life Assessment. *Journal of Clinical Epidemiology* **51**:933–44.

Kularatna S, Whitty JA, Johnson NW, Scuffham PA (2013). Health state valuation in low- and middle-income countries: a systematic review of the literature. *Value in Health* **16**:1091–9.

Li L, Wang HM, Shen Y (2003). Chinese SF-36 health survey: translation, cultural adaptation, validation, and normalization. *Journal of Epidemiology and Community Health* **57**:259–63.

Mahapatra P, Salomon JA, Nanda L (2002). Measuring health state values in developing countries—results from a community survey in Andhra Pradesh. In: Murray CJL, Salomon JA, Mathers CD, Lopez AD (eds). *Summary measures of population health: concepts, ethics, measurement and applications.* World Health Organization, Geneva, Switzerland, pp. 473–86.

Murray CJL (1994). Quantifying the burden of disease: the technical basis for disability-adjusted life years. *Bulletin of the World Health Organization* **72**:429–45.

Murray CJL (1996). Rethinking DALYs. In: Murray CJL, Lopez AD (eds). *The global burden of disease: a comprehensive assessment of mortality and disability from diseases, injuries, and risk factors in 1990 and projected to 2020.* Harvard School of Public Health, Cambridge, MA, pp. 1–98.

Murray CJL, Acharya AK (1997). Understanding DALYs. *Journal of Health Economics* **16**:703–30.

Murray CJL, Lopez AD (1994). Quantifying disability: data, methods and results. *Bulletin of the World Health Organization* **72**:481–94.

Murray CJL, Lopez AD, Jamison DT (1994). The global burden of disease in 1990: summary results, sensitivity analysis and future directions. *Bulletin of the World Health Organization* **72**:495–509.

Murray CJL, Salomon JA, Mathers CD (2000). A critical examination of summary measures of population health. *Bulletin of the World Health Organization* **78**: 981–94.

National Institute for Health and Clinical Excellence (2009). *Methods for the development of NICE public health guidance,* 2nd edn. National Institute for Health and Clinical Excellence, London, UK.

Sadana R (2002). Measurement of variance in health state valuations in Phnom Penh, Cambodia. In: Murray CJL, Salomon JA, Mathers CD, Lopez AD (eds). *Summary measures of population health: concepts, ethics, measurement and applications.* World Health Organization, Geneva, Switzerland, pp. 593–618.

Salomon JA (2003). Reconsidering the use of rankings in the valuation of health states: a model for estimating cardinal values from ordinal data. *Population Health Metrics* **1**(1):12. Available at: http://www.pophealthmetrics.com/content/1/1/12.

Salomon JA, Murray CJL (2004). A multi-method approach to measuring health-state valuations. *Health Economics* **13**:281–90.

Salomon JA, Mathers CD, Chatterji S, Sadana R, Üstün TB, Murray CJL (2003a). Quantifying individual levels of health: definitions, concepts and measurement issues. In: Murray CJL, Evans DB (eds). *Health systems performance assessment: debates, measures and empiricism.* World Health Organization, Geneva, Switzerland, pp. 301–18.

Salomon JA, Murray CJL, Üstün TB, Chatterji S (2003b). Health state valuations in summary measures of population health. In: Murray CJL, Evans DB (eds). *Health systems performance assessment: debates, measures and empiricism.* World Health Organization, Geneva, Switzerland, pp. 409–36.

Salomon JA, Vos T, Hogan DR, Gagnon M, Naghavi M, Mokdad A, *et al.* (2012). Common values in assessing health outcomes from disease and injury: disability weights measurement study for the Global Burden of Disease Study 2010. *Lancet* **380**:2129–43.

Salomon JA, Haagsma JA, Davis A, de Noordhout CM, Polinder S, Havelaar AH, *et al.* (2015). Disability weights for the Global Burden of Disease 2013 study. *Lancet Global Health* **3**:e712–23.

Sartorius N, Kuyken W (1994). Translation of health status instruments. In: Orley J, Kuyken W (eds). *Proceedings of the joint meeting organised by the World Health Organization and the foundation IPSEN.* Springer, Paris, France pp. 3–18.

Sommerfeld J, Baltussen RMPM, Metz Lm Sanon M, Sauerborn R (2002). Determinants of variance in health state valuations. In: Murray CJL, Salomon JA, Mathers CD, Lopez AD (eds). *Summary measures of population health: concepts, ethics, measurement and applications.* World Health Organization, Geneva, Switzerland, pp. 549–80.

Tan-Torres Edejer T, Baltussen R, Adam T, Hutubessy R, Acharya A, Evans DB, Murray CJL (2003). *Making choices in health: WHO guide to cost effectiveness analysis.* World Health Organization, Geneva, Switzerland.

Tsuchiya A, Ikeda S, Ikegami N, Nishimura S, Sakai I, Fukuda T, *et al.* (2002). Estimating an EQ-5D population value set: the case of Japan. *Health Economics* **11**:341–53.

Üstün TB, Chatterji S, Villanueva M, Zendeb L, Celik C, Sadaon R, *et al.* (2003*a*). WHO multi-country survey study on health and responsiveness 2000–2001. In: Murray CJL, Evans DB (eds). *Health systems performance assessment: debates, measures and empiricism.* World Health Organization, Geneva, Switzerland, pp. 761–96.

Üstün TB, Chatterji S, Mechbal A, Murray CJL, WHS Collaborating Group (2003*a*). The world health surveys. In: Murray CJL, Evans DB (eds). *Health systems performance assessment: debates, measures and empiricism.* World Health Organization, Geneva, Switzerland, pp. 797–808.

Wagner AK, Wyss K, Gandek B, Kilima PM, Lorenz S, Whiting D (1999). A Kiswahili version of the SF-36 Health Survey for use in Tanzania: translation and tests of scaling assumptions. *Quality of Life Research* **8**:101–10.

Wang H, Kindig DA, Mullahy J (2005). Variation in Chinese population health related quality of life: results from a EuroQol study in Beijing, China. *Quality of Life Research* **14**:119–32.

Ware JE, Keller SD, Gandek B, Brazier JE, Sullivan M (1995). Evaluating translations of health status questionnaires: methods from the IQOLA project. *International Journal of Technology Assessment in Health Care* **11**:525–51.

Wild D, Grove A, Martin M, Eremenco S, McElroy S, Verjee-Lorenz A, Erikson P (2005). Principles of good practice for the translation and cultural adaptation process for patient-reported outcomes (PRO) measures: report of the ISPOR task force for translation and cultural adaptation. *Value in Health* **8**:94–104.

World Bank (1993). *World development report 1993.* Oxford University Press, New York, NY.

Zuniga MA, Carrillo-Jimenez GT, Fos PJ, Gandek B, Medina-Moreno MR (1999). Evaluation of health status using the SF-36 survey: preliminary results in Mexico [in Spanish]. *Salud Pública de México* **41**:110–8.

Chapter 12

Conclusions: measurement and valuation of health

12.1 The variety of methods

In this book, we set out to address the main questions surrounding the measurement and valuation of health. Emerging from even a casual reading of this book is the wide range of ways available to address core questions involving: the definition of health, the techniques of valuation, who should provide the values, techniques for modelling health state values, and so forth. The last three decades have seen a substantial body of research seeking to address these questions and the development of new tools and instruments for putting the 'q' into the QALY (quality-adjusted life year). We hope we have fully reflected these developments.

This content begs the question of which combination of answers to these questions *should* be used. In economic evaluation, the precise choice of methods depends on normative judgements as well as technical considerations, and none more so than in the measurement and valuation of health. It is difficult to get a group of health economists to agree on whether the main outcome of health care is health or on a single definition of health, let alone who should value the states and by which valuation technique. International agencies using the results of economic evaluation are starting to develop a reference of preferred methods (to enhance comparability).

Economic theory might suggest that each individual has a well-established utility function in health that provides values for all sorts of health states. The methods described in this book are offering a different view. Whether or not a uni-dimensional latent scale exists, we know that the different methods themselves help fashion the value respondents provide. As Llewellyn-Thomas *et al.* (1984, p. 550) pointed out a number of years ago, it is ' . . . naive to think of any state of health as possessing a single utility or value. Rather, numerical values for health states are influenced by the state itself, the way in which information about the state is presented to a rater, the method used to elicit judgements and other circumstances of the rating task'. At the time of being asked, respondents are constructing their preferences over things they have given little thought to before the interview. Therefore, it is not surprising that their responses are influenced by the way they are asked. This problem is well recognized in psychology and has started to be taken seriously in health economics, but what is the solution?

One response might be that health state values are so labile and prone to external influence that they are largely meaningless. We would argue strongly that this is not the case. The values we obtain using different methods reflect the underlying views of respondents. It is important that researchers think hard about what they want to value, the theoretical basis of the technique (such as whether they want a choice-based technique like standard gamble or time trade-off rather than visual analogue scale), avoid obvious biases (such as from anchoring effects), and use modelling methods with the best predictive validity. There are also important options that require policy makers to make normative judgements. To inform resource allocation across a health care system (and beyond), it is necessary to achieve a degree of standardization in terms of the combination of key attributes, such as whose values, and the technique and variant of valuation (including the appropriate upper and lower anchors states). This was the approach recommended by the Washington Panel on Cost-Effectiveness in Health and Medicine (Gold *et al.* 1996) and later adopted by the National Institute for Health and Clinical (now Care) Excellence (2004). The extent to which this also requires a single descriptive system is more debatable.

12.2 **International Guidelines**

There are important differences in the methods adopted around the world and these have been changing over time (examples of the latest versions are NICE 2013; PBAC 2013; NOMA 2012; CADTH 2006; CVZ 2004; PBB 2003). Eight sets of guidelines are summarized in Table 12.1 to highlight the differences (though they are not comprehensive). They show that most guidelines currently permit a range of methods to be used. Some express a preference, but this does not seem to rule out other methods. Even where there is a preference between methods, there is no clear agreement between guidelines. However, it would seem that cost-effectiveness analysis or cost per QALY analysis is usually preferred to cost-benefit analysis, and that most agencies want general population values to be used for estimating QALYs, rather than patient values, or expert values. Beyond this, the specifics are often unclear. These guidelines are likely to be revised again in the near future and readers are advised to consult http://www.ispor.org/PEguidelines/index.asp regularly.

The adoption of a reference case does not imply that other methods are wrong. Any set of methods involves compromises and may be thought to work against the interests of some conditions and treatments that should be recognized. We still have much to learn about the measurement and valuation of health in the context of economic evaluation, such as: the role of descriptive systems; how values are influenced by the techniques and their variants; the development of new techniques for eliciting values (particularly in more vulnerable groups); the role of cross-cultural variation; why experience-based values differ from preferences; how best to econometrically model data; how best to incorporate values into economic models; and so forth. We cannot predict how the field is likely to develop over the next decade, but we are sure it will lose none of its intellectual challenge and controversy.

Table 12.1 Comparison of economic guidelines on valuation of benefits (as of January 2016)

Country	Agency	Measure of value	Descriptive system	Whose values	Method of obtaining values	Questionnaire recommended	Other information
Australia	Pharmaceutical Benefits Advisory Committee (2013)	CUA if incremental life years are gained and/or relevant direct randomized trials use a preference-based measure	None	Australian general population	SG or TTO	HUI2 or HUI3, EQ-5D, SF-6D, or AQoL	Hierarchy: recommended generic, patient own values, vignette, mapping, matching values, and literature
England and Wales	NICE (2013)	QALYs	Generic	UK general population preferences	Choice-based method	Preference for EQ-5D in adults	Where EQ-5D shown to be inappropriate can use alternative HRQoL measure
Canada	Canadian Agency for Drugs and Technologies in Health (CADTH, 2006)	QALY/monetary values	Justify selection	None	None	Mentions EQ-5D and HUI	
Ireland	Health Information and Quality Authority (2010)	QALYs	Generic	General population	Choice-based	EQ-5D or SF-6D	Direct patient values may be used
Norway	Norwegian Medicines Agency (2012)	QALYs or LYGs	Generic	Not specified	Not specified	None mentioned	Compulsory to perform a literature of values
The Netherlands	CVZ, Health Care Insurance Board (2004)	QALY where impact on QoL	None	Use random sample of the population		No preference	Can use representative patient population or literature to obtain values
New Zealand	PHARMAC (2015)	QALYs	Generic	General population	Choice-based	EQ-5D	Requests NZ tariff
Sweden	Pharmaceutical Benefits Board (2003)	CUA/CBA	None	Patient preferences	Choice-based	None	

Key to abbreviations: CBA = cost-benefit analysis; CUA = cost-utility analysis; CVZ = College voor zorgverzekeringen; HRQoL = health-related quality of life; HUI = Health Utilities Index; NICE = National Institute for Health and Care Excellence; PHARMAC = Pharmaceutical Management Agency; QALYs = quality-adjusted life years; SG = standard gamble; TTO = time trade-off.

References

Canadian Agency for Drugs and Technologies in Health (CADTH) (2006). *Guidelines for the economic evaluation of health technologies: Canada,* (3rd edn, 2006).

College voor zorgverzekeringen (CVZ) (2004). *Guidelines for pharmacoeconomic research in the Netherlands April 2006)* (Dutch version, 2004).

Gold MR, Siegel JE, Russell LB, Weinstein MC (1996). *Cost-effectiveness in health and medicine.* Oxford University Press, Oxford, UK.

Health Information and Quality Authority (2010). *Guidelines for the economic evaluation of health technologies in Ireland.* Available at: https://www.hiqa.ie/publication/guidelines-economic-evaluation-health-technologies-ireland

Llewellyn-Thomas H, Sutherland HJ, Tibshirani R, Ciampi A, Till JE, Boyd NF (1984). Describing health states: methodological issues in obtaining values for health states. *Medical Care* **22**:543–52.

National Institute for Clinical Excellence (NICE) (2004). *Guide to the methods of technology appraisal.* NICE, London, UK.

National Institute of Health and Care Excellence (NICE) (2013). *Guide to the methods of technology appraisal 2013.* NICE, London, UK.

The Norwegian Medicines Agency (NOMA) (2012). *Guidelines on how to conduct pharmaceutical analysis.* NOMA, Oslo, Norway.

Pharmaceutical Benefits Advisory Committee (PBAC) (2013). *Guidelines for preparing submissions to the Pharmaceutical Benefits Advisory Committee (June 2013).* PBAC, Canberra, Australia.

Pharmaceutical Benefits Board (2003). *General guidelines for economic evaluations from the Pharmaceutical Benefits Board (Sweden).* TLV, Stockholm, Sweden.

Pharmaceutical Management Agency (PHARMAC) (2015). *Prescriptions for pharmacoeconomic analysis: methods for cost-utility analysis.* PHARMAC, Wellington, New Zealand.

Glossary

Terms in italics are defined elsewhere in the glossary.

additive separability One of the conditions to be satisfied if the *quality-adjusted life years (QALY)* is to be interpreted as a representation of individual utility. It requires that the preference for a given state of health is not affected by the states of health that precede or follow it.

Bayesian method A branch of statistics that uses prior information on beliefs for estimation and inference.

best–worst scaling A variant of the discrete choice experiment. The best-known type of best–worst scaling presents respondents with a single profile at a time and elicits choices regarding which attribute is the best (most attractive) and which is the worst (least attractive), based on the attribute levels in the profile. (See *discrete choice data*).

bolt-ons An approach to extend the descriptive system of an existing health state classification system by adding a new dimension, or an extended descriptive system.

bootstrapping A simulation method for deriving non-parametric estimates of variables of interest (e.g. the variance in the C/E ratio) from a data set.

budget pie A technique for eliciting the relative social value of health (or health care interventions) where a respondent is asked to indicate how a fixed health care budget should be allocated between two (or more) competing programmes. The relative desirability of the attributes of each programme is then analysed using regression analysis. (Also see *weighed QALYs*.)

category rating scales Scales that are composed of distinct categories. The categories are often numerical, such as 0, 1, 2, . . ., 10; the phenomenon being rated must be assigned to one and only one category. Numerical categories often are treated as equal-interval in analyses. In psychology, sometimes referred to as the method of equal-appearing intervals.

compensation test In welfare economics, a gauge of the desirability of a programme and theoretical basis of cost-benefit analysis. In one (the Kaldor criterion), a programme is considered to be welfare enhancing if those who gain from it would be able to pay enough for their gains to compensate the losers. In the other (the Hicks criterion), a programme is not welfare enhancing if those who lose from it are able to pay enough to compensate the winners-to-be to forego the programme. Actual payments are not required. (Also *Pareto improvement*.)

condition preference-based measure An instrument for deriving health state values that uses a condition-specific health state descriptive system and a tariff or algorithm for assigning values to each state described by the classification (examples include the OAB-5D and EORTC-8D).

construct validity The ability of a measure to tap the construct of interest. It is established by examining convergence (e.g. the extent of correlation with other measures of the phenomenon being measured and known group validity). The ability of an instrument to discriminate between groups that have known differences.

contingent valuation A method of placing a monetary value on a good or service that is not available in the marketplace by determining, contingent on it being available in the marketplace, the maximum amount that people would be *willing to pay* for it (buying price) and/or the minimum amount that people would be willing to accept to part with it (selling price).

convergent validity The ability of an instrument to co-vary (in the fashion expected of a good measure for the construct or phenomenon of interest) with a number of other distinct measures, each of which is thought to be a direct or indirect correlate for some distinct aspect of the *construct* or phenomenon. The correlations between the instrument being evaluated and these other measures are conceived of as representing convergent lines of evidence for the *validity* of the instrument.

cost-benefit analysis (CBA) A technique of economic evaluation for estimating the net social benefit of a programme or intervention as the incremental benefit of the programme less the *incremental cost*, with all benefits and costs measured in dollars.

cost-consequence analysis A technique of economic evaluation in which the components of *incremental costs* and consequences of alternative programmes are computed and listed, without any attempt to aggregate these results.

cost-effectiveness analysis (CEA) A technique of economic evaluation in which costs and effects of a programme and at least one alternative are calculated and presented in a ratio of *incremental cost* to incremental effect. Effects are health outcomes, such as cases of a disease prevented, years of life gained, or *quality-adjusted life years*, rather than monetary measures as in *cost-benefit analysis*.

cost-effectiveness ratio The *incremental cost* of obtaining a unit of health effect (such as dollars per year, or per quality-adjusted year, of life expectancy) from a given health intervention, when compared with an alternative.

cost-minimization analysis (CMA) A technique of economic evaluation that compares the net costs of programmes that achieve the same outcome.

cost per QALY analysis A special case of CEA where the health effects of the intervention is represented in terms of QALYs. Also known as *cost-utility analysis*.

cost-utility analysis See *cost per QALY analysis*.

decision analysis An explicit, quantitative, systematic approach to decision making under conditions of *uncertainty* in which *probabilities* of each possible event, along with the consequences of those events, are stated explicitly.

decision tree A graphical representation of a decision, incorporating alternative choices, uncertain events (and their *probabilities*) and outcomes.

dimension(s) Component(s) of health status, also called health attributes.

direct preference elicitation A term used in the health economics literature meaning health state values obtained from patients for their own current state.

disability-adjusted life years (DALYs) An indicator developed to assess the global burden of disease. DALYs are computed by adjusting age-specific life expectancy for loss of healthy life due to disability. The value of a year of life at each age is weighted, as are decrements to health from disability from specified diseases and injuries.

discounting The process of converting future money and future health outcomes to their *present value*.

discount rate The interest rate used to compute *present value*, or the interest rate used in *discounting* future sums.

discrete choice data A kind of data generated by a respondent choosing between two or more alternatives, typically described by their levels along several dimensions of health and/or *non-health benefit*. For health state valuation, an attribute for duration of life can be added to estimate values on the zero to one scale.

discriminant validity The extent to which an instrument does not correlate with variables and measures thought to be unrelated to the *construct* being measured.

economic model An attempt to simplify reality into structure such a *decision tree* of *Markov* process in order to help with the application of one of the techniques of economic evaluation (e.g. *CEA, cost per QALY, CBA*).

effectiveness The extent to which medical interventions achieve health improvements in real practice settings.

effect size A standardized measure (some time known as a 'standardized' effect size) of change over time or between groups. For measuring change over time (such as in a 'before and after' design in a group or a difference in such changes between two groups), a commonly used version is the standardized response mean, which is the mean change divided by the standard deviation of changes across individuals.

efficacy The extent to which medical interventions achieve health improvements under ideal circumstances.

equity (in health outcomes) The absence of certain inequalities in health across different people that are judged to be unfair and normatively unacceptable. Also see *weighted QALYs*.

ex ante A situation viewed from beforehand, that is, before the event occurs, before an action is taken, or before an outcome is known. This is as opposed to *ex post*.

expected utility A quantity used to represent the relative desirability of a specified course of action(s) where the outcome of the action cannot be specified before the fact with certainty. Each potential outcome is assigned a *utility*, to represent its desirability, and a *probability*, to represent the likelihood of its occurrence if the course of action were adopted. The expected utility is the probability-weighted average *utility* of the potential outcomes.

expected utility theory A framework for analysing decisions under *uncertainty* positing that alternative actions are characterized by a set of possible outcomes and a set of *probabilities* corresponding to each outcome. The sum of the products of the *probability* of each outcome and the *utility* of that outcome is the expected value of *utility* and reflects the preferences of the decision maker. First axiomatized by von Neumann and Morgenstern in their 1947 book, *Theory of games and economic behavior*, the theory sets forth conditions under which there exists a numerical measure of subjective attractiveness of outcomes (called a *utility function*) with the following properties: (i) this function represents the *ordinal* preferences of the decision maker if outcomes were to be received with certainty; and (ii) the order of the expected utilities associated with various uncertain decision strategies represents the rankings of these strategies according to the decision maker's preferences.

experienced-based utility A form of utility concerned with a respondent's experience of the moment, in contrast to preference-based utility which concerns views about future states.

externalities The positive (beneficial) or negative (harmful) effects that market exchanges have on people who do not participate directly in those exchanges. Also called 'spillover' effects.

extra welfarism. See *non-welfarism*.

face validity A judgement of the *validity* or reasonableness of a measurement or model based on its examination by persons with expertise in the health problem and intervention being measured or modelled.

fair innings argument An egalitarian theory for equal lifetime health that reflects the feeling that everyone is entitled to some 'normal' span of health (i.e. a fair innings). It offers a theoretical basis for weighting QALYs by different characteristics such as age, social class, and severity. Also see *weighted QALYs*.

generic preference-based measure An instrument for deriving health state values that uses a generic health state descriptive system and a tariff or algorithm for assigning values to each state described by the classification (examples include the EQ-5D or HUI3).

health-related quality of life The impact of the health aspects of an individual's life on that person's *quality of life*, or overall well-being. Also used to refer to the value of a *health state* to an individual.

health state The health of an individual at any particular point in time. A health state may be modified by the impairments, functional states, perceptions, and social opportunities that are influenced by disease, injury, treatment, or health policy.

health status measures Systems used to define and describe *health states* (e.g. a multi-attribute health status classification system).

health status profile An instrument that describes the health status of a person on each of a comprehensive set of *dimensions*.

healthy-years equivalent (HYE) The number of years of perfect health (followed by death) that has the same *utility* as (is seen as equivalent to) the lifetime path of *health states* under consideration. It can be measured by two *standard gamble* questions or by one *time trade-off* question.

incremental cost-effectiveness (ratio) The ratio of the difference in costs between two alternatives to the difference in *effectiveness* between the same two alternatives.

inequality aversion The extent to which people prefer a more even distribution of the good in question (e.g. health) than a less even distribution.

inter-rater reliability A measure of consistency among multiple judges.

interval scale A scale on which equal intervals (e.g., 0.1–0.2, 0.8–0.9) have an equivalent interpretation. An interval scale may have two arbitrarily anchored points.

intrarater reliability A measure of the stability of the rating an individual judge gives to the same question presented more than once during the same or a subsequent administration (Also called test–retest reliability).

Kaldor–Hicks criterion See *compensation test.*

league table A table in which interventions are ranked by their (incremental) *cost-effectiveness ratios.*

magnitude estimation A technique from psychophysics wherein judges are asked to rate the magnitude of the sensation produced by one stimulus versus another as a ratio (e.g. '2.5 times as much').

marginal benefit The added benefit generated by the next unit consumed.

marginal cost The added cost of producing one additional unit of output.

marginal cost-effectiveness (ratio) The *incremental cost-effectiveness ratio* between two alternatives that differ by one unit along some quantitative scale of intensity, dose, or duration. (This term is often used incorrectly as a synonym for *incremental cost- effectiveness.*)

Markov models A type of mathematical model containing a finite number of mutually exclusive and exhaustive *health states*, having time periods of uniform length, and in which the *probability* of movement from one state to another depends on the current state and remains constant over time.

multiattribute utility theory An extension of *expected utility theory* by Keeny and Raiffa (1976) that uses an additional assumption that utility independence among dimensions (or attributes) can be represented by at least one of three forms (additive, multiplicaticative, or multilinear). Used to extrapolate values from a subset of states to all possible states defined by a descriptive system.

non-health benefit Benefits from health care that go beyond health.

non-welfarism An alternative approach to modern *welfare economics* that holds that judgements of *social welfare* can be based on information other than individual utility, such as their level of health, independently of how health is valued by the individuals themselves. Examples include extra welfarism, the decision makers' approach, and communitarianism.

normative theory A coherent group of general propositions or principles of which the objective is to define a norm or standard of correctness.

normative theory of social choice Any group of coherent propositions that lead to prescriptions about the choices society ought to make under well-defined circumstances.

objective function The summary quantity, expressed as a mathematical function of independent variables, that an investigator wished to maximize or minimize (e.g. total cost).

opportunity cost The value of time or any other 'input' in its highest value use. The benefits lost because the next best alternative was not selected.

ordinal preference elicitation techniques In relation to health, a ranking of two or more health states. See also *discrete choice datas*. These contrast with techniques such as *standard gamble* or *time trade-off* that elicit values on an *interval scale* at the individual respondent level. Some ordinal techniques are capable of generating interval scale values at the aggregate level.

parameter uncertainty *Uncertainty* about the true numerical values of the parameters used as inputs.

Pareto improvement A reallocation that makes at least one person better off and no one worse off.

Pareto optimality A distribution of resources such that any change in the distribution must make at least one person worse off.

perspective The viewpoint from which health state valuations are conducted (e.g. to judge own current or hypothetical health state as a private consumer, or to judge someone else's state as a social decision maker).

ping–pong method A method of eliciting preferences by converging to the final answer while alternating steps from both sides. For example, finding the difference *probability* in a *standard gamble* question by alternatingly asking about *probabilities* that are too high and too low while converging inward.

person trade-off A technique for valuing health states where a respondent is asked to indicate how many people (y) in health (x) state B are equivalent to a specified member of people in health state A. The undesirability of health state B is the ratio x/y times as great as that of health state A. It can also be used for the relative social value of health (see *weighed QALYs*).

point estimate A single estimate of a parameter of interest.

power See *statistical power*.

predictive validity The ability of a model to make verifiably accurate predictions of quantities of interest. A measurement instrument that has predictive validity is one that allows accurate predictions of future states of the *construct* being measured.

preference function A mathematical expression describing preferences or *utility function* of specific variables. See also *utility function*.

preference score See *preference weight*.

preference subgroup A group of individuals within a larger population whose preferences for particular *health states* are relatively homogeneous and differ systematically from the average preferences of the population.

preference weight A numerical judgement of the desirability of a particular outcome or situation. Also known as preference score or value.

present value The value to the decision maker now of outcomes occurring in the future.

prevalence The proportion of individuals in a population who have a disease or condition at a specific point in time.

probabilistic sensitivity analysis A method of *decision analysis* in which *probability distributions* are specified for each uncertain parameter (e.g. *probabilities, utilities,* costs); a simulation is performed whereby values of each parameter are randomly drawn from the corresponding distribution; and the resulting *probability distribution* of *expected utilities* (and costs) is displayed.

probability An expression of the degree of certainty that an event will occur, on a scale from zero (certainty that the event will not occur) to one (certainty that the event will occur).

probability distribution A numerical or mathematical representation of the relative likelihood of each possible value that a variable may take on (technically, a 'probability density function').

psychophysical methods Methods (or protocols) for asking judges to give numerical assessments representing the psychological perception or sensation produced by physical stimuli. These methods have been adapted to ask people to give numerical responses to represent preferences or degrees of preference for *health states*.

quality-adjusted life expectancy Life expectancy computed using *quality-adjusted life years* rather than nominal life years.

quality-adjusted life years (QALYs) A measure of health outcome which assigns to each period of time a weight, ranging from negative infinity (or negative one for one transformation) to one, corresponding to the *health-related quality of life* during that period, where a weight of one corresponds to optimal health, and a weight of zero corresponds to a *health state* judged equivalent to being dead; these are then aggregated across time periods.

quality of life A broad *construct* reflecting subjective or objective judgement concerning all aspects of an individual's existence, including health, economic, political, cultural, environmental, aesthetic, and spiritual aspects.

randomized clinical trial (RCT) A clinical trial in which the treatments are randomly assigned to the subjects. The random allocation eliminates bias in the assignment of treatments to patients and establishes the basis for statistical analysis.

recall bias Bias that arises when the study subjects are asked to report past events based on their memory. May arise because individuals with a particular exposure or adverse health outcome are likely to remember their experiences differently from those who are not similarly affected.

relative risk An estimate of the magnitude of an association between exposure and disease, which also indicates the likelihood of developing the disease among persons who are exposed relative to those who are not. It is defined as the ratio of incidence of disease in the exposed group divided by the corresponding incidence of disease in the non-exposed group.

relative social value of health The rate at which a unit health improvement increases social welfare. Standard cost per QALY analyses assume that the value of a QALY is constant ('a QALY is a QALY is a QALY'), but there are possible arguments to vary this for efficiency reasons and/or equity reasons. Also see *weighted QALY*.

reliability Consistency in repeated measures of a phenomenon by the same individual or across different groups of observers. The higher the reliability, the higher the test–retest correlation between replications of the measurement. Technically, the fraction of the variance in a measure that is the true value rather than measurement error. See also *intrarater reliability, inter-rater reliability*, and *test–retest reliability*.

response shift A change in the way a person perceives their *health-related quality of life* despite no objective difference over time in health status caused by changes in their internal standards, the way they weigh the life goals, and their very goals themselves.

risk aversion The extent to which an individual prefers a distribution of outcomes with a narrower spread to a wider one with the same expected value.

risk neutrality The risk attitude of an individual whose preference over different distributions of outcomes is determined by the expected value of the distribution and not affected by the spread.

social rate of time preference The rate at which the social decision maker is willing to trade-off present for future consumption. Frequently approximated by the real (inflation-adjusted) return on low-risk government investments.

social welfare An indication of how good or desirable a given state of affairs is for society as a whole. An *objective function* for society, which is a normative construct.

standard gamble In *health state valuation*, an approach to determining the *utility* of a particular outcome from a particular *perspective*. Judges are asked to compare life in a particular given *health state* that is 'a sure thing' to a gamble with a *probability P* that perfect health is the outcome and 1–*P* that immediate death is the outcome. The *probability P* is varied until the preference for the sure thing, the certainty of the particular *health state*, is equal to the preference for the gamble. The *probability P* for which the *expected utility* of the two choices is equal is then a measure of the preference for the *health state* and for all intents and purposes satisfies (by construction) the requirements for a *von Neumann–Morgenstern (nVM) utility*.

state-transition models Models which allocate, and subsequently reallocate, members of a population among several categories or *health states*. Transitions from one state to another occur at defined, recurring time intervals according to transition *probabilities*. Through simulation, or mathematical calculation, the number of members of the population passing through each state at each point in time can be estimated. State-transition models can be used to calculate life expectancy or *quality-adjusted life expectancy*.

statistical power The *probability* of detecting (as 'statistically significant') a postulated level of effect. Technically, the *probability* of (correctly) rejecting the null hypothesis, that is, the *probability* of rejecting the null hypothesis when in fact the alternative is true.

study arm A group of patients assigned to the same treatment (or control condition) in a controlled study.

subjective well-being Described under three headings: hedonism (well-being increases when an individual experiences more pleasure and/or less pain); flourishing theories (well-being increases when an individual fulfils their nature as a human being, or 'flourishes'); and life evaluation or life satisfaction (well-being increases when an individual positively assesses his or her life). Traditionally there are also objective list accounts of well-being including items such as literacy, accommodation, and ability to see and longevity, or health.

test–retest reliability The correlation between scores on the same measure administered on two separate occasions.

Thurstone's Law of Comparative Judgement One of the earliest methods for deriving psychological scales; it is based on paired-comparison judgements. Thurstone's law holds that stimulus differences which are detected equally often are subjectively equal.

time preference The rate at which the decision maker is just willing to trade present for future consumption of some commodity of interest. A positive rate of time preference means the decision maker is willing to forego some current consumption of the commodity in return for a sufficiently large gain in future consumption.

time trade-off A method of measuring *health state utilities* in which patients are asked to trade-off life years in a state of less than perfect health for a shorter life span in a state of perfect health. The ratio of the number of years of perfect health that is equivalent to a longer life span in less than perfect health provides a measure of the preference for that *health state*.

uncertainty A state in which the true value of a parameter or the structure of a process is unknown.

utility A concept in economics, psychology, and *decision analysis*, sometimes used to refer to the preference for, or desirability of, a particular outcome. In the context of *health-related quality of life* measurement, utility is used to refer to the preference of the rater (usually a patient or a member of the general public) for a particular health outcome or *health state*. For technical use in *decision analysis*, see *von Neumann–Morgenstern (vNM) utility*.

utility function An *objective function* for an individual. An algebraic expression stating that a decision maker's satisfaction is dependent on the types and amounts of commodities she consumes. Symbolically, $U = U(X1, X2 \ldots)$, where $X1, X2 \ldots$ are valued outcome attributes. According to *expected utility theory*, individuals behave so as to maximize the expected value of *utility*, subject to constraints.

utilitarianism A *welfarist* theory of social justice that holds the policies that produce the greatest good for the greatest number improve social welfare. This theory incorporates everyone's well-being into the social process by balancing the *utility* of persons who gain from a given policy with the *utility* of those who lose as a result of the same policy.

validity The extent to which a technique measures what it is intended to measure. See also *construct validity, convergent validity, discriminant validity, face validity*, and *predictive validity*.

value As in health state valuation, see *preference weight*.

valuation technique A technique (such as *standard gamble* or *time trade-off*) for valuaing health states, also known as preference elicitation technique.

veil of ignorance A philosophical construct in which a rational public decides what is the best course of action when blind to its own self-interest.

visual analogue scales Direct rating methods using a line on paper (or similar visual device) without internal markings; raters are asked to place a mark at some point between the two anchor states appearing at the ends of the line.

von Neumann–Morgenstern (vNM) utility A number representing relative desirability that satisfies axioms set forth by von Neumann and Morgenstern (1947) and suitable for computation of *expected utilities* to represent preferences among alternatives with uncertain outcomes.

weighted QALYs The outcome measure of a *CEA* when it is corrected to reflect various concerns implying that the relative societal value of health may differ depending on the circumstance. Weights can be applied to *QALYs* for equity reasons and efficiency reasons. Also see *relative social value of health*.

well-being How well an individual's life is going.

welfare economics A normative branch of economics concerned with the development of principles for maximizing social welfare and economic output.

welfarism The main school of thought within modern *welfare economics* that holds that judgements of *social welfare* must be a function of individual utility, as assessed by themselves. See also *non-welfarism*.

willingness to pay A method of measuring the value an individual places on a good, service, or reduction in the risk of death and illness by estimating the maximum monetary amount an individual would pay in order to obtain the good, service, or risk reduction.

years of healthy life (YHL) The duration of an individual's life, as modified by the changes in health and well-being experienced over a lifetime. Also called *quality-adjusted life years* or health-adjusted life years.

This glossary has drawn heavily on the Glossary presented in Gold *et al.* (1996), although any remaining errors are those of the authors.

Subject Index

Notes

Page numbers followed by *f* indicate material in figures, *t* tables and *b* boxed material
vs. indicates a comparison

The following abbreviations have been used in the index.

CSPBMs - condition-specific preference-based measures of health
DALYs - disability-adjusted life years
GPBMs - generic preference-based measures
QALYs - quality-adjusted life years
TTO - time trade-off
VAS - visual analog scale

Aballéa, S, 83, 238
Abásolo, I, 295
Abdalla, M, 117
Abellán-Perpiñán, JM, 69, 170
actuarially fair premium, 34*b*
Adamowicz, W, 131
ADHD (attention deficit hyperactivity
    disorder), 236
administration technique, GPBMs, 184
adolescents, GPBMs *see* generic preference-
    based measures (GPBMs)
Adult Social Care Outcomes Toolkit (ASCOT),
    245, 246–7*b*
  EQ-5D *vs.*, 214
Afzali, H, 275
age
  health state valuation data, 126
  weighted cost per QALY analysis, 290, 295
Ahmed, SM, 311
Akerlof, GA, 35
Al-Janabi, H, 222, 240, 241, 243, 244, 245*b*
Allison, PD, 137
amyotrophic lateral sclerosis (ALS), CSPBMs,
    223*t*, 227*t*
Anand, P, 240, 309
anchor-based methods
  sample size in health state valuation data, 263
  well-being, 242–3
Anderson, JP, 50, 109, 110, 113, 148
Anderson, RT, 311
Apajasalo, M, 191, 197
AQL-5D, 216
  derivation of, 218
  EQ-5D *vs.*, 230, 231*f*
AQLQ (Asthma Quality of Life Questionnaire)
    see Asthma Quality of Life
    Questionnaire (AQLQ)
AQoL *see* Assessment of Quality of Life
    (AQoL)
Ara, R, 213, 264, 277, 279

area under the curve method, QALY
    estimation, 267
Arrow, KJ, 34
ASCOT *see* Adult Social Care Outcomes Toolkit
    (ASCOT)
Assessment of Quality of Life (AQoL), 148
  AQoL-6D Adolescent, 195
  AQoL-8D, 172, 174
    descriptive systems, 149*t*, 172, 173*f*
    valuation, 149*t*, 172, 174
  empirical validity evidence, 187
  performance levels, 188
  practicality, 180–1
  selection of content, 183
  TTO variants, 59
  valuation
    decomposed approach, 110
    methods used, 179
assessment timing, health state valuation
    data, 260–2
asthma, CSPBMs, 223*t*, 225*t*, 227*t*, 228*t*
Asthma Quality of Life Questionnaire (AQLQ),
    216, 218
atopic dermatitis, CSPBMs, 225*t*, 228*t*
Attema, AE, 67, 70
attention deficit hyperactivity disorder
    (ADHD), 236
Audit of Diabetes-Dependent Quality of
    Life, 216
Augustovski, F, 57, 59, 66
Australia, 8
  health state valuations, 321*t*
aversion to inequality, 38, 38*b*

Badia, X, 125, 162
Balaban, DJ, 125
Baltussen, RMPM, 313
Bansback, N, 59, 66, 132, 139, 142–3, 162, 170,
    258, 260
Baron, J, 260